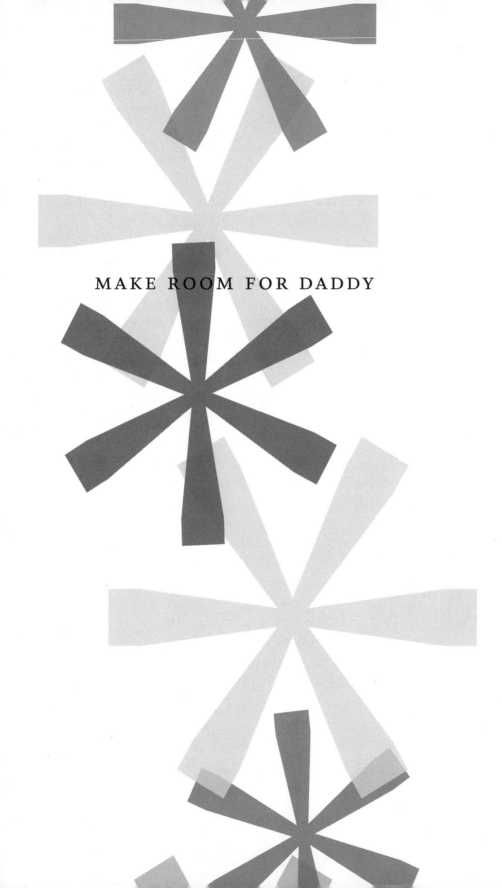

MAKE ROOM FOR DADDY

JUDITH WALZER LEAVITT

MAKE ROOM FOR DADDY

THE JOURNEY FROM WAITING ROOM TO BIRTHING ROOM

THE UNIVERSITY OF NORTH CAROLINA PRESS * CHAPEL HILL

© 2009

THE UNIVERSITY OF NORTH CAROLINA PRESS

*

All rights reserved * Manufactured in the United States of America
Designed by Courtney Leigh Baker and set in Whitman with
Futura display by Tseng Information Systems, Inc.

The paper in this book meets the guidelines for permanence and
durability of the Committee on Production Guidelines for
Book Longevity of the Council on Library Resources.

The University of North Carolina Press has been a member
of the Green Press Initiative since 2003.

Library of Congress Cataloging-in-Publication Data
Leavitt, Judith Walzer.
Make room for daddy : the journey from waiting room
to birthing room / Judith Walzer Leavitt.
p. cm.
Includes bibliographical references and index.
ISBN 978-0-8078-3255-4 (cloth : alk. paper)
1. Childbirth—United States—History—20th century.
2. Fatherhood—United States—History—20th century. I. Title.
[DNLM: 1. Labor, Obstetric—history—United States. 2. Father-Child
Relations—United States. 3. Fathers—psychology—United States.
4. History, 20th Century—United States. 5. Infant, Newborn—
United States. 6. Parturition—United States. WQ 11 AA1 L4m 2009]
RG652.L38 2009 * 392.1'2—dc22 * 2008050473

13 12 11 10 09   5 4 3 2 1

To the fathers in my family,

PAST, PRESENT, AND FUTURE

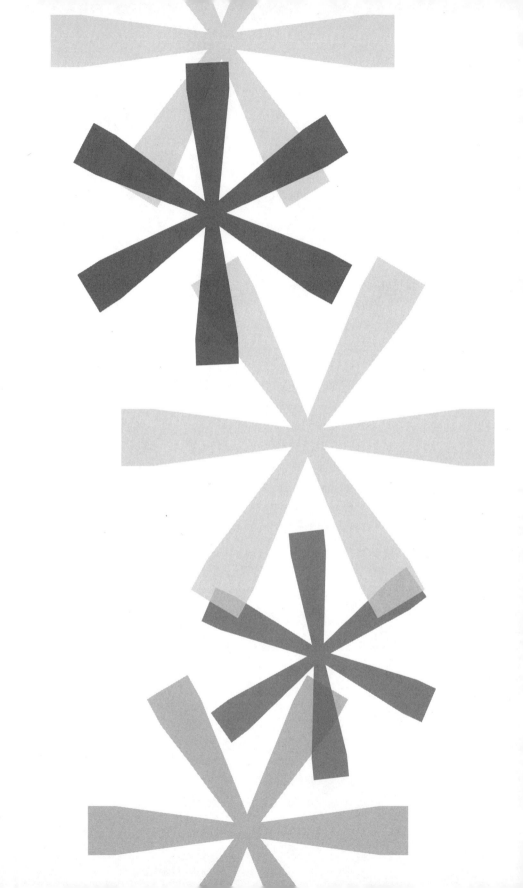

CONTENTS

Preface * ix

Introduction * MEN MATTER * 1

1 * ALONE AMONG STRANGERS * 21

The Medicalization of Childbirth

2 * KEEPING VIGIL * 48

Fathers in Waiting Rooms

3 * THE BEST BACKRUBBER * 86

Fathers Move into Labor Rooms

4 * HE WANTS TO KNOW * 120

Prenatal Education for Fathers

5 * PEACEFUL AND CONFIDENT * 156

Mothers and Fathers in Labor Rooms

6 * SIDE BY SIDE * 195

Men Move into Delivery Rooms

7 * WE DID IT * 236

Together in Delivery and Birthing Rooms

Epilogue * EXPECTANT FATHERS' EXPECTATIONS * 284

A Note on Sources * 297

Notes * 299

Acknowledgments * 367

Index * 371

PREFACE

Until fairly recently, historians have treated childbirth as if it were a story only about midwives, physicians, changing technology, and medical advances. Then it became clear that labor and delivery could not be understood without the birthing woman's perspective and experience. After all, she was the main actor, the one doing the hard physical work, of course with the help of birth attendants and medical knowledge. For the most part the history of childbirth has entirely neglected the fathers-to-be.[1]

I am one of the historians of childbirth who previously ignored the fathers; in earlier work my emphasis has been on birthing women and their experiences.[2] So it is natural to ask why a women's historian would want to write a book about men and childbirth. The answer is that the more I studied the history of medicalized childbirth, the more I realized that it is impossible to understand women's experience without also addressing all the participants involved in the birth of a child—including the men—and without analyzing the place in which most births of the period occurred, the hospital. Because it is both a biological and a cultural event, childbirth illuminates evolving power relationships, the importance of place, and the disparities of both race- and class-based privilege. In order to understand women's childbirth experiences in the five decades from 1935 to 1985, it is essential to consider the men and the hospital context.

Even though I had not written about fathers and childbirth before launching this project, I have been attuned to the subject for a long time. When I was growing up, my mother often told a story about her labor before the birth of my brother in the mid-1930s in a New York City hospital. During labor in a semiprivate room, the woman in the next bed would scream out with every contraction—and here my mother would raise her arm in the air and shout, mimicking the woman: "God damn you, Seymour!!" Over and over again the suffering woman repeated this phrase at the top of her lungs, blaming her husband for her pains: "God damn you, Seymour!!" Imprinting itself on my mother's birth experience, the phrase has resonated with me, too, over the years. Had Seymour done any more than the obvious to warrant such abuse? The next morning, after both women had delivered healthy babies, Seymour himself appeared, with flowers for his wife, who welcomed him warmly without any of the previous day's vitriol.

My mother's story about Seymour, with emphasis on the woman's screams during labor blaming her husband and with some hilarity about Seymour himself, whom my mother portrayed as looking rather henpecked and meek, stayed with me. As a historian, however, I did not see its significance in my previous writing about childbirth, which occurred during the height of the women's movement when my focus primarily was the birthing woman herself. The births of my own two children in the 1970s, during which my husband accompanied and helped me throughout labor and delivery, proved the point of men's importance ever more strongly. Now moving my research focus into the mid- to late twentieth century, I have come to understand how in that period men played vital roles in hospitalized childbirth as supporters of birthing women, and even as decision makers, and that their roles evolved over time.[3]

The men who form the major focus of this book were starting their families in a period dominated by the aftermath of World War II, the Korean conflict, and the Vietnam War and by fears of the atomic bomb and the Cold War. Television situation comedies, like *Ozzie and Harriet* and *Leave It to Beaver*, portrayed the 1950s as a decade of happy nuclear families with a breadwinning father, a stay-at-home mother, and happy children living in suburban bliss. Yet family historians have identified this period as one filled with significant changes that are relevant for understanding changing roles for new fathers and new birth options.

The celebration of Father's Day is a good indicator of changes within the family and within society that are reflected in the changing practices of childbirth between the postwar period and the mid-1980s. The holiday was first recognized by a joint resolution of Congress in 1956, and then in 1972 President Richard Nixon established a permanent national observance of Father's Day to be held on the third Sunday of June. This public recognition of men's new family roles can be seen, too, in the 1980s when Bill Cosby published his extremely popular book on fatherhood and a new magazine called *Fathers Magazine* appeared because, in the words of its editor, "fathers were showing a new interest in themselves."[4]

Men's participation in hospital-based births can be conceptualized along a space-time continuum. Fathers-to-be found their place in hospital childbirth in four chronologically sequential spaces. These spaces—the waiting room, the labor room, the delivery room, and the birthing room—significantly shaped and held the men's experiences and thus influence the organization of this book. These rooms illustrate the expanding scope as well as the limits and boundaries of the men's participation at different points in time: men first bonded as a group in maternity waiting rooms in the 1940s and 1950s; as they moved from the waiting room to the labor room in the 1960s and ultimately to the delivery and birthing rooms in the 1970s and 1980s, they became individually more integral to the birth experience, and their influence over events expanded.

Fathers not only supported the birthing mothers; they also acted for themselves, from a separate, emotionally distinct, and very poignant place. In so doing, they created and defined a historically new domestic role for men. This book tells their story.

MAKE ROOM FOR DADDY

MEN MATTER

On December 8, 1952, American television audiences watching *I Love Lucy* saw a prime-time first: a pregnant actress playing the part of a pregnant woman. Lucille Ball and Desi Arnaz, her real-life and television husband, along with the show's producer, had decided to address directly a subject that had previously been taboo. Although women had been getting pregnant and having babies for millennia, television shows in the early 1950s routinely acknowledged that fact by producing a baby without the nine-month preliminaries. Arnaz, already the father of little Lucie, wanted it to be different this time: "I wanted to talk about my child. I didn't want to put Lucille in a closet for nine months. Having a baby is a perfectly natural happening."[1]

CBS initially balked at the idea, worried that its audience would find pregnancy and childbirth subjects of questionable taste for television. The show's sponsor, Philip Morris, also took some convincing. The cigarette maker ultimately agreed but insisted, ironically, that Lucy not smoke in the episodes about her pregnancy. Jess Oppenheimer, the show's producer, recalled: "We felt certain we could extract all the inherent humor from the situation while staying within the bounds of good taste." To ensure that nothing offensive escaped notice, the network arranged for a priest, a minister, and a rabbi to vet the scripts.[2]

In the popular situation comedy, Arnaz played Ricky Ricardo, a Cuban nightclub singer and orchestra leader, and Ball was Lucy Ricardo, a housewife with ambitions for a career beyond the confines of domestic life. Starting with the episode that aired in early December 1952, the series dealt with familiar prenatal topics and played up two different gendered responses. In the first episode, Ricky learned he was going to be a father. After a number of botched attempts to tell him the good news in private, Lucy went to the Tropicana Club to tell Ricky in public. Overwhelmed with happiness, Ricky sang of his—and their—joy: "We're having a baby. My baby and me! We're adding a limb to our family tree. While pushing that carriage, how proud I will be."[3]

For television, the pregnancy was telescoped into seven episodes. Throughout the shows in which Lucy was "enceinte" (writers used the French word along with "expecting" to describe Lucy's condition),[4] the series took on various quirks of pregnant women, including food cravings, unpredictability, and preoccupations. Not only did these episodes open the door for television to look humorously and more frankly at experiences that most American women faced at least once during their lives, but they also allowed a comedic prime-time spoof of that other person involved with and affected by a pregnancy, the "expectant" father.

Television critics and scholars of popular culture have tended to focus on Lucy's role in the maternity episodes.[5] To focus on Ricky, however, and through him on the millions of new fathers to whose condition he gives voice and humor, reveals not only a different point of view but the stirrings of cultural change. Ricky wants to be a father, but he is not sure how to react when the fact of his wife's pregnancy seems to dismiss his importance or to ignore him completely. In one episode, Ricky laments explicitly, "It's very hard to be an expectant father." Pregnancy and childbirth, it seems, are conditions women know about and share in their particular gender-linked ways; in contrast, men have to learn and grow into their roles.

Even as Ricky declared he was thrilled with his wife's new status, the show also portrayed his own more ambivalent feelings and confusions, playing his responses off against hers. For example, as they debated possible names for the baby, Lucy changed her mind frequently, and Ricky tolerantly went along with every suggestion. Lucy admitted wanting a girl, to dress up in frilly clothes, and Ricky wanted a boy, to play football and box.

In one episode, Ricky suffers from what its title calls "Labor Pains." Lucy is so preoccupied with baby clothes, diapering and bathing a doll for practice, and daydreaming about the baby that she seems not to notice him. She pays little attention to his needs and forgets her usual domestic tasks like cooking dinner. Finally Ricky takes to bed with stomachaches and pains, unconsciously mimicking Lucy's physical changes.* The doctor, who understands what is happening, secretly advises Lucy to find a way to make Ricky again the center of domestic attention. Lucy and her friend Ethel plot to have Ethel's husband, Fred, throw Ricky a "daddy shower," which turns out to be a great success and puts Ricky back on top. At the end of the episode, however, Ricky finds out the whole thing was a setup and at 4:00 A.M. joins Lucy in her craving for pistachio ice cream with hot fudge and sardines.

Ricky makes jokes about expectant fathers' anxieties and humorously demonstrates his worries about impending fatherhood. In the process he faces the very real changes of life that happen to the man as well as to the woman during the months leading up to delivery. Ricky worries about having enough money to raise and properly educate the child, and he shares Lucy's concerns about being a good parent. As the father-to-be, Ricky shows audiences how to laugh about the sometimes inane, sometimes poignant role of the man whose wife gets all the attention as her body changes. He also depicts the ways in which a man can help a woman through pregnancy and childbirth when he humors Lucy's whims, picks up after her, and carefully plans every detail of their trip to the hospital so they will be prepared "when the time has come."

---

*Anthropologists have uncovered such practices in most of the world's cultures; called couvade, it refers to a man's physical reactions to his wife's pregnancy and childbirth.

The final episode of the pregnancy series aired on January 19, 1953 (the day Lucille Ball actually delivered her second child), and was watched by an audience estimated at 70 percent of television viewers—44 million Americans. In "Lucy Goes to the Hospital," Ricky, Fred, and Ethel rehearse their plan calmly: to call the doctor, remember to take the pre-packed suitcase, support Lucy, call a cab, and get her to the hospital. They practice it a few times and perfect all the logistics. When Lucy announces that she is really ready to go to the hospital, predictably and hilariously everything falls apart. The doctor's phone line is busy, Ricky and Fred drop the suitcase, emptying its contents onto the floor, and the three rush out of the apartment leaving Lucy to fend for herself. By the time they arrive at the hospital, Ricky is in the wheelchair, and Lucy is walking behind, carrying her own suitcase.

Like real-life men in this period, Ricky is not permitted beyond the maternity ward's reception area, where he signs all the necessary papers and provides the money while Lucy goes off into the labor room. Ricky is relegated to the fathers' waiting room, where he paces, constantly checks his watch, and tries to imagine what is happening beyond the closed door. There is one other man in the room with Ricky, but he is experienced in the waiting business and remains calm while Ricky paces. Labor is slow, and Ricky finally has to leave to go to work. He dresses up in his nightclub "voodoo" costume in the waiting room before leaving for the Tropicana. In the middle of his club act, he learns that Lucy has delivered, and he rushes back to the hospital without changing out of his costume, ultimately scaring the nurses and getting into trouble with the police until Fred and Ethel rescue him.

The scene portrayed Ricky prancing around the waiting room with face paint and a wig, looking completely alien.[6] In addition to spoofing the situation of the father-to-be, the writers accentuated Ricky's Cuban ethnicity and exaggerated his otherness by adding the voodoo costume.[7] The decision to have Ricky in such a costume demonstrated how uncomfortable the television producers thought viewers might be with the whole subject of childbirth. The producers hoped that by portraying the scene as so far out of the ordinary it would become more palatable for their mostly white television audience.

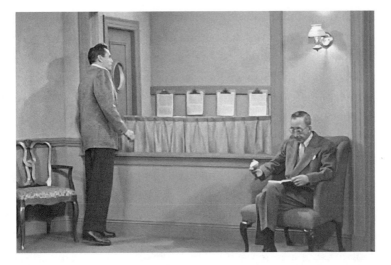

Ricky paces nervously in a fathers' waiting room as he awaits the news of the delivery after Lucy was admitted to the hospital and put in a labor room. His only companion in the room is a man who had been through the experience before and remains calm. From *I Love Lucy*, January 19, 1953. Courtesy of CBS Broadcasting Inc.

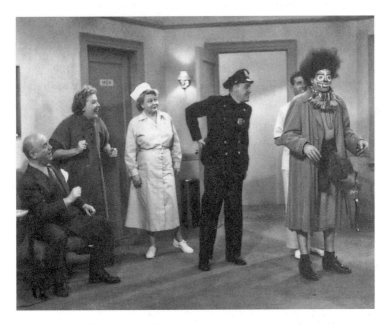

Ricky in his nightclub costume in the fathers' waiting room, where his appearance causes the hospital staff to call the police. From *I Love Lucy*, January 19, 1953. Courtesy of CBS Broadcasting Inc.

In the context of the history of childbirth in this period, the costume also has to be seen as a demonstration of Ricky's outsider status with regard to motherhood itself. He was not the one giving birth; he was not included in labor and delivery; he paced in the waiting room apart from the action because birth is women's work. The costume emphasized this outsider status for all fathers even as it played on Ricky's specific ethnic and racial otherness. Men were supposed to wait outside while women did the real work of labor and delivery.

It is useful to examine these episodes of I Love Lucy in part because they were the first of their kind on television and had a very large audience. Even more important, the series demonstrates that not just motherhood but also fatherhood had become an acceptable public topic by the early 1950s. The men represented by Ricky's escapades were becoming newly aware of their impending fatherhood and of their separation from their birthing wives. They were beginning to want to do something to change hospital childbirth practices. They did not like sitting alone and apart and were starting to flex their muscles about this subject; Ricky's dilemmas were theirs.

In ways that scholars have previously noted, situation comedies address subjects of interest in the lives of their viewers. They reflect that interest at the same time that they sometimes move it in new directions. The fact that I Love Lucy could portray a pregnant woman and her expectant husband underscores the judgment of the show's network and sponsor that American television-viewing audiences in the early 1950s were open to those portrayals and were ready to examine how what they saw on the screen might somehow reflect on their own lives. Television's portrayals can be seen as important to understanding the cultural perceptions of the period. In the words of critic John Fiske, "Television often acts like a relay station: it rarely originates topics of public interest . . . ; rather, what it does is give them high visibility, energize them, and direct or redirect their general orientation."[8]

Like I Love Lucy, most examples of television shows and films that addressed childbirth in the mid-twentieth century (as we will see elsewhere in this book) were among the most popular of the domestic situation-comedy genre and had some impact, even if not a direct one or a conscious one, on how society saw expectant fathers. Robert Price, an African American writer who described his own behavior during his wife's delivery in 1975, wrote, "Despite hundreds of TV comedies about the antics of expectant fathers, all of which I despise, I was acting just like one."[9] Shows like *I Love Lucy* indeed may have helped to determine how men responded to labor and delivery; at the least, they were part of the filter through which many of those men viewed their own behavior.[10]

Lucille Ball's actual delivery, a prearranged cesarean section on the morning of the day the show's waiting-room episode aired, was outwardly much calmer than the television portrayal. Desi Arnaz waited in the fathers' waiting room with one reporter, and when he received news of the birth of his son, Desi Jr. (Little Ricky on TV), he ran out of the waiting room shouting, "It's a boy! It's a boy!" Referring to the couple's eighteen-month-old daughter, he pronounced, "Now we have everything!" The television and real-life event was momentous enough that in his regular national news broadcast that week, which also saw the presidential inauguration of Dwight D. Eisenhower, ABC commentator Walter Winchell announced: "This was a banner week—the nation got a man and Lucy got a boy."[11]

*

In the chapters that follow, expectant fathers, both real-life and fictional figures like Ricky Ricardo, hold center stage in the exploration of twentieth-century childbirth in American hospitals. Fathers form a crucial facet of the story of childbirth even, maybe especially, in the period when most American women gave birth in hospitals under the supervision of physicians.[12] In the popular culture and popular literature these fathers were usually caricatured and ridiculed as hapless and helpless, ignorant fools pacing in the hallways and waiting rooms of hospitals. They were not a serious part of the event.

The story of childbirth provides a telling example of how each generation of historians asks its own questions, changes how we tell history, and changes its meaning. The traditional history of obstetrics, full of great doctors and their scientific innovations, morphed into the history of childbirth, emphasizing birthing women's role in the process. Along the way, historians added research on midwives and on obstetric nurses, on the hospital, and on the state. We set the experience into its social and political context. We understood childbirth as both a medical and a women's experience. And now, as our consciousness about how gender analysis must include and illuminate men's experiences, we add fathers-to-be as vital players in understanding childbirth's history. An examination of all the participants in the twentieth-century childbirth story provides a fuller and more complex picture and changes our understanding of who wielded power and how the basic narrative changed over time.[13]

The five middle decades of the twentieth century, approximately 1935–85, represent the historical period when the medicalization of childbirth achieved its firmest grip. In 1938 half of American women delivered their babies in hospitals, attended by physicians and increasingly by obstetric specialists, and the proportion of hospital deliveries rose dramatically thereafter. By 1955, 95 percent of all births in the United States occurred within hospital walls. By 1985, the essential outlines of early twenty-first-century childbirth were well established: the vast majority of American women of all races and economic circumstances delivered their babies in hospitals, attended by physicians and nurses and often accompanied by family or friends.

There were significant variations in hospital birth experiences, and many of them will be explored in this book. By the mid-1960s, for example, 99 percent of white births took place within hospitals, of which there were more than seven thousand throughout the country, but only 85 percent of nonwhite births were hospitalized. About 25 percent of all live births took place in hospitals with fewer than one hundred beds, and half of these in very small hospitals not accredited by the American Hospital Association. The length of hospital maternity stays also varied and changed over time. In the 1940s, women might remain in the hospital for seven to fourteen days after delivery; by the 1960s, this had decreased to four to five days; and by the 1980s a two- to three-day stay was typical.[14]

During these five decades, physicians and hospitals came to define how most American women delivered their children. Hospital routines and rituals set the parameters of most women's experiences, which became considerably more homogeneous than birth had been at home in the sense that marked differences by race, class, and culture at the beginning of the period had by 1985 become more similar. From the 1930s into the 1960s, the women who went to the hospital to have their babies often likened birth in the hospital to factory assembly lines. Reform groups, such as those that formed the natural childbirth movement by the 1970s, worked to make the hospital birth experience less medical and impersonal and more family friendly, and these efforts are a part of the story that follows. Parents, including fathers, played key roles in effecting those reforms. The men acted not just to improve their wives' experiences but also on their own behalf. They contested hospital spaces and medical authority to find a place for themselves and, in so doing, created unprecedented new roles for themselves. Fathers responded to childbirth by seeking considerable participation and increasing authority at the very height of medical definition and regulation of the event.

An examination of the evolution of fathers' place in hospital childbirth from the waiting room to the labor room to the delivery room and the birthing room, reveals that these spaces literally situate the men's actions and become frames through which to understand the progression of their activities and concerns. The rooms themselves — the actual physical spaces — thus form an important component in defining men's roles in the birth process. The rooms and the process by which the men moved in and through them also help us to understand that men at the beginning of the twenty-first century are still defining their own place in the drama of childbirth.

Chapter 1 provides background to the chapters that follow by situating hospital childbirth historically. Chapter 2 focuses on the men in the waiting rooms and examines how they felt as they waited for the births of their children and bonded with one another. Chapter 3 follows the men as they take their first steps out of the waiting room and into the labor room to be with their wives during the 1940s and 1950s. Because most hospitals required that men take prenatal classes before becoming active participants in hospital birth, Chapter 4 looks at those classes, which were also places where men found reassurance from the presence of other men. Chapter 5 looks at hospital labor rooms during the 1960s and 1970s, when fathers become a routine presence during this first stage of the birth experience. Once they were active participants in labor, many men wanted to continue to be involved in birth, and they sought entrance into hospital delivery rooms, a process described through the 1960s in Chapter 6. Chapter 7 describes men's increasing participation in delivery and presence in the ultimate hospital spaces, birthing rooms, starting in the 1970s. The Epilogue examines what men in the early twenty-first century expect from their experiences with childbirth.

Hospital spaces reflect power relations in those institutions. There have been and remain two strong sources of power in the hospital: administrative and medical. Administrative power is arguably the most potent because of the importance of financial stability to expanding the hospital patient base or medical and surgical treatment options. Bottom-line finances thus undergird all hospital planning.[15] The focus in this book is on the second form of hospital power, that which relies on science and technology and is personalized in the physician and the specialist. Outside of administrative offices, hospital spaces with the greatest show of technical equipment often represent procedures of the specialists who earn the most money and wield the greatest influence. In obstetrics, delivery rooms, with their sophisticated machines and equipment, are the heart of the important work. Labor rooms are places where women's bodies slowly prepare themselves as the cervix effaces and the womb opens, but it is in the delivery rooms where the hard work of getting the babies out occurs.

In tracing the story of childbirth practices, it is useful to think of three "Ps"—place, privilege, and power. Along the continuum of five decades of change, these axes not only give meaning and complexity to the story but also provide a lens through which to view larger issues of twentieth-century medicine and its inequalities.

Place defines. The hospital itself mattered. Those women who could get access to and afford to deliver in private hospitals had earliest access to flexibility in birth practices. Place within the hospital—the geography of labor and delivery—shaped and influenced men's birth experiences over the mid-twentieth-century years examined here. In the waiting rooms, men were physically removed from the birth action, but within those distant rooms, they communicated meaningfully with one another and collectively helped to figure out ways to participate more actively in labor and delivery. From the waiting rooms, men moved into labor rooms, those bare rooms where they could share the experience of labor with their wives and help them cope. Being alone together in labor was a significant step for the couples, many of whom waxed eloquent about how much it meant to them to share those intimate hours. In the labor rooms men had access to nurses and physicians, they learned more about the birth process, and many of them eagerly became part of it. The next step, moving into the delivery room, completed the quest. Men, in traveling from the periphery of the waiting room to the center of delivery room, had gained their own place in birth. Combined labor-delivery rooms, or birthing rooms, became a spatial monument to men's success in entering and becoming connected to the hospital childbirth experience. The fathers, by their very presence and by their activities, changed the activities within the rooms. Still in flux at the beginning of the twenty-first century are the myriad ways men might yet define and practice that place.

The power of place is evident in the geography of the hospital. The physical spaces themselves first let the laymen know their place: they were outsiders, present only at the pleasure of the medical staff. They did not have a place for themselves. But ultimately the men learned to make the spaces less alien and more accommodating; in fact, some men found ways to use the spaces to increase their own comfort, activity, and even authority alongside the physicians.

Privilege counts. Hospital childbirth practices varied widely in the twentieth century. Hospitals in rural areas with small patient loads had a high degree of flexibility, and individual stories revealed relatively relaxed practices. But hospitals, once built (often with federal funds), could not easily be rebuilt, and space limitations often made reformed practices, such as allowing men into labor or delivery rooms, difficult or impossible. Urban hospitals serving paying patients were the first to change systematically, but there, too, architecture sometimes demanded restraints on such reforms. Furthermore, urban hospitals' high population density sometimes restricted reforms. One would need a hospital-by-hospital review to quantify and map the different levels and rates of change in this period.

Nonetheless, overall patterns emerge. Segregation by social class was a significant organizer of hospital spaces, with private or semiprivate rooms for those who could pay for the privilege and multibed wards for the others. White middle-class women—those who wanted to adopt natural childbirth and who wanted their husbands to accompany them through labor and delivery—accomplished their goals first. Race and class restrained others who might have wanted such practices. At mid-twentieth century, many hospitals around the country remained racially segregated. At least 98 of the 7,750 hospitals and clinics receiving federal funds under the 1946 Hill-Burton Act did not accept black patients at all, and most of the ones that did maintained racially segregated wards. According to David Barton Smith, "Until the 1960s, health services and providers were segregated in the South and in most northern cities." In Alabama, for example, Hill-Burton funds helped construct racially segregated or separate hospitals and clinics in all but two of its sixty-seven counties. In the South, not only were floors labeled "colored" and "white," but sheets, gowns, and thermometers also were not shared between the races. In the North, racial segregation practices included hospital rooms and maternity floors. Not until 1963, when a landmark court case, *Simkins v. Moses H. Cone Memorial Hospital*, established that the equal protection clause of the Fourteenth Amendment to the Constitution applied to all hospitals— public and voluntary—and prohibited them from such discrimination, did such practices begin to disappear.[16] The anti-discrimination decision was reflected in the 1964 Civil Rights Act, and in 1966 Medicare systematically operationalized it and finally, in the words of two historians, "broke the back of segregated health services."[17]

Both race- and class-based privilege influenced Cook County Hospital in Chicago, as an example. In the 1950s, 96 percent of Chicago births took place within hospitals, but two-thirds of area hospitals did not admit African American patients. Black women ready to deliver could go to four Chicago hospitals, two predominantly black voluntary hospitals and two public hospitals. Fifty-four percent delivered at Cook County Hospital, compared with 2 percent of whites. In that overcrowded hospital, women frequently labored in hallways, alone in public spaces. Choices about methods of birth or attendants did not exist for those women.[18] By the 1970s and 1980s, birth options had expanded for middle-class women of color, whereas poor black and white women's options still were constrained. Men sharing labor and delivery in the 1970s and 1980s were still mostly middle or upper class. Childbirth reform in this sense was a movement of the privileged.

Power shifts. Decision-making power and authority followed their own trajectory concurrent with the men moving into and through the four rooms. Power over childbirth activities historically lodged with birthing women and their female friends and relations. When birth left its traditional home setting and became a hospital event, decisions about birthing procedures moved significantly to the health care professionals, mainly physicians. Then, over time, because of combined factors of women's collective demands, the childbirth reform movement, and a gendered masculine bonding between the male physicians and the fathers-to-be and among the laymen themselves, decision making became more of a shared process. By the late twentieth century, birthing women, their partners, their physicians and nurses, and ultimately other family members joined in planning the birth event. The changes examined in this book reside almost exclusively with married men in traditional heterosexual couples. Of course, unmarried women and lesbians found themselves in hospital birthing rooms concurrently. But their systems of support did not receive recognition in hospital policy and did not become evident in the records until many of the formal changes had already occurred and until a broader definition of the family emerged at the end of the five decades under study.

At midcentury physicians and specialist obstetricians were at the pinnacle of their labor and delivery powers. They provided modern medical and surgical procedures aimed at making birth scientific and safe. Nurses strongly felt that they worked in tension between their obligations to hospitals, birthing women, and physicians. For their part, birthing women had lost much decision-making authority when they no longer delivered in their own homes and went instead to hospitals to give birth. Their husbands had had some traditional authority—based in the patriarchal family structure—sometimes in choosing the birth attendant, for example, but in the hospital, men in waiting rooms deeply felt their lack of control or even connection to the events of birth. They were present in the hospital but separated from the action. As they moved from the periphery to the center, from the waiting room to the delivery room, men become more involved and gained in their ability to intervene in the birth process.

Physicians continued to wield a lot of power throughout this period, the power that came with knowledge and expertise as well as tradition and status, and even as they learned to share some of it over time, they did not lose this commanding position. Just as physicians in other specialties learned the power of consumer demands, so too did obstetricians.[19] They shared it in part by including laymen in discussions, and they shared it in communication with both birthing women and their partners, in collaboration with obstetric nurses, and in their participation in community organizations. Power shifted as men moved to a participatory role in childbirth: decisions about specific procedures and methods were shared more widely. Even so, fathers' participation did not create an egalitarian environment; rather, it often reinforced both their own authority as head of the household and physicians' authority as medical experts. Men's involvement in their wives' labors and deliveries did not challenge traditional hierarchies.

The basic patterns of changing spaces and evolving authority showed great variation in the United States, differing according to geographic region, rural or urban setting, socioeconomic class, and race. Changes that moved fathers into more active birthing roles were first implemented by those institutions that catered to white middle- and upper-class women and men, who could afford the services, whereas predominantly black hospitals and financially limited public hospitals, as well as many hospitals in the South, did not incorporate changes sometimes until decades later. Thus, this history of men's involvement in childbirth, which might at first appear to be a rather narrow issue of concern—relevant to men and women only during the few moments in their lives when they are having children—actually becomes a window into larger issues of twentieth-century medicalization and its inequalities.

*

Even before the 1950s, suburban living changed men's roles in the home as much as it defined women's domestic life. Historian Margaret Marsh calls the changes for men associated with the move to the suburbs "masculine domesticity," which before the second wave of feminism "prompted husbands to take on increased responsibility for the emotional well-being of their children, to spend their leisure with their wives rather than male cronies, and even to take on limited domestic duties."[20] This change did not promote an equal sharing of domestic tasks or resemble a feminist vision of equality of opportunities in the larger society, but it did extend men's roles especially with regard to their children, as experts advised men to participate in "nightly feedings and bedtime stories."[21] Even Dr. Spock, whose child-rearing handbook dominated middle-class thinking about parenting at midcentury and who advocated women staying home to raise their children, similarly advised that men play a larger domestic role.[22] Men's increasing interest in childbirth is closely connected to this notion of an increased masculine role in training up the next generation. Indeed, one early proponent of this domestic masculinity, in advocating that men should share in the rearing of their children, explicitly noted that men should begin this involvement by attending their children's births.[23]

The decade of the 1950s, during which many of the changes described in this book began or accelerated, instead of representing a romantic family utopia, was the beginning of a volatile era in family history. During the Second World War, of course, many women, epitomized by Rosie the Riveter, worked outside the home participating in the war industry and taking the places of men who were in the military. During the postwar period many women continued working outside the home. In 1950, still one-quarter of married women were in the paid workforce, often moving from their husbands' old jobs into sales and clerical positions in suburban banks, corporations, and retail shops. Married women made up more than half of the total number of women working outside the home. Nonetheless, historian Stephanie Coontz reminds us, "Nearly 60 percent of kids—an all time high—were born into male breadwinner–female homemaker families."[24] The suburbs—where nuclear families owned their own homes—might have epitomized the white middle-class ideal (in the 1950s also realized by many of the skilled working class), but life in them was not uncomplicated.[25]

Indeed, from its start the decade of the 1950s was already a period of flux. The popular 1955 novel and subsequent movie *The Man in the Gray Flannel Suit* caught some of the changing moods and anxieties.[26] The male protagonist returns from the war and searches for purpose; ultimately he turns down a high-pressure job in order to spend more time with his family. Men and women felt the strains of meshing work and home life in this period. There were more married women (including pregnant women) in the workforce, and many suburban stay-at-home women found their lives unfulfilled, a situation popularly recognized in 1963 by Betty Friedan in her book on the "feminine mystique."[27] Historian Jessica Weiss, in her study of postwar families, finds that Friedan's description "hid the vast diversity of women's experiences behind the full skirts of the bored middle-class homemaker. The picture is much more complicated."[28] Women's and men's search for more satisfying childbirth experiences must be seen within this fluid and complex cultural context of family redefinition and flux. Much childbirth reform activity was rooted in suburban living and changing family structures.

Black families and black masculinity in this period followed a somewhat different trajectory. Housing covenants often segregated African Americans or entirely kept them out of the suburbs and many middle-class neighborhoods. In contrast to what was pushing white suburban men to increase their family-oriented activities, one strand of cultural values that emerged in the African American community was epitomized by the "strong black man." It focused attention on men providing financial support and discipline for the family but in the postwar period did not call for a more domestic role for the father and head of the household. Not until the 1970s and later did competing ideas incorporating notions of masculine domesticity, including valuing a more systematic participation in domestic tasks and child rearing, find significant support among black men as they turned to more varied notions of black masculinities.[29] Resistance to such behavior remained strong. As Mark Anthony Neal, a scholar of black cultural studies, put it, "Models of black masculinity that ventured too far beyond the 'Strong Black Man' are seen as suspect: not quite black enough, not quite man enough, not quite blackman enough."[30]

Yet in the 1970s and 1980s many individual African American men withstood this kind of criticism and adopted a broader notion of masculinity that included an important domestic role. *The Cosby Show*, which first aired in 1984 and ran for eight seasons, capitalized on depicting domestic fatherly roles for middle-class African American men and provided a public model for increasing black men's domestic activities.[31] And as hospitals integrated during the same decades, black couples found that being together during the births of their children fostered this new role in the family for African American men.[32]

Compounding the situation, the suburbs themselves became more diverse in the 1960s and 1970s, and the domestic housewife's way of life came under the critical scrutiny of the feminist movement. These changes also impacted childbirth reform and other twentieth-century efforts to make hospitals more responsive to consumer desires.[33] One expression of how a feminist point of view about childbirth affected childbirth practices came in 1973 when U.S. representative Martha Griffiths, a Democrat from Michigan, introduced a bill to allow fathers to accompany the mothers of their children into the delivery room and to be there when their children were born. The language of the bill expressed the women's movement's emphasis on equality for women. Certainly many women saw the right to determine the methods and circumstances of childbirth—to exercise choice—as important to women *as women*; this was one aspect of the basic issue of gender equality, along with reproductive rights, access to employment, and equal pay.[34]

It is noteworthy that the childbirth reform movement ultimately melded both feminist and nonfeminist parts. Childbirth reform overlapped the women's movement when it supported women's voices in choosing birthing methods and attendants; yet, in contrast to the women's movement, it accommodated rather than challenged medical authority, and it accepted cultural gender norms. Women and men across the political spectrum, community organizations, and physicians and nurses worked together to bring about change within the system.[35] The language of childbirth education and reform emphasized the heterosexual nuclear family more than it did women's rights. The reforms served men's interests as well as women's—just as the reformers were both men and women—and enhanced the power of men to help determine events.

Those who brought about the changes that form the core of this book represented a diverse group, but the majority of them were people who were willing to work within prevailing power structures. It was a movement of the advantaged; most of the activity led first to changes in private hospitals and private wings of community hospitals that served paying white middle-class couples. Minority middle-class couples entered the fray next and also gained access to shared birth experiences. Working-class and poor women (both white and women of color), single mothers, and others who delivered in public hospitals had more limited choices in childbirth throughout the midcentury period.

The postwar period was extremely fraught. According to historian Jane E. Levey: "The stresses of war, the uncertainties of the ensuing peace, and the emerging relationship between ideologies of the family and American national identity together lent an unparalleled ambiguity and anxiety about family life."[36] While historians have argued that many eras of American history were filled with anxiety and that masculinity was challenged at various historical moments, it is still the case that in the middle decades of the twentieth century men's roles in the family were of great cultural interest and their fatherhood became a focus of substantial public comment.[37] Men in this period articulated their worries about the state of the world at the same time they tried to overcome their fears and prepare for fatherhood. In the process, they demonstrated emotional vulnerability and worries about whether and to what extent they would be up to their new roles. Caught as they were at the cusp of new familial relationships, they took their coming parenthood very seriously. Impending fatherhood, as it played out around the event of childbirth itself and as it was becoming publicly articulated as in the *I Love Lucy* episodes, reveals much both about how the men themselves internalized the period's ambiguities about masculinity and their roles within the family and about how men resolved the issues for themselves. In so doing, they helped to change hospital childbirth practices.

Men were not always happy with their experiences or with the changes they helped to bring about, and they could not necessarily laugh at themselves in the ways that Ricky Ricardo did on television. Real life, after all, does not directly imitate art. Nonetheless, Ricky's comical ways of coping with Lucy's reactions to pregnancy and his public acknowledgment of the importance of impending fatherhood help us to understand that whether humorous or serious, emotionally charged or ambivalent, men's diverse responses to childbirth matter.

1 * ALONE AMONG STRANGERS

The Medicalization of Childbirth

The vast majority of American women (99 percent) currently deliver their babies in hospitals, accompanied by their physicians, nurses, and midwives and often by their husbands, partners, family, and friends. The hospital routine is fairly standard, although variations exist among hospitals, and medical protocols have been developed for most exigencies. Many women discuss the possible procedures in advance with their physicians and midwives and, within prescribed limits, make birth plans outlining their choices about what might happen to them during labor and delivery. Once labor begins, however, some women find that their desires are ignored, either because a different physician happens to be on call or because the course of their labor necessitates unexpected specific interventions. Because of the need for medical assessment on the spot, often more decisions are left to the hospital and the physician than to the woman or her family.[1]

This kind of "medicalized" childbirth is relatively new, a product of the twentieth century. Even though we have come to accept it as typical, the historical record is very clear on how recent a phenomenon it is for physicians to be in control of labor and delivery and for women to bow to their expertise. Before settling in with the fathers for the rest of the book, this chapter reviews the broad trends in American childbirth and examines how and why and under what conditions such hospital-based, physician-directed, medicalized childbirth evolved. In the process, it lays out why mid-twentieth-century birthing women came to want their husbands to accompany them through labor and delivery in the hospital.

Traditional Childbirth

For most of human history, childbirth was exclusively a woman's event. When a woman went into labor, she "called her women together" and left her husband and other male family members outside. "I went to bed about 10 o'clock," wrote William Byrd of Virginia in the eighteenth century, "and left the women full of expectation with my wife."[2] Only in cases in which women were not available did men participate in labor and delivery, and only in cases in which labor did not progress normally did physicians intervene and perhaps extricate a dead fetus. A midwife orchestrated the events of labor and delivery, and women neighbors and relatives comforted and shared advice with the parturient.

Ebenezer Parkman wrote in the middle of the eighteenth century of one of the twelve times his wife was "brought to bed": "My wife very full of pain. This Morning I sent Ebenezer for Mrs. Forbush. . . . A number of Women here. Mrs. Hephzibath Maynard and her son's wife, Mrs. How, Mr. David Maynard's wife and his Brother Ebenezer's, Captain Forbush's and Mr. Richard Barns's. My son Ebenezer went out for most of them. At night I resign my Dear Spouse to the infinite Compassions, all sufficiency and sovereign pleasure of God and under God to the good Women that are with her, waiting Humbly the Event."[3]

Mary Louise Fowler wrote to her pregnant sister Nettie in 1863, when Nettie was in Europe with her husband: "I think of you in anticipation of your coming trial. I know you will have all that can be procured under the circumstances, but it would relieve me of great anxiety if you were in our best bed-room where I could nurse you as only a *mother* or a *sister* can."[4] The ethic of a proper childbirth was, for the overwhelming majority of women in the United States, rich or poor, and over a long period of time, a home birth attended by caring, concerned women relatives and friends. One mid-nineteenth-century woman put it this way: "A woman that was expecting had to take good care that she had plenty fixed to eat for her neighbors when they got there. There was no telling how long they was in for. There wasn't no paying these friends so you had to treat them good."[5]

To this women's world husbands, brothers, or fathers could gain only temporary entrance. In one instance, a new father was invited in to see his wife and new daughter, but then, "Mrs. Warren, who was absolute in this season of female despotism, interposed, and the happy father was compelled, with reluctant steps, to quit the spot."[6]

The women's world around the home birthing bed that is revealed in letters and diaries represents the existence of a specific female group identity among women. Women could write and speak to each other about intimate details of confinement-related care; they could confide their innermost thoughts about their coming motherhood. While nineteenth-century conventions did not permit discourse about such private matters in public, among themselves, in private, women could and did speak more freely. In their private writings and around the confinement bed, women identified with each other's concerns, shared their wisdom, and united, as women, in the knowledge that they were not alone in their problems. The roles women played for one another were not just psychological support but also involved very specific duties to aid labor and delivery along, such as applying olive oil and perineal massage.[7] In the words of one observer, women could be counted on to "know what to do without telling."[8] Another wrote, "Only a woman can know what a woman has suffered or is suffering."[9]

Physician-Attended Home Childbirth

Despite the very female nature of the childbirth experience, women in eighteenth-century American cities who could afford medical aid began inviting male physicians to attend them during labor and delivery. They did so because they thought doctors could improve on their chances of survival and comfort. They had no intention at that time to give over decision-making authority to the doctors. They wanted medical help and sought it in very specific ways. For a long time historians assumed that, when male doctors began attending normal births, women's birthing networks disappeared.[10] But more recent research has shown that women continued to help each other and to control childbirth events until birth moved to the hospital.[11]

The "medicalization" of childbirth did not occur in the eighteenth century, when physicians first attended obstetrical cases; nor did it develop in the nineteenth century as physicians became established figures in the home birthing rooms of most middle- and upper-class American women. Childbirth was not medicalized, in the sense that we use the term today to mean under physician control, until birth moved to the hospital.

In the home-birth period, physicians entered women's world around the birthing bed, and they learned how to act within a domain that was not their own. Some doctors learned it better than others as they tried to create a place for themselves in women's domestic world. One physician realized that "obstetrical practice is an intimate intrusion into family affairs."[12] Some doctors fit right in. "Dr. Marsh stalked into the room," wrote one birthing woman, "like an easy old friend. In a few minutes he was playing with Louisa [a child] and talking to me about the new baby. . . . He did what was expected of him, ate a bite of breakfast with Kate [her friend in attendance], then made himself so much at home, he put us all at ease. He took Louisa on his lap, and soon had her speaking pieces and singing."[13] Dr. Daniel Cameron, who practiced medicine in Wisconsin in the 1850s, told of one of his obstetric calls: "Wednesday, a week ago, was called on to confine Mrs. Conklin. . . . Sat up all night and talked *scandal* with some Cornish women in attendance."[14] Successful physicians were those who learned to relax and interact with the birthing woman's female attendants.

In the eighteenth century, physicians used opium and bleeding to help ease labor's discomforts, and by the end of that century they applied forceps to help along a protracted labor. In the mid-nineteenth century they added anesthetics, primarily ether and chloroform, for effective pain re-

lief. The possibility of a difficult delivery, which women fearfully anticipated, and the knowledge that physicians' remedies could provide relief
and successful outcomes encouraged women to seek out practitioners
whose obstetric armamentarium included drugs and instruments.[15]

Throughout the nineteenth century, the decision of whether to em-
ploy a physician remained where it had been traditionally, with birthing women and their female relatives and friends. Often the women consulted with their husbands, who paid the bill. The birthing woman, her
midwife, and her assistants might have decided to call a doctor after labor
had begun, and they then gave or withheld permission for each procedure
suggested. Home birthing rooms usually contained the traditional female
attendants right alongside the newer medical attendant, and these people
all discussed and decided what procedures might be employed during the
labor and delivery, the doctor adding his voice to the others. William Potts
Dewees, for example, wanted in one case to take blood from a laboring
woman: "I represented to the friends of the patient, the danger of her
case. . . . They agreed to the trial."[16] Although male physicians had broken
the gender barrier and birth was no longer exclusively a women's event,
women, by making their own choices about attendants and procedures,
continued to hold the power to shape events in the birthing room.

As new obstetrical techniques became available—especially forceps
and anesthesia—they worked to the advantage of physicians, who held
a monopoly over their use.[17] Centuries of female traditions and the domestic environment in which those traditions operated, however, continued to work to the advantage of women. Both women and physicians
had an expertise about childbirth, physicians' based on textbooks and
theory and women's based on experience. Some physicians welcomed
the knowledge of the birthing woman and her attendants. Chicago physician Morris Fishbein admitted that when he was a medical student in the
second decade of the twentieth century, he "received better instruction"
from a poor Irish woman whose eighth birth he attended than he ever
had in any classroom. "She was thoroughly familiar with every step of the
process."[18] Others found well-informed women intimidating. One physician recalled, "A young doctor, fresh from medical college, can pass many
embarrassing moments in the presence of the neighborhood midwife."[19]

As advisers in women's homes, physicians had to learn that while their words could be added to the other voices in the room, their views might or might not predominate. Sometimes considerable tension resulted from differences of opinion. An Oklahoma physician explained to his fellow doctors, for example, that he would never try to shave a patient's pubic hair (a procedure associated with the understanding of germ transmission at the end of the nineteenth century) even though he thought it would help prevent infection. "In about three seconds after the doctor has made the first rake with his safety [razor], he will find himself on his back out in the yard with the imprint of a woman's bare foot emblazoned on his manly chest, the window sash around his neck and a revolving vision of all the stars in the fermament [sic] presented to him. Tell him not to try to shave 'em."[20] Similarly, Dr. J. H. Guinn of Arkansas City, Kansas, wrote of the impossibility of achieving sterile conditions in urban or rural homes "in which there are five or six neighbor women, and, perhaps, the mother of the patient—all mothers of large families of children." The doctor could not, he thought, under such observation, "strip his patient and go at her with soap and scrub-brush, lather and razor."[21] Another practitioner put it bluntly: a doctor, he wrote, "has his living to make and cannot be too insistent with his patient over whom, usually, he has no control."[22] Doctors could offer advice, but they did not have the freedom of action in women's homes that they later achieved in hospitals.

The pressures some physicians felt in home birthing rooms did not abate as long as birth remained a home event. Dr. Samuel X. Radbill, who delivered babies in Philadelphia in the 1930s before limiting his practice to pediatrics, remembered the discomfort of working under the close observation of parturients' female friends and relatives. In one delivery he attended, the birthing woman's mother, who, after two days of labor, was extremely anxious for her daughter's welfare, "came rushing in in a rage, brandishing the [kitchen] knife and yelling, 'Doctor, if my daughter dies, I kill you!'" Radbill reported with great relief that shortly after that "the baby was safely delivered and everybody was as delirious with joy as they had been frantic with terror before."[23]

Under such conditions physicians had to keep a cool head and a steady hand. Radbill was relieved when a nearby hospital opened a maternity ward, where he could deliver his patients outside their homes and away from the pressures of the woman's family. From such examples, it is clear that physicians did not have the kind of control they came to want in obstetric cases until birth moved to the hospital. Home birth was medicalized only as much as women wanted it to be.

Birth Moves to the Hospital

In the twentieth century, birthing women and the growing number of physicians who specialized in obstetrics increasingly found fault with these home-based childbirth practices. Application of the new knowledge about bacteriology and germ transmission made home deliveries, even under the best of conditions, difficult to manage. Bacteriology was only one of five forces that pushed both birthing women and their physicians to try to modernize birth by moving it to the hospital.

The first factor propelling birth into the hospital was a continuation of fears about the dangers of childbirth; in the words of nineteenth-century women, it was the "shadow of maternity," a burden women carried through their reproductive years. The burden grew from high fertility rates and the ever present possibility of death or debility that concerned women as soon as they found themselves pregnant.[24] Women worried throughout their nine months of pregnancy that they would not survive the ordeal or that they would be maimed in the process. Clara Lenroot confided in her diary when she found herself pregnant in 1891, "It occurs to me that possibly I may not live. . . . I wonder if I should die, and leave a little daughter behind me, they would name her Clara. I should like to have them." Three days later she again worried, "If I shouldn't live I wonder what they will do with the baby! I should want Mamma and Bertha [sister] to have the bringing up of it, but I should want Irvine [husband] to see it every day and love it so much, and I should want it taught to love him better than anyone else in the world."[25] Lillie M. Jackson recalled her 1905 confinement: "While carrying my baby, I was so miserable. . . . I went down to death's door to bring my son into the world, and I've never forgotten."[26]

The shadow of maternity, which repeatedly darkened women's lives, moved women to seek to improve and make safer their maternity experiences. It led women to seek medical expertise in their confinements and helped them to appreciate, especially after germ theory was understood, the promise of the new medicine. They anticipated improving their own conditions by calling in doctors, and this growing faith in medicine ultimately led women to want childbirth to move to the hospital, where seemingly cleaner and safer conditions prevailed.

A second prominent factor leading women to put increasing trust in medical science was bacteriology, the science of the study of microorganisms, many of which cause infectious diseases in humans. The beginnings of bacteriology are usually associated with the work of Hungarian physician Ignaz Semmelweis, who instituted cleansing the hands and instruments used on laboring women during the 1840s, and the French chemist Louis Pasteur and German physician Robert Koch, whose investigations from the 1860s through the end of the century led to the identification of specific microorganisms and an understanding of their role in causing infection and disease. In obstetrics, the practical application of these discoveries took the form of physicians trying to keep a clean birth environment and minimize the transmission of bacteria that could cause postpartum infection, the single most significant killer of birthing women. By the end of the nineteenth century, physicians routinely tried to use sterile techniques when attending childbearing women in their homes; because they could not always achieve the desired cleanliness, physicians increasingly argued that childbirth would be safer in the hospital, where the environment could be better controlled.

Many physicians complained in this transition period that it was hard to persuade birthing women and their attending friends of the necessity for sterile environments. While it is no doubt true that some women did not understand why such extreme precautions for "scrupulous cleanliness" had to be taken, others very quickly took up the language and promise of the new science and worked hard to help physicians and nurses in their efforts. Whatever their feelings about bacteriology and its impact on obstetric practice, women found that the new prescriptions for cleanliness were hard to follow in their own homes. Thus both physicians and birthing women understood that the hospital offered the kind of environmental control that would allow for routine sterile deliveries and lessen — potentially — the danger of infection. One impact of the new medicine was to provide a compelling reason to centralize obstetrics practices within hospitals, where women's voices became weaker.

If promises and hope pulled women toward medical institutions in the early twentieth century, an equally potent force pushed them away from their traditional confinements. A third factor in the move to the hospital was the breakdown of the strong women's network that had existed through much of history. As America industrialized and urbanized, it became harder and harder for women to have at their beck and call a group of women who could offer the kinds of assistance they needed at the time of labor and delivery. The hospital thus beckoned the growing number of women who found their home births logistically hard to manage. Hallie Nelson's experiences in rural Nebraska emphasized some of the reasons women had begun to dread the ordeal of childbirth at home. Recalling when she was pregnant with her fifth child in 1936, Nelson wrote, "We had been at wit's ends to find a woman to take care of me and the baby and to help take care of the children." While she had been relatively successful in finding neighboring friends and relatives to attend her during her first four births, this time Hallie lamented, "The Clines had left the hills. . . . My sister Beulah was not available. . . . The other neighbors had children of their own to care for."[27]

The traditional woman-centered event in the home, called "social childbirth" by historians, had been predicated on women being available when parturients needed them. With the increased mobility of the population and subsequent physical isolation from families and friends, women found it more and more difficult to obtain the help they needed. Helen Whiting of Winchester, Virginia, believed that "if there are other children, the mother cannot have the peace and rest she needs [at home]."[28] Getting out of the home for confinements seemed the only way of coping with the stresses that developed when a woman was ready to deliver her baby.

The fourth factor that encouraged increased medicalization of childbirth at the turn of the century period was the use of new technology.

Throughout American childbirth history, two trends have been evident: one, women's awareness of the dangers of childbirth for their own lives and postpartum health, and two, the attempts to improve the level of safety for both mother and child through the use of new drugs and new instruments and the application of new technology. Bleeding techniques and opium derivatives were used in the colonial period to help women through labor; forceps were welcomed by the end of the eighteenth century; and in the nineteenth century anesthesia use increased to alleviate the pains of labor. Physicians modified and improved forceps innumerable times. Yet not until the twentieth century did the use of such innovations begin to work in the direction of increasing more exclusive medical authority over childbirth.

The relationship between the new technology and growing medical authority can best be seen through an examination of cases of difficult delivery—for example, cephalopelvic disproportion, in which a woman's pelvis is too small or misshapen to allow the passage of the fetal head. In such cases, physicians intervened, using forceps and other implements to attempt a live delivery, but often could not succeed. When forceps did not work—a situation more common in the past because of the prevalence of rickets, a vitamin D deficiency resulting in abnormal or weak bone growth—physicians tried to perform a craniotomy. By puncturing the fetal cranium and removing its contents, physicians reduced head size, facilitating delivery and saving the mother's life. By the end of the nineteenth century, a series of improvements on the cesarean section and new surgical procedures like the symphysiotomy or pubiotomy—procedures in which the pelvic opening was increased through the surgical separation of the pubic bones—offered a real chance for both mother and child to survive problematic deliveries. It was this potential that allowed physicians to transform their participation in such cases into a new, more active and authority-wielding role in the birthing room. Prefacing his argument with the remark "It would seem hardly necessary for me to emphasize the fact that the obstetrician alone must be the judge of what is to be done," Dr. George McKelway explained why such cases demanded medical control:

The preference of the ignorant or prejudiced parents or of the friends, the disposition on their part to save the life of one being from any added risk at the expense of the other being, or any sentimental considerations on their part of any nature, for or against either life at the expense of the other, should not weigh at all in the obstetrician's mind or decide his course. The responsibility is his for his conduct in the case, and he cannot answer to his own conscience if he does that which he believes to be inadvisable or wrong, simply because someone else prefers that he should.[29]

Obstetricians, for the first time in history, tried to take command on their own terms rather than respond to the problems as others defined them. It was in such high-risk cases requiring surgical interventions that physicians found their first true voice in the birthing room; they later learned to use the new authority in all birthing rooms, especially as childbirth moved out of women's homes and into medical institutions.

The fifth factor that led to increased medicalization in the early twentieth century was the hospital itself, the institution and what it came to stand for, and the public monies that became available to help some women pay for their hospital stays. The hospital attracted physicians who were trying to maintain a sterile environment, and it attracted those women who supported their efforts. The hospital became more attractive to women as their homes seemed less able to accommodate childbirth disruptions. The "hospital is equipped with every modern device for the safe delivery of babies," wrote one mother; "nursing and medical attention is available at any hour of the day or night. How much simpler—and more restful—to be in the hospital where babies are an accepted business."[30] Another woman found that her stay in the hospital "was like a lovely vacation."[31] Most important, the hospital came to symbolize what the new medicine had to offer. Whether the new medicine yet delivered on its promises (which, in the case of obstetrics, it arguably did not), women traded on the promises and hoped that the miracles of modern medicine would help them through a dangerous time.

Perhaps even more significant was the federal government's new willingness and ability to pay for medically aided maternity care. Arguing that childbirth was women's battleground in the same way as the Great War had been men's, advocates of the proposed Sheppard-Towner Act argued in 1921, "During the nineteen months we were at war, for every soldier who died as a result of wounds, one mother in the United States went down into the valley of the shadow and did not return."[32] The argument was powerful. Under the act, which was in effect from 1921 until 1929, federal funds became available for maternal and child health, and some of these were used to allow women who otherwise could not afford hospital care to go into the institutions for their deliveries. More wide ranging, the 1935 Social Security Act provided federal money for maternal and child health projects, which served to increase the medical attention received by pregnant and childbearing women.

The confluence of these five factors in the early twentieth century propelled childbirth into the hospital. For millennia women had controlled childbirth practices. But in a relatively short time in the twentieth century, women gave up what they had had for something even better: safety and security to survive the dangerous experience of childbirth. Women relinquished their own collective decision making, the traditional ways of helping one another deliver their babies, and participated actively in transferring their own authority to the medical experts, to those they hoped would save them from the dangers that had plagued childbirth throughout history.

Birth moved into the hospital very unevenly in the early twentieth century. Although half of all American women delivered in a hospital by 1938, the numbers varied widely by race and geographic area. In rural areas during the 1930s it was still common practice to deliver babies at home. In the South, especially among black women, hospital childbirth was rare, and almost all deliveries took place under the supervision of African American midwives in women's homes.[33] In the farm families living around Prescott, Wisconsin, the father would arrange for a "medical doctor and a neighborhood lady to be present. . . . Dad's participation was to call the doctor, ensure he arrived, call in a neighborhood lady, and stay out of the way."[34] Hospital births were more common in the cities because of proximity: by 1940, 84 percent of urban births took place in hos-

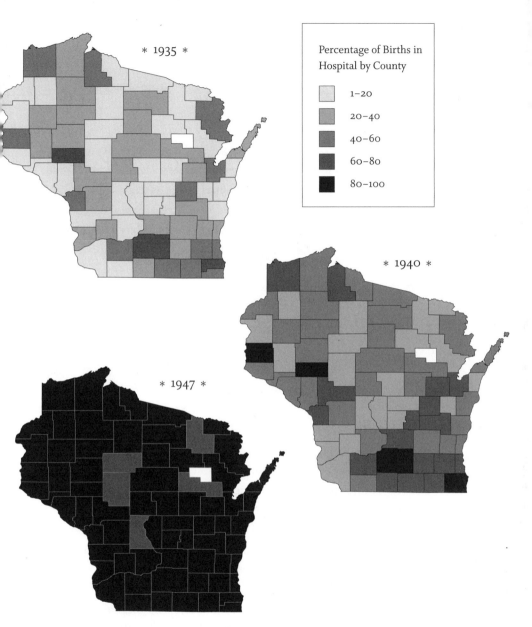

Maps showing changing percentages of births in the hospital in Wisconsin counties, 1935, 1940, 1947. The transition from home delivery to giving birth in the hospital, first in urban areas and then more generally, occurred relatively quickly over this twelve-year period. (There are no data for one county.) Thanks to Kendra Smith-Howard, who constructed the maps from statistics in the state board of health records in the Wisconsin Historical Society Archives, Madison. Maps are now in the collection of the Department of Medical History and Bioethics, University of Wisconsin, Madison.

pitals; in the same year only 25 percent of rural women had their babies in hospitals. Sixty percent of white mothers delivered in hospitals in the same year, but only 25 percent of black women. For black rural women, the numbers were even smaller: a mere 3 percent of black rural women delivered in a hospital.[35]

This transition occurred in Wisconsin in the twelve years from 1935 to 1947. At the beginning of the period, women living in or near urban Milwaukee and Madison and other population centers used hospitals heavily, but others in the state did not have such access. The changes came quickly. By 1947, the large majority of women in all parts of the state went to the hospital to have their babies.

Birth in the Hospital

The bargain that women had counted on when they made the move into the hospital did not occur quite as they had anticipated. The hospitals in the 1930s and 1940s were not as safe as they had been promised to be; maternal mortality did not drop as a result of the move to the hospital. It was not until the development and use of antibiotic drugs following the Second World War that postpartum infection rates fell significantly. In addition, women found that they had given up more than they had expected by moving out of the home for childbirth. "The cruelest part of [hospital] childbirth is being alone among strangers," wrote one woman.[36] Women soon realized that the physical move from their own homes to the physicians' institutions shifted the balance of power. Birth was no longer part of the woman's domain, as it had been throughout history. It became, instead, a medical affair run by medical professionals. Women were no longer the main actors; instead, physicians acted upon women's bodies. Women who entered the birthing rooms of medicine were captured by the routine and by the expertise surrounding them, but they missed the companionship that had been theirs at home, and they often felt alone and alienated by the sterile and impersonal hospital environment. Perhaps they could not have predicted ahead of time that the domestic comforts would not be replicated in the hospital, but they missed them when they were gone. Upon entering the hospital, many women found that hos-

pital routine put them on an assembly line and took away their individu-
ality. The experience helps us to understand why so many women wanted
their husbands to stay with them through hospital labor and delivery.

Not all mothers-to-be, however, viewed modern hospital childbirth as
an upsetting experience. Many women appreciated the streamlined—
medicalized—twentieth-century hospital birth, one that took place
under the observation and control of specialist nurses and doctors. Some
hospitals were so enticing that author Betty MacDonald, giving birth in
the 1920s, recalled, "The prospect of two weeks in that heavenly place
tempted me to stay pregnant all the rest of my life."[37] Mothers-to-be
learned that, to some extent, they could plan when they would have their
babies because doctors could induce labor, and doctors could predict the
course of labor because they controlled it with drugs and instruments.
"The old way [of having a baby] was no fun," wrote one father about the
1916 birth of his first daughter. Twenty-two years later, in 1938, his second
wife gave birth to another daughter, who "was born the new way—the
easy, painless, streamlined way." His second wife reflected in the general-
interest periodical *Reader's Digest*, "It's a good hour's ride by auto from
our house in the country to the hospital in New York and for weeks I
had nightmares of a mad dash in the dark over a sleety road, and all the
stories I'd ever read of babies being born in taxicabs filled me with terror.
So it was with vast relief I heard the doctor say: 'Come in to the hospital
next Tuesday night and you'll have your baby Wednesday.' Just like that.
It was like ordering something from a store." She and her husband took
in a matinee and dinner before she checked into the hospital. The next
morning the new medications Pituitrin induced her labor, Nembutal and
scopolamine deadened her perceptions and memory of it, and the doctor delivered her baby. "Why, I wouldn't mind having another baby next
week," she said, "if that's all there is to it."[38] Maternity wards and maternity hospitals promised women the ultimate in modern and safe hospitalized experiences.[39]

As hospitals attempted to carry out these promises, childbirth in the
mid-twentieth-century lost some of the diversity of experience evident in
the home deliveries of earlier years; it seemed to become homogenized
as hospital policy and medical protocols determined the succession of

events.[40] In typical hospital deliveries in the 1930s and 1940s, women left their family and friends at the door of the labor room and faced their birthings alone, as this account described:

> Arriving [at the hospital], she is immediately given the benefit of one of the modern analgesics or pain-killers. Soon she is in a dreamy, half-conscious state at the height of a pain, sound asleep between spasms. . . . She knows nothing about being taken to a spotlessly clean delivery room, placed on a sterile table, draped with sterile sheets; neither does she see her attendants, the doctor and nurses, garbed for her protection in sterile white gowns and gloves; nor the shiny boiled instruments and antiseptic solutions. She does not hear the cry of her baby when first he feels the chill of this cold world, or see the care with which the doctor repairs such lacerations as may have occurred. She is, as most of us want to be when severe pain has us in its grasp — asleep. Finally she awakes in smiles, a mother with no recollection of having become one.[41]

The use of analgesics and anesthetics to reduce or eliminate a laboring woman's discomfort and the use of forceps to deliver the baby became routine in hospitalized childbirth during the 1930s and 1940s, as did putting women in the lithotomy position — on her back with her legs in stirrups. The drugs and the position reduced women's involvement in and awareness of their births. A nurse who graduated from nursing school in 1946 and worked in obstetrics in Madison, Wisconsin, remembered, "The trend in those days was not for patients to know what was going on and of course, the fathers were . . . no where near. . . . [The women were] real calm. . . . The majority of women had 100 [milligrams] of Demerol and 100 [micrograms] of scope [scopolamine] and then probably a repeat on it. And then, of course, they also had general anesthetic."[42] One historian of the subject concluded: "Indeed, by the end of the 1940s, virtually every physician who wrote on the subject of pain relief in childbirth believed that it was the moral and professional obligation of all physicians to relieve pain."[43] In the 1940s physicians applied forceps in 70 percent of births they attended.[44]

During this period, then, many women labored woozily in a semicon-

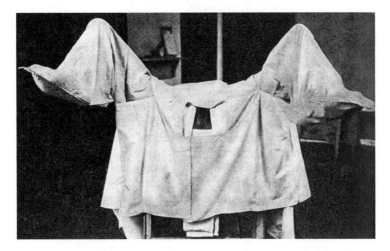

Birthing woman in lithotomy position and fully draped for a forceps delivery, 1920s. The woman received general anesthesia. Reprinted with permission of Scribner, an imprint of Simon & Schuster Adult Publishing Group, from *Obstetrical Nursing* by Carolyn Conant Van Blarcom. © 1922 Macmillan Publishing Company, copyright renewed.

scious or unconscious state. Separated from their family supports and familiar surroundings and confined instead to stark private, semiprivate, or ward settings, women in labor were virtually alone, with nurses checking in on them only as frequently as their schedules and other duties allowed. They were willing to give up their traditional decision making and bodily control, however, because they believed that going to the hospital provided protection to them and their babies; the new benefits seemed more important, and they had fewer of the fears of death and debility that had haunted generations of their foremothers.

Yet the routine use of analgesics and anesthetics as well as instruments — especially forceps — and surgical procedures in these years led physicians to a reconsideration of their safety. As early as the 1930s, the New York Academy of Medicine questioned the safety of the new procedures and noted that maternal mortality remained "unnecessarily high" as birth moved into the hospital. The physicians who wrote the 1933 report thought that birth in the hospital contributed to maternal risk with a "high incidence of operative interference during labor . . . undertaken when there was no indication or a plain contra-indication." They concluded, "Clearly a reduction of the mortality rate can be achieved through a reduction in operative interference."[45] In 1926, drawing on his long experience as an obstetrician in Chicago, Joseph B. DeLee attributed the continuing high maternal death rate to infection, which did not decrease as it should have as birth moved into the hospital: "The maternity ward in the general hospital of today is a dangerous place for a woman to have a baby." In 1933 DeLee wrote, "The increasing preference of the hospital as a place of delivery, one of the most marked changes that has taken place during the last few years and is growing, seems not only not to have bettered the results but seems actually to have made them worse[,] . . . increasing maternal mortality and morbidity."[46] Despite these worries, medical interventions continued apace in American hospitals.

Women knew little about the debates within medicine about hospital safety. But many of the women who went into hospitals did know — even if they did not associate the loss with the traditional domestic supports of home and family — that they did not like their lonely hospital experience. Although, as discussed earlier, some women appreciated the hospital and did not voice any disappointment with it, many others complained about the bustle of starched skirts, the thermometer poked in their mouth at odd hours, and the whispers of strange people speaking among themselves. One woman remembered her 1935 confinement as a "nightmare of impersonality," during which she felt "helpless" and "like a pawn in a strange game." Others remembered being "all alone," "abandoned," and "lonely . . . knowing no one." Hospitals seemed unable to provide a supportive atmosphere for women in labor; perhaps more significant, hospital staffs did not notice that such an environment was needed or desired by their maternity patients. Women felt too intimidated by institutionalized medicine to make their feelings known; doctors and nurses did not show a personal empathy for women's ordeals; and routines and schedules did not encourage providing the comforts of home. One woman found her hospital experience so traumatic that, she wrote, "months later I would scream out loud and wake up remembering that lonely labor room and just feeling no one cared what happened to me, no one kind reassuring word was spoken by nurse or doctor. I was treated as if I was an inanimate object." For many American women in the 1930s and later, giving birth in the hospital was no blessing at all. It was still dangerous, perhaps more dangerous than being at home because of the potential for cross infection, and it was psychologically alienating.[47]

The women who gave up their home deliveries and went to the hospital to give birth faced the psychological costs of leaving their own domestic world and entering a strange environment controlled by others. When they got to the hospital, said goodbye to their husbands and family, and went to the labor rooms alone, many women did not feel comforted by the efficiency of the hospital. A woman from Elkhart, Indiana, wrote to the *Ladies' Home Journal*, which exposed some of the impersonal conditions in the 1950s in two widely read articles, "So many women, especially first mothers, who are frightened to start out with, receive such brutal inconsiderate treatment that the whole thing is a horrible nightmare. They give you drugs, whether you want them or not, strap you down like an animal." A woman from Columbus, Ohio, concurred that a new mother was "foiled in every attempt to follow her own wishes."[48]

Not only did physicians continue routinely to use analgesics and anesthetics and forceps when they attended women in hospital deliveries, but hospital routines during the 1950s and 1960s often included interventions such as labor induction and augmentation and episiotomy; in the 1970s electronic fetal monitoring joined the list. Robbie Davis-Floyd, a cultural anthropologist who studied hospital birth patterns, describes how women, in assembly-line lockstep, moved through the regimented model of this period: "The vast majority of women giving birth in American hospitals are dressed in a hospital gown, placed in a hospital bed, hooked up to an electronic fetal monitor, and ordered not to eat; they have an intravenous needle inserted into their arm, are anesthetized to some degree, receive the synthetic hormone Pitocin if their labor is not progressing rapidly and regularly, and have an episiotomy."[49] There was little room for individual variation in the regimen.

Inducing or accelerating labor with Pitocin, the synthetic version of oxytocin, a natural hormone released during labor that helps the cervix to dilate, expanded significantly in this midcentury period. With this drug, physicians could schedule deliveries by inducing labor, and, if labor had already begun, they could increase the intensity of contractions that were

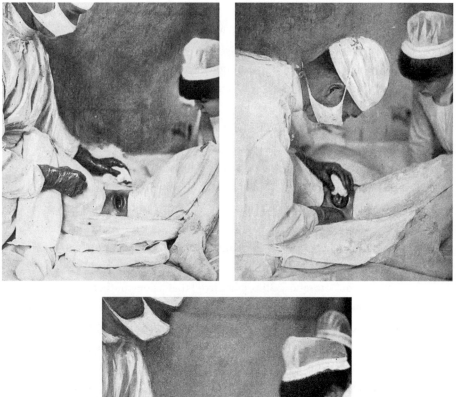

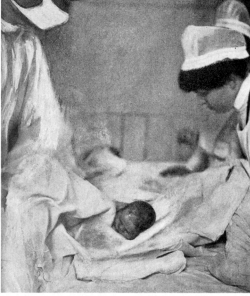

Three images of delivery: the head crowning, the physician holding back
the head to prevent tearing, and the birth of the head and external rotation.
Reprinted with permission of Scribner, an imprint of Simon & Schuster Adult
Publishing Group, from *Obstetrical Nursing* 2/e by Carolyn Conant Van
Blarcom. © 1928 Macmillan Publishing Company, copyright renewed.

not productive. Even though Pitocin-induced contractions are usually more painful than natural ones, women often requested the medication. Induction rates were much higher for private patients, from 10 to 20 percent; ward services reported much lower rates during the midcentury period.[50] The process took away some of the anxiety of awaiting labor and allowed women and physicians to plan ahead.

Many times physicians planned inductions, urging the women to agree. One physician described his methods: "I never insist on induction, but explain the procedure and if there are any objections the matter is dropped. However, acceptance of and belief in induction is growing, and mothers plan on that method of delivery."[51] During these midcentury years, women mostly did not question medical advice. "I think most of us never thought to question the doctor," one woman wrote. "We just did what the doctors and nurses told us to." She wrote about her 1954 delivery, which was induced: the physician "told her to come to hospital next morning and he would induce her." He gave no reason, and she asked for none.[52] As a woman said about her second and third labors, which were induced, "I really trusted my doctor. I didn't really give it [induction] any thought. I figured he knew what he was doing and I figured he wouldn't do it if it wasn't safe."[53]

Carolyn Splett, an obstetrical nurse who began her career in the 1960s in Daniel Freeman Hospital in Los Angeles, told how some of the physicians there decided on inductions: "The way they were done, was usually it made it possible for the OB-GYN to have an 8:00 to 5:00 practice, and a lot of those doctors had a reputation as this was the kind of practice they wanted to have and they scheduled their inductions for Thursday or Friday mornings, so they weren't going to be bothered on the weekend. . . . So it wasn't unusual at all to have a whole slew of inductions on Thursdays and Fridays."[54]

Once labor was progressing, physicians could monitor the fetal heart rate and health with the use of the electronic fetal monitor, which was either attached to the fetal scalp or fastened with a belt around the mother's abdomen. Rates of use soared. From 2 percent of births at Columbia University's Sloane Hospital in 1970, continuous fetal monitoring rose to 85 percent in just five years.[55] By 1980, according to historian

Margarete Sandelowski, 70 percent of all American hospital births included the use of fetal monitors. Birth attendants, physicians and nurses, found the monitor a more reassuring instrument than the stethoscope because it was more precise and continuous.[56] But birthing women found their movements restricted once the monitor was applied, and they could no longer get out of bed to walk around or use the bathroom.[57]

Despite the relatively rapid adoption of electronic monitors, Sandelowski found that some hospitals responded to the new technology slowly and initially used them only on women having difficult labors. Sandelowski demonstrated a wide variation in use: in some rural hospitals, there were no monitors at all during the 1970s, and some physicians wouldn't tolerate their use. Yet during that decade, nurses came to prefer the instruments because they made it easier to trace the progress of labor and to know when to call the physician. The machines, in fact, helped to put the nurses at the center of diagnosing, since they were the ones to monitor the monitors.[58] Some men who were with their wives during labor came to like the machine, too, seeing it as providing an "objective window" into the labor process that allowed them to experience it "without mediation by mothers or manuals."[59] Physicians came to appreciate the monitors for their help in possible lawsuits, since the tracings throughout labor could be used in court to justify their interventions.[60]

Episiotomy, the precise surgical cutting of perineal tissue to allow the baby's head to emerge without ragged tearing, was developed early in the twentieth century and became a common routine procedure in the 1950s.[61] According to Barbara Bridgman Perkins, some individual hospitals reported episiotomy rates as high as 85 percent at midcentury, and in the following decades national rates generally exceeded 70 percent.[62] Physicians became convinced that the surgery would prevent excess stretching and was beneficial despite many women's protestations that the incision, made with scissors and extending deep into the musculature, was painful and interfered with postchildbirth sexual activity.[63]

Some women felt physicians did not sufficiently consider their wishes when deciding on an episiotomy. Jayne F. related that her doctor told her, "So just plan on having one. And that was the end of the subject. I mean, he is the one who has delivered babies for 20 years. Who am I to say, 'No, you cannot give me an episiotomy.' All he'll have to do is march out all his evidence and horror stories of women who tore horribly. . . . Well, you have to have some faith in this man. . . . If I would have argued with him up and down, he probably still would have done it the way he did." She described the scene in the delivery room:

> The thing that struck me, even in my disorientation and pain, that it was a room full of people. There were people everywhere. I don't know if they belonged there or were just passing through. But they were all in green scrubs, and were all wearing masks and hood. So I could sort of make out who was male and female, but other than that it was a room full of strangers. There were probably 5 or 6 people there including the doctor. They put me on the table. . . . He did a huge episiotomy. . . . While he was sewing it up, he said to C. [husband] kind of jokingly, he said, "Well I put an extra stitch in for you." Meaning that he sewed me up tighter than I probably was before. And so it was [for] C's benefit.[64]

Such stories fueled women's resistance to the routine adoption of episiotomies.

Much of the habitual use of these interventions can be traced to ideas about normal childbirth introduced by obstetrician Emanuel Friedman in the 1950s.[65] Friedman mapped out average times for the various stages of labor, identified "ideal" labor, and defined as normal those labors that fell within the averaged limits on each curve. Depending on how a particular woman's labor developed, physicians could intervene to control its course and put it more in line with expectations. Determining interventions based on such averages added to the idea that a woman's body was a machine that could be regulated. Davis-Floyd found that many American women wanted just this kind of birth (which she calls technocratic birth), one they would not suffer through or perhaps not even remember and one that used medical techniques to help them take home a healthy baby.[66]

Hospital architecture and geography accommodated the increasingly technological births. The standardized stages of birth needed specific spaces. Thus, when a woman first entered the hospital, she went to a "prep" room, where nurses provided enemas and shaved the perineal area. Then she would go to a labor room, where her contractions started, accelerated, and got stronger. Delivery, as the baby pushed its way into the world, needed to take place in a different room in which the most technologically sophisticated equipment could be called upon to help. Postpartum recovery necessitated yet another room. Hospitals were advised to help the new obstetrics by providing "proper sequential arrangement" of maternity units. The American Hospital Association called for a "maternity center designed for 'assembly-line' efficiency" and sought the "continuous operational flow" of patients.[67] Architectural historian Roslyn Lindheim concluded that postwar hospitals tried to rationalize obstetrical suites in much the same way that wartime munitions factories had done: "Approached like any other industrial process, hospital maternity procedures were designed to keep the flow of patients moving—to avoid crowding and possible back-up." Lindheim quoted a 1964 hospital design text that advised the "conveyor belt concept . . . [that] emphasizes the repeated transference of a mother (as in motor-car assembly) from place and to place," rendering birth, in Lindheim's words, "increasingly mechanized and dehumanizing."[68]

Some women had complained individually and privately about their hospital deliveries during the 1930s and 1940s, but there was a much greater public outpouring of such unhappy sentiments in the 1950s as these interventions and practices became more commonplace. The medical institutionalization of birth took away parts of the birth experience that had previously been under women's control, and it left women vulnerable and alone. The move to the hospital, which turned birth into a physician-directed medical and surgical event, although appreciated by some women, encouraged many others to search for ways to improve the situation.

Birthing women frequently blamed obstetric nurses for their dissatisfaction with hospitalized labor and delivery. The *Ladies' Home Journal* revealed some of the fault lines in its 1958 exposé. One woman wrote about her experiences in a suburban hospital outside Chicago: "I wonder if the people who ran that place were actually human. My lips parched and cracked, but the nurses refused to even moisten them with a damp cloth. I was left alone all night in a labor room. I felt exactly like a trapped animal. . . . Never have I needed someone, anyone, as desperately as I did that night." Another woman wrote, "I remember screaming, 'help me, help me!' to a nurse who was sitting at a nearby desk. She ignored me." Another woman noted, "I have listened to nurses laughing at other new mothers who were crying out in pain, I have heard other mothers being slapped and threatened with dead babies and misfits. I heard these things while I waited for the births of my second and third babies. What happens to the women who are threatened this way and then do deliver a misfit or a stillborn? Do they spend the rest of their lives blaming themselves? Do the words of these sadistic nurses . . . forever ring in their ears?"[69]

Some registered nurses added their voices to the chorus of complaint in the popular women's magazine. One related, "I have seen nurses . . . become impatient (or worse) with a patient and express their feelings, often within her hearing. 'She got herself in this fix and now is a poor time to change her mind.'" Another nurse admitted, "I have seen careless and callous treatment of obstetrical patients, along with indifference and discourtesy. . . . I have seen nurses be careless in screening patients from public view during procedures requiring their bodies to be exposed, to the outrage of the patients' feelings of modesty. I have heard such un-thinking remarks as 'You had your fun, now you can suffer' made by a nurse to a mother in great distress."

Certainly not all nurses were to blame for women's loneliness in hospital labor rooms, and certainly not all women felt this alienated from their hospital births. Many were happy to give up the bother of needing to make arrangements and decisions that home birth represented and instead surrender to the new, more passive hospital routines. They wanted to go home with healthy babies without having the stress of concerning themselves with how the event itself took place. As one woman declared, "Actually I didn't even want my husband around. . . . It was just something that I wanted to do, get it over with, and that's fine."[70]

But most of the women who articulated their feelings in this mid-twentieth-century period instead voiced frustration, loneliness, and help-lessness, and they wished things could change. Many of the women who left their husbands to wait in the maternity ward waiting rooms and went by themselves up to the labor rooms described their experiences in ways that made it clear how alone they felt. Katherine Egan, who delivered at Boston Lying-In Hospital, related that decisions "were pretty much taken out of my hands": "The birth of a baby should be a happy experience, not a nightmare of impersonality. . . . I was given an enema (very unpleasant), shaved with a dull, rusty razor blade (very unpleasant), and put to bed in a darkened labor room with six or eight moaning, groaning screaming women (very unpleasant). . . . Nurses were only in the room part of the time. We were not allowed to walk around or even get out of bed."[71] Another woman described how she felt when her husband was directed to the fathers' room to wait out her labor and delivery in 1951: "'We'll keep you posted on her progress,' the nurse promised him and she pointed out the 'Father's Room.' But that was no comfort to me. I wanted Jim! I wanted to cry on his shoulder, to squeeze his hand, just to feel him near; but hospital routine and rules must come first so Jim went."[72] Another woman described her fifteen-hour 1952 labor at Manhattan General Hospital in New York City: "I had no preparation, was irrational, screamed and felt very lonely. My husband could not see me in labor."[73]

To ease their concerns, the women begged: "Let us have our husbands with us."[74] One woman, who understood from her own experience how husbands could help, wrote, "Only from personal experience can you comprehend the loneliness of lying 17 hours alone."[75] In this controlled hospital environment in which many birthing women felt alienated from the childbirth experience and miserably alone during labor and delivery, the women's husbands, people they knew and trusted, had a potentially important role to play. But in this period the men sat, also alone, a few rooms away, in maternity waiting rooms.

Women had not always wanted their male partners to be with them during labor and delivery. Traditionally, in home births, they had chosen other women—family members and friends who had been through the birth experience themselves and knew what to expect—to be with them during labor and delivery. Now, though, in the lonely and strange mid-twentieth-century hospital, birthing women called out for their husbands rather than their women friends. This change is in part a reflection of the trend toward emotionally closer marriages in which men and women shared intimacies that they had not earlier shared. Although historians writing about men and fatherhood during the middle of the twentieth century emphasize the men's preoccupation with their work, especially following the Great Depression, and their concerns about the Cold War and the hydrogen bomb, they also recognize men's growing interest in family life.[76] Men's preoccupations with their families went well beyond worrying about financial security; married men's growing desire to become involved in their wives' pregnancy, labor, and delivery demonstrates the widening scope of their domestic interests. Not all men wanted to be included in events such as birth, but increasing numbers found their physical separation from their wives during labor and delivery in the hospital frustrating and unsatisfactory.

2 * KEEPING VIGIL

Fathers in Waiting Rooms

As the hospital came to be the preferred setting for childbirth in the mid-twentieth century, some of the men who accompanied their laboring wives returned home to await news of their child's birth. Others may have retired to a nearby bar or restaurant to drink and eat their worries away. Still another alternative was to wait stolidly in hospital hallways, on hard benches and chairs, with few amenities. Most often, however, the men sat in "stork clubs," "husbands' rooms," or "fathers' rooms," hospital waiting rooms located near maternity suites and newborn nurseries reserved exclusively for them. At the middle of the twentieth century, most hospitals provided these separate waiting rooms for prospective fathers, where the men would sit, pace, smoke cigarettes, listen to the radio (or, later, watch TV), read, sleep, talk on the pay telephone, and commiserate with one another as they awaited updated information about their wives' condition.[1] These waiting rooms have been the butt of many jokes, and few scholars have previously paid serious attention to them. However, fathers' waiting rooms provided the spaces for intense self-reflection, serious worrying, and some very significant sharing of experiences that ultimately led the men to help transform the purpose and use of the rooms themselves.

In 1949 new father Dale Clark published an account in the men's magazine *Esquire* detailing his experience of sitting in a fathers' waiting room during his wife's labor and delivery. At the time, not very many other men articulated agreement with his views of resistance to hospital policies, but this point of view was on the horizon:

> Framed on the inner side of the corridor door, a printed notice directed the husband to the waiting lounge on the floor below. . . . Half a dozen expectant fathers were gathered there — just like in the movies, and in fiction, and the cartoons. The lounge was a comfortable place. Its tall-stemmed lamps shone down on a divan, padded armchairs, and reclining chairs that were almost beds. Here a man dozed, there one thumbed a magazine, and yonder a third chainsmoked. You never in your life have seen an unhappier set of poor devils. Each started visibly when, just as I entered, the telephone rang. The nearest man — I learned later that his wife had been in labor twenty-eight hours — snatched at the instrument. But the call was for another chap, who, after listening, exclaimed, "I only brought her in half an hour ago! That's what I call a woman getting it over with quick!" And away he rushed, to peer through a glass pane at his newly arrived son. Just like in the movies, there was something sad and a little ridiculous about these waiting men, perspiring, suffering, and useless as they were. That, after all, was the way I myself had expected to participate in our child's birth. I'd managed to live forty-three years without ever hearing of a husband's doing anything else. . . . The specialized modern age seemed to have progressed to the point where an expectant father was not needed, or even *allowed*, beyond the waiting lounge of the urban hospital. . . . Every man in that room might have been upstairs with his wife — where, it seems to me, a man should not only be allowed to be, but where, for sound physiological and psychological reasons, he is imperatively needed. . . . It's about time for all husbands — the whole crowd in the waiting lounge — to grab hatchets and chop through the partition.[2]

Only a few men actually wanted to grab hatchets and actively resist hospital policies in 1949. In the decades of the mid-twentieth century, most men worried and paced in hospital waiting rooms without many thoughts that things might be different. They spent long hours sitting in one room while their wives were laboring in a different one, sometimes only a partition away. The men did ultimately become an eager part of a movement to break through the walls and share directly in their wives' labor experiences, a movement that included lay groups as well as other concerned parents. In hospital waiting rooms, men's restricted movement germinated the changes that were to come.

Fathers' Waiting Rooms

Beginning in the 1920s, as increasing numbers of American women went into the hospital to have their babies, general hospitals established obstetrical departments, and in some communities hospitals were built that were dedicated solely to maternity care. Many, although not all, of these new or refurbished wings of hospitals contained separate waiting rooms for the fathers. St. Luke's Hospital in New Bedford, Massachusetts, had a "Men's Waiting Room" on one of its two maternity floors. Chicago's Lying-In Hospital, designed in consultation with famed obstetrician Joseph DeLee, provided a "Husbands' Room."[3] Increasingly in the 1930s and 1940s, hospitals provided such spaces for the waiting expectant fathers. If they did not, the men could wait in general hospital waiting rooms, prowl the public hallways near the maternity units, or leave the premises altogether.

Norman Rockwell captured the mood of a maternity waiting room for the *Saturday Evening Post* in 1946, illustrating the various ways men might have behaved while their wives did the active work of delivering babies.[4] Rockwell drew men in multiple attitudes: the frightened novice, the magazine shredder, the believer in the worst, the hearty salesman, the chain smoker, the pacer. (That Rockwell's fathers-to-be were all white reflected his particular artistic emphasis and the majority of the readership of the magazine. It also reflected the period's racially segregated hospitals.)[5] Rockwell's popular image of expectant fathers showed men

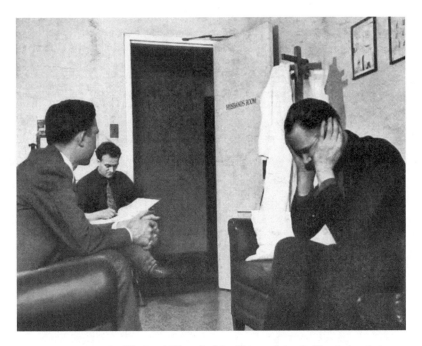

Men waiting in the "Husbands' Room" of the Chicago Lying-In Hospital as their wives labor and deliver elsewhere in the hospital. The photograph shows the potential for the men to talk to each other and offer mutual support as they share the anxious time together. "Birth of a Baby," *Hygeia* 16 (May 1938): 419. Photograph by Wallace Kirkland; reprinted with permission of Mary Glenn Kirkland.

who were extraneous to childbirth; they were funny and even pathetic hangers-on. Such renderings of men as outsiders reveal how deeply that representation permeated the American mind-set. Often overstating men's real experiences and poking fun at them, the portrayals nonetheless tell us a lot about what images were in the minds of the men who waited when their wives went into labor in the hospital.

As hospitals became the most common venue for American women to have their babies, most fathers-to-be did not challenge the rules that made them sit and wait in their separate areas, and they usually followed what doctors and nurses told them to do and when to do it. They did not know very much about the process of labor and delivery or what their wives were going through, and they did not voice missing that knowledge. Yet even as they waited outside, much as they had done in an earlier

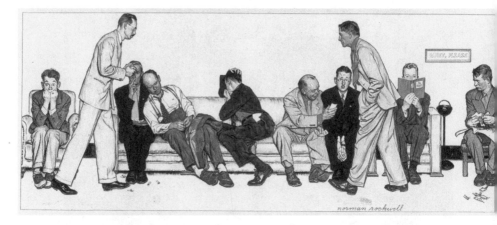

Norman Rockwell's depiction of a maternity waiting room, illustrating the different ways men showed their nervousness. "Maternity Waiting Room," *Saturday Evening Post*, July 13, 1946, 12. Thanks to Jean von Allmen for help in locating this illustration. Photograph courtesy of Martin Diamond Fine Art, New York. Reprinted with permission of the Norman Rockwell Family Agency. © 1946 Norman Rockwell Family Entities.

period when birth occurred at home, the fathers were not necessarily passive in their pacing. Men found ways to participate in, comment upon, and ultimately influence the birth experiences of their wives even from their exile in hospital waiting rooms.

The physical space of the fathers' waiting rooms worked against any father's involvement in the birth process. Usually the rooms were located away from the action of labor and delivery; if they were more integral to the maternity rooms, the men were cut off from any interaction. Sociologists William Rosengren and Spencer DeVault discovered in their analysis of maternity-floor spaces that the physical spaces determined the status and importance of activities. They found that the fathers' room in the hospital they observed in 1958 was "suggestive that the father is regarded as the least important person in the process. By its sparseness of furnishing, its physical isolation, and its small size, this room seemed to communicate symbolically the idea that the fathers are unnecessary and functionally peripheral."[6]

Hospital floor plans reveal just how cut off men were from the action of labor and delivery. The rooms themselves were sometimes located on a different floor than were the labor and delivery rooms; more often, the rooms were situated off the small "public corridor" near the elevator or staircase on the maternity floor itself and separated by doors from the labor and delivery suites.[7] The men who sat in the waiting rooms were physically separated from any activity around labor and delivery. Their access was to the elevator and stairway, a public hallway, a restroom, and, sometimes, the nurses' workroom. Standards for hospital maternity suites in this period recommended that waiting rooms for fathers be located "as remote as possible from the delivery unit."[8]

Between the waiting room and the rest of the maternity floor were doors that physically barred the men from access to their laboring wives or to direct knowledge of what was happening to them. Sometimes they might hear the cries of women in labor, but that was the closest they could get to directly experiencing what the mothers of their children were going through. David Gruener related that in 1959 he was "sent to the father's waiting room. Three or four nervous fathers-to-be smoked, paced, and worried together." Occasionally a nurse arrived with news for one or another of the men.[9] Well into the 1960s these waiting rooms continued to be holding spaces for the men.

Some fathers' rooms were in close proximity to the nursery, "through the show window of which you can gaze in on a mad paradise of 30 or 40 babies in bassinets and incubators, almost all of these little upstarts howling their heads off."[10] Stuart Price left his wife in the delivery area of an Evanston, Illinois, hospital in 1964 and waited in such a fathers' waiting room. "Probably a dozen chairs lined the outside walls and a coffee table with assorted, out-dated magazines made up the furnishings. There were 4 or 5 other guys waiting. . . . The only sound was one woman screaming very loudly in the delivery area. . . . Dads got to see their children through the window."[11]

Many men found the waiting room, or "Stork Club" as Wesley Memorial Hospital in Chicago called it, comforting. "Pretty nice place, this stork club," wrote one father-to-be. "Soft music now playing on the radio."[12] Others found a lot to complain about in the physical space. "Sadists planned this torture chamber," wrote one frustrated man during a hot summer night. "No air! Plenty of heat!"[13] "The damn radio won't work,"

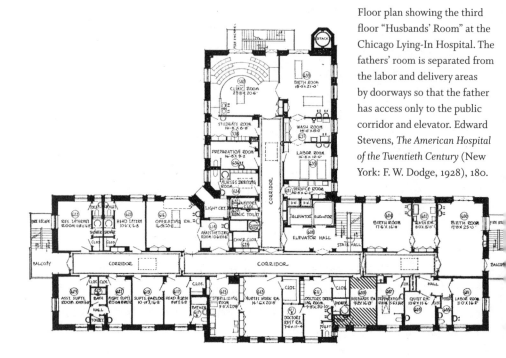

Floor plan showing the third floor "Husbands' Room" at the Chicago Lying-In Hospital. The fathers' room is separated from the labor and delivery areas by doorways so that the father has access only to the public corridor and elevator. Edward Stevens, *The American Hospital of the Twentieth Century* (New York: F. W. Dodge, 1928), 180.

Cartoon of a nurse showing the father that he can wait in the Stork Club; it reinforces the image of fathers-to-be as nervous and intimidated by the hospital. Robert S. Kleckner, "Jottings from 'Stork Room' Diary," *Chicago Sun-Times*, May 4, 1952, sec. 2, 2. Cartoon by John (Jack) Ryan. As published in *The Chicago Sun-Times*, © 1952 The Chicago Sun-Times LLC. Reprinted with permission.

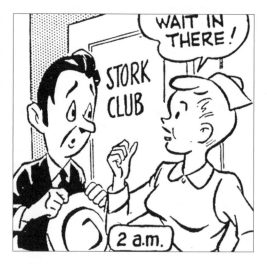

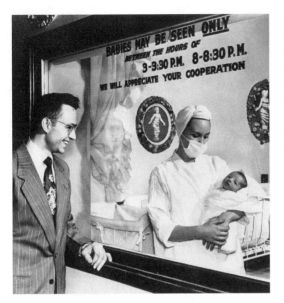

This new father could see his child only through the nursery window and only during very limited hours, Abbott Hospital, Minneapolis, Minnesota. Used with permission of the Minnesota Historical Society.

complained another, "and I can't sleep."[14] Another man commented, "The magazines are old. . . . There are no soft seats in the club room. . . . The room is to[o] small for my long legs. . . . These hours of anxiety sure drag by."[15]

During these hours — or through long days and nights — the men learned very little about how their wives' labors were progressing. Their main source of information was the nurse or occasional doctor who entered the room or called on the telephone to announce a birth. In at least one hospital, the telephone switchboard attendant delivered the news.[16] Joseph DeLee, a prominent Chicago physician and author of popular obstetrics textbooks, one for doctors and one for nurses, advised that a father "should spend most of his time downstairs in the waiting room and should not haunt the birth room corridor. . . . [He] should be informed at intervals regarding the progress of his wife's case — and as soon as the baby is born he should be told of it to relieve his anxiety and give him joy."[17] Another textbook clarified whose duty it was to keep fathers informed: "If the policy of the institution does not provide for the husband to be with his wife during labor, the nurse must keep him well informed of his wife's progress at frequent intervals."[18]

Many examples of fathers' hearing little or no word from labor or delivery indicate that this advice was not always followed. One father recalled his experience this way: "All the nurses seemed so busy. One told me to be patient, that I'd be informed when there was news. Finally I called a friend to get some support. He congratulated me and told me that he had called the hospital and received the announcement that mother and son were well. The nurses had forgotten me."[19] Another father submitted to his local monthly magazine this vivid account:

Of course they gave me one look and whirled her quickly away, putting me in the decontamination room at the end, where I lighted a cigarette and opened [a] magazine to the first story. I'd finished the book and cigarettes by noon and was beginning to sag in the middle from hunger but I was afraid to leave the floor for fear little Joe or whoever it was would put in an appearance and Momma would never forgive me as long as she lived for not being there when my child arrived. So I hung on for another hour till I was able to snag a nurse and ask her about my wife. "Oh, I'd say about another twelve hours," she said airily, so I went down and had two milkshakes just to kill time. For the rest of the afternoon I stood looking out of the window and watching the doctors pull out of the driveway for a round of golf. I was also thinking of several of my friends who had given up and gone home to bed when the doctor called to say the baby had arrived. I had promised my wife faithfully I would not leave. But six o'clock came around and I had read even the women's advertisements in the magazine and smoked two more packs of cigarettes and pulled all the hairs out of my overcoat and called both families five times.[20]

John Gould, whose wife had a baby in 1947, complained about the waiting-room experience to *Esquire*. He wrote about "the vigil—that dark hour when the husband hands his wife to the wonders of modern medical science and sits outside on an uncomfortable bench. . . . The greatest blot on the escutcheon of the medical profession is its failure to alleviate the suffering of the borning father." Gould said that after his wife gave birth, her doctor, on the run, shook his hand and the nurse beamed at him as she hurried down the corridor. He couldn't see his wife until the next day.

He noted that "reception rooms for prospective fathers get little attention." His account, meant to be humorous, had an edge to it.[21]

Nurses did not have a lot of time to spend with laboring women or to inform the husbands with any frequency of their wives' progress. One nurse described midcentury nursing as including an "incredible amount of other duties that we had to accomplish to keep the place running." She listed folding and wrapping all the linen packs, peri-drapes, and leggings; washing all the gloves in green soap; and powdering and drying them and sterilizing them, in addition to checking on patients and administering medications.[22] Nursing time was strictly regimented.

An obstetrical nurse from Indiana admitted that there was certain comfort in having a strictly defined system that did not allow the fathers to be involved: "Under the conventional system all of us had always worked . . . fathers waited in some far-removed spot in the hospital during the long hours of labor and delivery. Most of us were quite satisfied with this situation, for we felt that the routinized program of care, even with certain apparent disadvantages, was nevertheless the best and most practical. . . . We made our system of care ever more rigid."[23]

The rigidity with which hospitals maintained the separation between waiting father and laboring mother varied significantly around the country. (There is not sufficient extant data to identify specific regional variations.) Some hospitals allowed fathers to visit the laboring women briefly during prescribed times; others kept them out altogether. Hospitals in rural communities seem to have been the most flexible, possibly because of smaller patient volume and closer ties to the community. During a 1947 delivery in Sioux Falls, South Dakota, for example, the mother later remembered, "My spouse and my mother came in to chat with me from time to time during labor and this provided cheer and welcome distraction."[24]

In some places, not only were the men not allowed to visit the laboring women in their rooms, but the women were also not allowed to visit their husbands in the waiting room. At Wesley Hospital in Chicago, for example, around midcentury, a notice was posted on the fathers' room door: "Patients are not allowed in Stork Club—for 'waiting fathers only.'"[25] But other hospitals permitted some men to receive visits from their laboring wives as they sat in the waiting rooms. One woman wrote of her 1952 labor and in the process revealed the practice of reverse visiting in her hospital:

> Since no visitors were allowed in the labor room I received permission to join David in the waiting room at the other end of the floor. We sat and chatted . . . wondered whether the next few hours would bring us a boy or a girl . . . had a final talk about the baby-to-be's name . . . spoke of important matters and trivia. . . . I stayed with David until about 3:00 am [two hours] but as the waiting-room chair (even padded with bed pillows) was not too comfortable and certainly not ideal for relaxing, I decided to be practical rather than romantic and to return to that wonderful comfortable bed in the labor room.[26]

Usually, when hospitals allowed the practice at all, women in labor could visit their husbands in the waiting room only if no other men were there at the time, and the visits were kept short. In Milwaukee in 1946, for example, a woman was "allowed to go to the 'fathers' room to visit with him for a few minutes." She was then "put to bed and given a sedative."[27]

In Shreveport, Louisiana, black women who went to the hospital were delivered in a "colored ward," and the segregated waiting room sometimes became the site of a "family occasion." As one historian described, "The relatives gathered in the waiting room with lunches and drinks, and the doctor would join them off and on to announce the progress of labor."[28] Unlike in so many other waiting rooms, in this case the anxious fathers-to-be had company; their wives, however, labored without any family support. Hospitals that provided racially integrated waiting rooms and labor wards sometimes maintained separate delivery rooms for black and white women.[29]

Coffee and cigarettes provided some measure of comfort to the waiting men but more frequently led to more complaints about dry throats and stale air. "Two packs of smokes are now butts," admitted one father-to-be. "3 cigars from other papas have long since gone up in smoke. I am hungry. . . . Going out for more cigarettes."[30] One of the men summed it up this way: "The wait is on! Guess I feel the same as anyone . . . as I sit, wait, walk and wait, smoke and wait. Waiting for what, a look, a spoken word from your wife's doctor about the greatest moment of your life. . . . Still waiting. Cigarettes almost gone."[31]

The high level of cigarette smoking in fathers' waiting rooms deserves some comment. Midcentury was a time when Americans significantly increased their habit of cigarette smoking. A good deal of the increase was connected to soldiers in combat, according to historian Allan Brandt, because they were issued cigarettes while in the service and returned home and introduced the practice to others. Smoking quickly became a part of social interactions and also frequently was connected to nervousness. Many believed cigarettes could calm jangled nerves. By midcentury more than half of all American men indulged in the habit.[32] Cut off from food and alcohol, expectant fathers often turned to smoking to ease their worries about labor and delivery. Smoking may have been a way for the men to bond in those cases in which a group of men waited together, or it may have just been the most convenient activity. Smoking cigarettes (and handing out cigars) characterized the waiting-room experience so much that cartoon artists usually depicted fathers' waiting rooms as smoke-filled rooms containing nervous men.

Humorist Russell Baker remembered his experiences as a father-to-be, and his recollections reveal how smoking fit the cultural conception of what waiting fathers did. He wrote: "All I knew about the glorious experience had been learned from the movies. . . . I knew [fathers] were supposed to sit in waiting rooms and smoke cigarettes, drink coffee, loosen their neckties, perspire heavily and rush into the corridor periodically to ask, 'How is she, Doc?' That's what I did. It seemed absurd but I did it anyway because nobody had told me anything else to do. And didn't Jimmy Stewart do the same thing whenever he had a baby?"[33] The male role during childbirth as depicted in television and film of the 1950s and 1960s—as in *I Love Lucy*—was characterized by men's complete lack of knowledge about labor and delivery, their banishment to fathers' waiting rooms, and their nervous and often inane behavior.[34]

One of the most charming examples was aired just before Father's Day in 1958 when NBC television ran a short skit on *The Steve Allen Show* starring Allen and his guest Henry Fonda, playing first-time fathers-to-be in a

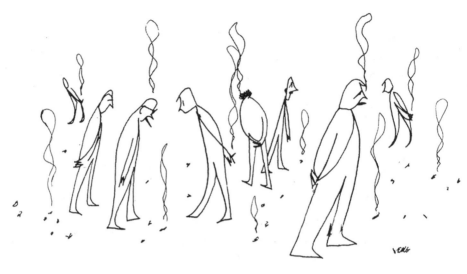

Cartoon of men pacing and smoking as they await news of their wives' deliveries.
Greer Williams, "I Was a Father Once Myself . . . ," *Modern Hospital* 84
(January 1955): 68. Reprinted with permission of Modern Healthcare.

Paternity Pains

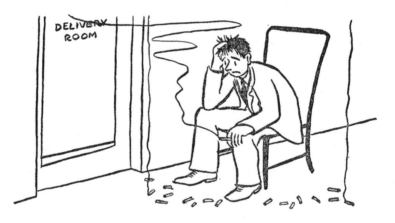

"Paternity Pains." Cartoon showing the stereotypical man
as he nervously smokes and waits for news of his wife's delivery.
David Victor, *Father's Doing Nicely: The Expectant Father's
Handbook* (Indianapolis: Bobbs Merrill, 1938), 92.

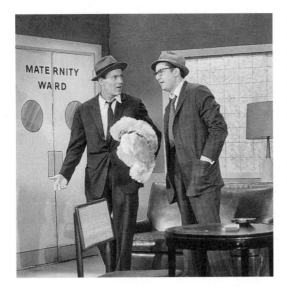

Henry Fonda and Steve Allen in a Father's Day television skit. They pace around a fathers' waiting room, showing their discomfort by wearing their hats indoors and with constant comedic banter. Fonda holds a stuffed animal. *Steve Allen Show*, June 1, 1958, NBC. Photograph from the *Steve Allen Show* provided by Meadowland Enterprises, Inc. All rights reserved. Used with permission.

maternity waiting room.[35] The introduction to the piece noted that even a man who is a successful industrialist will turn into a "bumbling incompetent wreck" when facing his wife's delivery, and the skit delivered on that premise. The two actors—who wore their hats inside the waiting room during the entire skit, indicating they were always ready to leave this place where they were so uncomfortable—paced up and down in a small fathers' waiting-room set, using every clichéd line to great comic effect.

Fonda carried a huge stuffed teddy bear, he said for his boy, Charles. Allen asked why he was so sure the baby would be a boy, and Fonda replied that Charles would be a silly name for a girl. Fonda asked Allen for a cigarette, and Allen littered the room with them before finally giving Fonda a bent one. But when Allen offered a light, Fonda replied that he didn't smoke. Fonda offered Allen chewing gum, which he put in his mouth with the paper wrapper still on. They offered congratulatory cigars to each other. Allen said he had been waiting ten and a half hours because his wife "is a very stubborn woman." Allen then responded to Fonda's anxiety by saying there was nothing to worry about, since cab drivers, police, and firemen deliver babies. Fonda retorted, to great studio laughter, "Yeah, but I'm using a doctor!" They played cards without knowing what game they were playing, and with Fonda holding his cards back-ward. The biggest audience laugh came when a third man entered the room and sat down calmly, saying this was his sixth and he did not worry any more. When the nurse came to inform him of the delivery, he merely asked, "Boy or girl?" and then got up and left. The skit ended when the nurse informed Allen that his wife had delivered an eight-pound boy and Allen replied, "I'll take it." Fonda asked, "What about me?" The nurse answered, "Who are you?" and then noted, "Didn't anyone tell you? Your wife went home yesterday." Fonda fainted.

The scene contained most of the classic tropes of awkward, blunder-ing, jumpy, ill-informed men who stayed outside the female and medical world of delivering babies and knew little about it. It was not kind to hos-pital practices, showing the nurse forgetting to tell Fonda of his wife's de-livery. The men knew they were supposed to be nervous, and they were. They had done nothing to inform themselves about labor and delivery and seemed to have very little connection beyond waiting for news of the result. TV-watching Americans laughed at the scene because of its famil-iarity and the basic truths it held about men's distance from childbirth experiences. To outward appearances, many expectant fathers resembled Allen and Fonda: confined to spaces outside the maternity ward, pacing and smoking, anxious and edgy.

Another classic portrayal of a man fidgeting in a maternity waiting room while his wife labored and delivered was the popular film *Rock-a-Bye Baby*, released in 1958, starring Jerry Lewis. Lewis believed that comedy was "nothing more than a mirror we hold up to life."[36] His role in the movie stretched the usual role of the father to a much more domestic care-taking role. But during the birth itself, Jerry was the stereotypical nervous wreck, smoking and pacing in the maternity waiting room.[37]

As these representations demonstrate, it was common in the middle of the twentieth century for men not to see their wives from the time they dropped them off at the hospital admissions unit until after the delivery of their babies.[38] Katherine Egan, who delivered in Boston in 1935, wrote, "I kissed my husband goodbye in the lobby and went upstairs to face it, exhilarated but frightened and lonely."[39] Similarly, Deb B., referring to her birth experience in Michigan in the 1940s, said, "My husband took

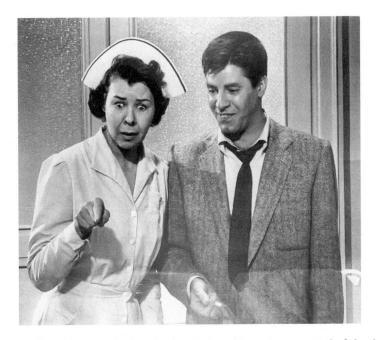

In the film *Rock-a-Bye Baby*, Jerry Lewis waited, smoking and nervous, in the fathers' waiting room while his wife labored and delivered; then, with Lewis still smoking, the nurse showed him his babies through the nursery glass. Photograph from *Rock-a-Bye Baby* released in 1958 by Paramount Pictures; used with permission of Photofest NYC.

me to the hospital. They took me in and he went to sit in the waiting room while I went up to the labor room because they weren't allowed with us."[40] Perhaps episodes like my mother's with the screaming woman in the next bed who blamed Seymour for all her difficulties reveal one reason that hospitals excluded men from the scene. Indeed, one woman wrote that during her labor in a city hospital in the 1950s nurses encouraged the women to blame their husbands for their agony, and many did scream bitterly against their husbands with each pain.[41] Shirley Ricketts remembered her 1945 labor at Columbia Presbyterian Hospital in New York City: "I was alone, except for the nurse. I wasn't scared or nervous, I didn't scream as the woman in the next room, who was not only screaming but cursing her husband for getting her pregnant."[42]

Women's partners probably did not hear such screams, and they might have had no way of knowing how the women felt about being alone during labor as they sat in the waiting rooms. They no doubt heard later how much their wives missed them. This might have contributed to the men's growing desire to share the labor experience. Even more important, the men talked to each other as they waited and together came to want more participation in labor and delivery, in part to enhance their own experiences of impending parenthood.

A Grace–New Haven Hospital study of first-time parents provides some insight into how men and women felt about stringent hospital regulations. The researchers reported in 1948: "During labor and delivery many of the mothers and fathers wanted to be together. They felt timid in the strange hospital with unknown doctors and nurses. The waiting in the hall on 'The Bench' distressed the father. The cries of other women in labor upset the mother. If she was left alone her fear increased. . . . Mothers were rebellious against hospital regulations. . . . Fathers spoke of fear, loneliness, need for professional explanation and reassurance."[43] Sentiment was building for reactions such as Dale Clark's—which opened this chapter—to try to change hospital practices.

Fathers' Books

Probably in an effort to provide solace to the men who spent so many hours in the waiting rooms (there is no direct evidence about motivation), many hospitals, like Wesley Memorial Hospital in Chicago and St. Mary's Hospital in Madison, Wisconsin, kept "Fathers' Books" in the maternity waiting rooms, blank journals in which the men could read what other waiting fathers had written and add their own remarks.[44] The fathers-to-be took time to write in the books as they waited, revealing much about their thoughts and worries; fathers' books are an enormous help in understanding the hospital childbirth experience at midcentury. In addition to this rich source, although hospital policy manuals reveal little of what actually occurred in the waiting rooms, medical and health journals and popular magazines in this period frequently addressed labor and delivery, as did oral histories, interviews, and personal letters. Thus, a multitude of sources exist to help us understand what was happening within the walls of the fathers' rooms that ultimately helped to change the face of hospi-

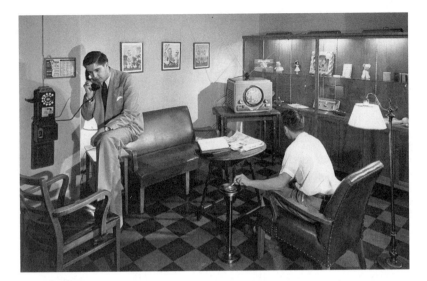

Two men wait in the "Stork Club" at Wesley Memorial Hospital, Chicago,
ca. 1950; the Fathers' Book occupies a prominent place on the table.
Hedrich Blessing Photographers, HB-16555-P, Chicago History Museum.

tal childbirth by the 1960s and 1970s. These diverse sources reveal that the expectant fathers, although not necessarily wielding hatchets, played active roles in bringing about the changes that moved the men from the periphery of the waiting rooms into the labor rooms and finally to the center of birthing activity in the delivery rooms of American hospitals.

The men who wrote in the Wesley Memorial Hospital Fathers' Books represent a diverse group of new fathers in the post–World War II period (extant books cover the years from 1949 through 1965). The hospital, associated with Northwestern University Medical School, was located on Chicago's near north side. The large majority of Wesley Memorial's patient population was white, working and middle class, what one writer called "the deserving middle class."[45] Some higher-status families that had moved from the city to the suburbs also used this hospital, along with smaller numbers of new immigrants — Italian, Hispanic, and Chinese — and African Americans.[46] A very small number of its patients were non-English-speaking. Physicians in this hospital delivered approximately four babies a day to a diverse group of women, including some who were referred from the Chicago Maternity Center, which was located on the south side of the city.[47] Started by Joseph DeLee, the Chicago Maternity Center was a training site for medical students and interns; it served an impoverished community and provided a home-delivery service for most of the women. When complications arose, the women would be admitted to the Chicago Lying-In Hospital or brought to Wesley and delivered there. The area in which the Maternity Center was located was largely an ethnic white immigrant neighborhood when the center opened in 1895, but by the middle of the twentieth century many of the women it served were African American. The Maternity Center clients and some black women who lived in the area formed the 15 percent of the city's African American hospitalized childbearing women who delivered at Wesley.[48] (Most of the other 85 percent gave birth at Cook County Hospital.)

Despite their diversity, the waiting Chicago fathers had many of the same fears and feelings regarding the momentous event happening yards away, and they tried to voice these feelings by writing in the books. "Well, the butterflys [sic] started fluttering down in the pit of my stomach," confessed one man awaiting the birth of his first child.[49] "I suppose that it is just as well that we, who sit and wait, be denied the ability to know the future," penned another author. "I think that any man that denies the fact that he is worried is either a darn liar or flat nuts. . . . My stomach just will not relax."[50] "Tanya is on the cross now," another husband confided. "How can I ever know how much I love her and how much she loves me? She is suffering so. . . . Write what you are thinking," he advised future stork clubbers; "it helped me."[51]

This last comment is especially telling. The men—many of whom might have been alone in the room—found solace in communication with other worrying expectant fathers through writing in these books. They learned what other men were thinking and were comforted by the fact that they were not alone in their concerns. It was through such written interactions (and oral ones as men found themselves in the company of others) that men bonded and realized more communally that they wanted to change their circumstances and participate more actively in labor and delivery.

In a New York hospital (not named in the source), fathers wrote poetry in the waiting-room fathers' books. One man expressed his anxiety in this way:

Confession
Am supposed to be a hardboiled construction man
Have handled jobs in every clime
But here I sit and wring my hands
Waiting for Wife to release that Baby of mine.[52]

Another, signed "Cabinet Maker," penned:

Ode to the Men's Labor Room
Mental labor is the worst
For news of Her my mind doth thirst
How long will my feeble brain distort?
I'll lay down on the davenport.[53]

Some men, perhaps not wanting to show their true feelings, hid behind a flippant approach: "Nothin' to it, once its over with."[54] Others felt sorry for themselves: "Women are so inconsiderate," wrote one impatient man; "they make a man wait so long for the delivery."[55] Two days after that entry, in response, another restless father-to-be combined the two emotions and exclaimed, "They say the women suffer thru childbirth!! What the heck do you call what I'm going thru right now."[56] Television personality Bob Newhart, with humor, remembered that when his wife delivered in the 1960s "fathers waited in the fathers' room. It's sort of a torture chamber they devised to drive the fathers nuts while their wives are having the babies." He was thankful his wife labored only four hours, which made his wait shorter than most.[57]

Although some expectant fathers' comments were sarcastic or humorous, most men writing in the waiting-room books showed what today might be called their "feminine" side. Instead of trying to sound stereotypically masculine—brave and strong—they revealed vulnerabilities and fears and reflected on how much the experience of bringing new life into the world affected them. One man recognized this explicitly: "All of the cynicism and hardness, with which we provide ourselves in order to survive, disappear before the brilliance of a little baby girl."[58] Public demonstration of masculinity might have demanded hiding vulnerabilities, but in this private space of the fathers' books, supposedly shared only with others in the same situation who had already revealed their fears and hopes, men could be more honest and reflective. Their sometimes raw statements conveyed an openness and honesty that revealed that this was a stirring time for the men. Two of the waiting men became veritable philosophers. One wrote:

> Expectant fathers have been the source of many gags. They seem to have a slightly hollow ring now. Perhaps I'll laugh with them again but not for some time I assure you. While reading through this book the thing that strikes me . . . [is that birth] makes you really get down to fundamentals. . . . Gives us a bond with the past . . . [and] a bond with the future—not even the H bomb can change it—Perhaps a change of our ideals back to things that don't change with fad would be a good thing.[59]

The other expressed similarly weighty thoughts:

> Reproduction is one of the richest experiences available to man. It gives one the full feeling of participation in life's wonders and of contribution to the stream of life—the feeling of fulfillment—the feeling is so strong that it outweighs all the pain, doubts, & fears for the projected environment of the new little one. In times like these when plans for wholesale destruction are being formulated even one small step in the other direction seems worthwhile. It is our obligation as parents to strive with all energy to produce—if not a comfortable place to live—at least one that is safe from the ravages of war and pestilence—so that the little ones we bring into the world will be allowed to mature and achieve their fulfillment in life's richest experience.[60]

The men combined their concerns about the risky times in which they lived with their concerns about their own impending fatherhood. Even if they had not been the ones who fought in the wars directly, many of them internalized the dangers of living during the Cold War as they thought about their obligations as parents. They certainly appreciated the magnitude of bringing new life into the world. The fathers-to-be who placed their comments in the context of the hydrogen bomb and the Cold War in these years help us understand the seriousness with which they approached bringing new life into the world.[61]

These quotations from fathers' contemplations about the meaning of the childbirth experience for themselves and their growing families also suggest how seriously many fathers took their entries in the Wesley Memorial Hospital's Fathers' Books. One man looking back from 1999 to his entry fifty years earlier said, "I was very serious when I wrote that, and I think probably in most if not all cases all of the men who wrote in that book were writing some of the most honest statements they have ever or ever will make. It's a very emotional time. I really never thought about anybody reading it other than fathers who came into the room."[62] Indeed, most hospitals that kept journals in fathers' waiting rooms destroyed them.[63]

Expectant fathers demonstrated most strongly and most frequently their concern about their wives' and babies' health and safety. Almost every entry in the fathers' books I have examined included some worry about the physical ordeal of childbirth. "God I do hope she's alright — that the delivery is normal — that the baby is a healthy normal tyke!" exclaimed one father.[64] "Will Dora be alright — will the baby be alright — thoughts really swim in the back of a persons mind," another penned in the fathers' book as the new year 1950 dawned. "Its torture to see a loved one suffer, no matter how mild a pain can be. . . . It really helps to be able to write at this time."[65]

Religious faith helped a lot of the men through the waiting time. "Dear God, make it a fine baby and keep Betty safe," wrote a father as he waited all night for his daughter.[66] Echoing the sentiment, another father penned, "I seldom pray but I'm praying right now. May God watch over her & keep her through this ordeal."[67] Another realized: "Experiences such as these should develop many good Christian fathers here in the Stork Club. I prayed as I waited and thank the Lord my wife made it fine."[68] One waiting dad put it very succinctly: "Stork Club empty. God and I are keeping a vigil."[69] Another addressed his fellow waiters in a way that summed it up for many: "I know some mighty prayers and appeals have been made in wherever you fellows worship but I dare say none has been as fervent or heaven shattering as those made in this little room."[70]

A journalist looking at these entries concluded, in an expansion of the famous saying about people turning to God in times of crisis (attributed often to Ernie Pyle but of unknown origin), "If there are no atheists in foxholes, there are also few in fathers' rooms."[71] The vast majority of the religiously inclined writers in the Wesley Hospital Fathers' Books represented one of the Christian denominations. A few Jewish men entered their pleas to God, and one Muslim man entered only this brief remark: "To Allah I give my thanks for our little girl."[72]

Clergy were among the most eager to evoke God while sitting in the waiting room. Sigurd T. Lokken, the pastor of the Lutheran Church in Moscow, Idaho, who shared some of the labor experience with his wife in 1953, sat out the delivery in a fathers' waiting room. He wrote an account of it at the time for his son: "The nurse came out to tell me that we had a *boy*! . . . Thank you dear God for presenting to me both my wife and my child. All is well. Thou has done all things exceedingly well. . . . I should write that during this time I have been reading cases out of 'Childbirth without Fear' [by Grantly Dick-Read] and *praying*. Thank you again, God."[73] A minister looking back at his wife's delivery in 1962, when he was a seminary student, wrote, "I believe that birth is a theological experience. I felt close to God sharing this event [he was with his wife in labor], and I wish I could have been in the delivery room with my wife." When they rushed his wife into delivery, he said, "I felt lonely and left out of this important experience. I did not know what was going on in the delivery room. After about an hour, an intern went by and he turned around and asked if anyone had told me I was a father. He then told me that my daughter had been born an hour before."[74]

Most of the men who praised God also praised the doctors and nurses. "God has been so kind to give me such a wonderful little wife. But he didn't stop there. He guided us to the doctor of his choice," wrote a grateful father after the event. "Both my wife Velma and I are grateful to God and Dr. Bradburn for their wisdom and work."[75] A comrade echoed,

"Thank God, the Doctor of the Year Dorr and Wesley's fine staff of nurses. Praise God from whom all blessings flow. Amen."[76]

A few men remembered God even when experiencing loss: "My son was born dead," wrote a grieving father. "I guess it can't be helped but I thank God that my wife, Bernice, the baby's mother, is out of danger and will recover."[77] Others echoed the sentiment when their wives were spared but their newborns were not. "I thank God a million, million times for letting me still keep my loving wife," emoted one man.[78] "Our Rose is doing fine," related another, already the father of a toddler. "Had to take our baby. . . . But we feel that God you knew best and are thankful you spared Rose, for little Billy needs you & so do I honey."[79] As the entries indicate, infant mortality rates were higher than maternal death rates in this period, although both had decreased over the previous decade.[80]

Many of the men waiting in fathers' rooms thought about the possibility of death as their wives labored and they paced and worried. One New York man wrote a poem he called "Gloomy Vista":

They call it the Valley of the Shadow
Which chills me to the very marrow
How long will Selma be in there
While I, depraved, just pull my hair?[81]

A Chicago man put men's worried thoughts into words this way:

Many fathers in the past, as do I, have thanked God for a successful delivery into this world of their child, and for the well being of their wives after such an ordeal. How lucky we are, how truly fortunate we are to have been blessed with sons and daughters to love and cherish always. How lucky we are to have "mama" go home too. But for those of us who have this good fortune, there are others who do not fare quite so well. How many are there, fathers, I mean, who have left this room sick to their stomachs with anguish and grief—knowing that they'll be going home alone—with no wife and no baby. . . . If you read this, don't you recall wondering and praying that all will go well? As I saw my wife in the agony of labor I could not help feeling how terrible it would be for her if she were to endure all the suffering of this morning and not survive in the end. She did survive, but what if she hadn't, or if the baby hadn't? I pray for anyone who is ever faced with this situation. . . . [signed] a thankful father.[82]

This last entry especially illustrates how the waiting room and the fathers' books played a crucial role in linking men to other men through this experience of waiting together while their wives labored alone elsewhere. The empathy this man exhibited toward other men he did not even know was strong and powerful. The rooms provided the waiting men with companionship throughout the long hours and connected them through a common bond that grew around the birth experience, especially during the years when the men did not attend the actual labor or delivery. Sharing their worries and expressing their concerns in writing, the men felt close to one another and felt free to express these feelings. Perhaps it was this closeness that developed men's interest in helping to change hospital policies that had been designed to exclude the expectant fathers from the process of labor and delivery and redirect them to include men in these events. As men moved out of the waiting rooms, they lost this cramped, intense physical space that had fostered their collective emotion and the sharing of their feelings. The waiting experience became instead an event they shared with their wives.

This mid-twentieth-century generation of men faced the births of their children with a high degree of faith in modern medicine. Although fearing death during childbirth was not as common for this generation as it had been for previous generations, it was not completely absent from their thoughts. The men who wrote in the fathers' books voiced a lot of optimism that, despite the dangers inherent to childbirth, medicine could save the day. While acknowledging that mortality for infant or mother was still a possibility, most men who wrote in the fathers' books looked to medicine to save their wives unnecessary suffering and to conquer any potential dangers. Although this attitude may represent in part the feeling of working-class men in awe of medicine, there was no discernible pattern of race, class, or religion among the men regarding their views on this subject. Most of the men's comments in the books mirrored the respect for medicine held by society in general in the middle years of the twentieth century.[83]

As the fathers-to-be sat waiting, the men gave special praise to their doctors. "Dr. Bradburn says we'll have a baby tonight. What a wonderful guy."[84] Indeed, physicians reading through these books at the beginning of the twenty-first century who might be feeling underappreciated by their patients would be heartened to see repeated, over and over again, "Dr. Bradburn is a great man."[85] "Loads of thanks to a great doctor & a wonderful man who made it so lovely for my wife."[86] "No words, no matter how well put, can inscribe a father's feeling—thank you Dr. Benaron. . . . Your golden hands are more than human."[87] The men demonstrated over and over again respect and appreciation for what modern medicine had to offer; they did not often challenge medical authority or medical treatments. A manual for fathers underlined this sentiment and advised fathers-to-be: "While you are pacing the floor, talking with other expectant fathers or otherwise trying to occupy the time, your wife will be in the hands of a carefully trained and highly coordinated delivery room team prepared to cope with any situation."[88]

The induction of labor with medication like Pitocin provides an example of the degree of men's faith in medicine and their lack of inclusion, while in waiting rooms, in making decisions about what was being done inside the maternity suite. Medical personnel wielded most of the decision-making authority about induction, as they did with other interventions at midcentury. One physician said that in his practice he induced patients "who have rapid labors, live at a great distance from the institution, and have poor transportation facilities, or for other reasons in which it might be desirable and convenient to have the onset of labor planned by schedule." He thought, "Surely, no one would object to convenience to the obstetrician if it can be accomplished without jeopardy or hazard to the mother of the baby."[89]

Usually the women's husbands, sitting in the waiting room, were not consulted, and some not even informed, about labor induction: "Saw Doctor Chung after he gave June another inspection. He decided to give the wife medication to induce labor."[90] Another explained, "She was put into induced labor and was out for the count."[91] While it was not always clear whether the father had been or wanted to be consulted about an induction, it was certain that often at midcentury the men approved of procedures that they interpreted as means to help their wives have an easier and shorter labor. One father wrote, "[They] proceeded with induced labor solution. . . . I recommend this for all mothers—a gift from medical science to deliver gifts from God. What a wonderful country we live in."[92]

Birthing women voiced similar feelings. One woman remembered that her 1947 labor was induced: "Doctor preferred to deliver six lb. babies, so labor was induced almost a month early according to my calculations."[93] When her last child was born, a different woman remembered, without any rancor, "Our doctor was ill and we had an associate. He persuaded me to go in for induction for his convenience."[94]

This faith in medicine that led men and women not to question such medical decisions and procedures makes it all the more clear that when the men chose to challenge hospital policy and break down the barriers to their presence in the labor and delivery rooms, they did not act as radicals or as doctor bashers. When they grabbed their "hatchets," as Dale Clark put it, they did so in concert with their wives and with lay groups that believed in the value of couples sharing the birth experience—to gain what came to be called "family centered childbirth"—not as revolutionaries trying to break down the institution of the hospital or the authority of medicine.

Before we leave the waiting rooms, it is necessary to examine a major preoccupation of the waiting dads-to-be and the new fathers who often returned to the waiting room to write about the outcome of their particular cases: the sex of their baby. So many of the men who wrote in the fathers' books commented strongly about their preferences that this subject becomes part of the gestalt of the midcentury childbirth experience. Their consciousness about sex roles underscores the men's acceptance of midcentury cultural norms.

Overwhelmingly the men voiced a preference for a boy, a male heir to the family name. "I do hope it is a boy," wrote one father.[95] "Miracle of miracles," wrote another. "A BOY!! Gosh what a thrill. (I was expecting a girl.) . . . Now I can go home and dream of my swell little son."[96] Another asserted, "A boy—my wife wouldn't dare to have anything else."[97] "Third try and at last I have my boy," trilled one delighted father. "Our family is now complete."[98] Two other fathers put it in particularly gendered terms: "Manhood has again been demonstrated," one penned after the birth of a 7 ½-pound boy; the other, "It's a boy. Takes a man to make a man."[99] But yet another went home sadly: "I wanted a little boy, but I got a little girl, so what is the use of hoping?"[100] A father in Madison, Wisconsin, wrote after learning that his wife delivered a girl: "I'll never put her through this ordeal again, at least not for a couple of weeks when we start working on a boy!"[101] A Chicago man summed it up this way: "O boy, o boy, o boy, o boy, o boy, o boy, it's a boy!"[102]

Most new fathers settled happily enough when their wives delivered daughters. As one put it: "All I wanted was a boy—and I didn't even know I really wanted a girl. But she came at 9:25 am, and she's gorgeous!"[103] Singer-entertainer Nat King Cole had thought he wanted a boy, but when Natalie was born in 1950, Cole assured his wife, "Girls stick closer to home . . . and truthfully, the moment I heard it was a girl, all the past feelings went away. I'm happy."[104] Many men were delighted to welcome daughters. One claimed to be "the happiest man in the earth" when his daughter was born, adding, "I hope she will like Chgo [Chicago]."[105] Many of the new fathers wrote of their desire for a balanced family: if they already had a daughter, they wanted a son, and vice versa.

Even so, the preference fathers voiced for male children was intense. One man asked for advice: "Got myself a harem. This is the fourth girl born. . . . Anybody got a suggestion on how to get a boy?"[106] Another wrote, using a phrase echoed elsewhere in the fathers' books, "This makes girl # 3. . . . I was hoping for some outside plumbing."[107] One man put it starkly: "It's a (ugh!) girl."[108]

Whatever the sex of their babies, the new fathers voiced strong gender-role expectations: boys would be interested in or play sports; girls would be domestically inclined. Using such stereotypical language, a new father concluded, "Was going for a football team but now settle for a sewing club."[109] Another man wrote: "I am happy to say a baby girl was blessed to us to complete a fine little family one boy and one girl which should

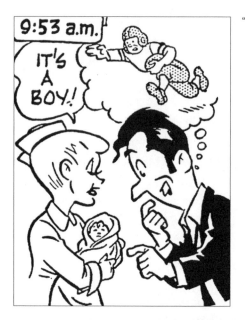

"It's a boy!" Cartoon showing how happy the father is with a boy who might someday play football. Robert S. Kleckner, "Jottings from 'Stork Room' Diary," *Chicago Sun-Times*, May 4, 1952, sec. 2, 2. Cartoon by John (Jack) Ryan. As published in *The Chicago Sun-Times*, © 1952 The Chicago Sun-Times LLC. Reprinted with permission.

"That's my Baby," says a happy Nat King Cole as he gazes proudly at his new daughter. *Ebony*, June 1950, 33. Photograph by Larry Barbier, M.P. & T.V. Photo Archive.

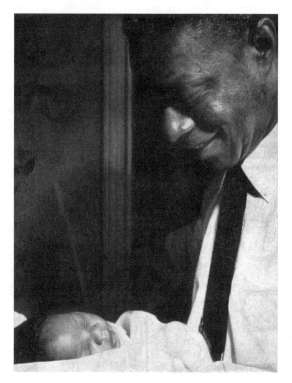

give my Darling some of the pleasure of raising not only a guy that looks &
acts like his father, but a gal to dress and play with."[110] "A girl!" exclaimed
a new father. "Well, my sewing circle gets larger. . . . Be back soon; trying
for a boy."[111] Another man bluntly wrote, "It's a Boy. . . . After two girls
what a relief to get the change—where's those boxing gloves?"[112]

Men's gender preferences sometimes received the attention—and re-
inforcement—of male obstetricians. In Manhattan, Kansas, in 1959, a
member of the faculty of Kansas State University sat in the waiting room
until he was allowed to see his wife, just coming out of anesthesia. David
Gruener related, "While I held her hand and comforted her, the obstetrician stuck his head in the door and said he had bad news. 'What is it?'
I asked, shocked. 'It was just a girl, he said, but she looks healthy.' I told
him we were glad to have a girl, and we did not see him again." A different physician delivered their next baby, this time with Professor Gruener
watching in the delivery room.[113]

The gender stereotyping voiced when fathers declared their preferences for boys or girls was frequently echoed in the military and sports
analogies and metaphors in the language they used to express themselves.
Dubbing the event the "battle of the stork," one father set the scene:
"Captain smoking cigarettes in the ward room. Chief engineer is with
Executive officer who is busy trying to produce a new crew member. . . .
Speed increased to 20 knots. Much smoke resulted. . . . New crew mem-
ber arrived aboard (had no uniforms or gear with him; Bos'n will have
to fit him out in something borrowed.) Exec doing fine," he expanded.
"Captain thinks Chief Engineer did a fine job."[114]

Men who did not have military experience often used sports language
to express their feelings. As one wrote, "There is only one trying point in
the ordeal the father goes thru and that is the last ½ hour when the one
you love is on the delivery table. It is like the feeling a coach goes thru
in the last few minutes of a game & you are behind by one touchdown &
there is a chance for a win or a loss. Well in this big game we won . . . first
member of my all girl baseball team."[115] "We're hoping for a Jr. 'Mickey
Mantle,'" wrote one man, "still waiting . . . no runs, no hits, no errors
yet."[116] In the company of men, the men who wrote in the fathers' books
used mutually understood gendered language.

The men's wishes about the sex of their baby were fostered in the collective nature of the waiting rooms, encouraged by the existence of the fathers' books themselves, as men read what other men had written and then added their own accounts. That is, not only did men bond with the men with whom they shared the space of the waiting room, but they also felt connected to the men, now gone from the spaces, who had occupied the rooms earlier. Just when women lost their gendered network of supporters as they went to the hospital to give birth, men gained a team of supporters in the hospital waiting rooms. The male bonding that developed in those spaces helped the men want to seek more control in the birthing process—ultimately helped them move out of the confined fathers' rooms and into labor and delivery rooms, where the main action of birth took place. One of the subjects the men bonded about was their feelings about the sex of their babies.

Marvin Muhlhausen described a fairly typical scenario of the fathers' waiting rooms at midcentury. His wife delivered their first child at Holy Cross Hospital in Silver Spring, Maryland, in 1969. The couple had attended a prenatal class together, but he had "fainted at the beginning of a movie on childbirth and was removed from the room. Of course, I had no interest in being present during the birth of my child. I have always believed, and still do [in 2005], that this is best left to the professionals." He described what happened when she went into labor:

> I drove my wife to the . . . hospital where hospital staff took charge. I was directed to the "father's room." There I waited for about three hours with other fathers. . . . The father's room was down the hall and around the corner from the delivery room(s) and nursery. I arrived at about 6 A.M. and found two other fathers-to-be waiting. One had been waiting for about 20 hours. . . . The other father had been waiting 7 to 8 hours. They related their experiences—their anxieties and what their wives were going through. . . . We talked about complications that can happen at childbirth. I was sorry for their long wait and hoped my wife had a quick delivery.[117]

Howard Johnson told a very different waiting-room story, one that must have been extremely rare, if not unique. In the mid-1960s, in Sioux

Valley Hospital in South Dakota, he waited while his wife delivered their third child. He was alone in the waiting room when the nurse brought out his baby and left father and son together. The baby was wrapped in a blanket but not yet washed. "We just sat there and bonded. I rather enjoyed it. We cannot understand to this day why that occurred. I may have had the baby with me for a half an hour or so."[118]

Beginnings of Change

Despite — and in part because of — the gendered sharing and bonding and other favorable aspects of the experiences that occurred in fathers' rooms as men waited together, many fathers by the 1950s and through the 1960s began voicing significant displeasure with hospital policies that separated them from their laboring wives. One published article about fathers put it this way: "During the hours of labor he sits helpless in the waiting room, weighed down by a very real sense of inadequacy. He is responsible for this baby. He should be by his wife. . . . He feels there must be some part in this for him. . . . He knows his wife needs him . . . wants him with her . . . but he sees no way."[119] Another publication drew a stark contrast between a man's take-charge heroic activity during war — a common image in the period — and his helplessness in the maternity ward, again pointing to a main question with which this generation grappled, namely, how the big issues of war and world safety intruded so often into private family lives: "This thin little fellow who paces up and down the waiting room floor, such discontent on his face when he asks why he cannot be with his wife — this is the boy who blasted age-old cities and the population off the face of the earth. This man gazing through a glass window at his day-old son — irritation, annoyance and frustration keeping him silent — this is the man who crashed through barriers of steel in a blazing tank."[120] It was difficult to understand how men who had demonstrated their masculinity and bravery when they were soldiers at war returned home and behaved more meekly. But this lack of initiative that men seemed to have as they waited in their separate spaces in hospital maternity suites was changing. Dale Clark's position about chopping down the partition was beginning to gain more advocates.

During the 1950s, men's discontent with their banishment from labor and delivery became a more common lament. Journalist, social critic, and author Vance Packard, whose best-selling book *The Hidden Persuaders* would later become a cultural staple, wrote in 1952 about his children's births: "Each time, I was shunted into a darkened hospital waiting room to pace and wring my hands, and listen for distant screams. Whenever I sought information I was repulsed as a nuisance by frowning nurses. To me, as well as my wife, the whole process of having a baby was a frustrating and painful one."[121]

As men got information about possible alternatives to the separation from their wives, especially about natural childbirth, complaints about their dissatisfaction with being left out of the birth process increased further. Jack Pollack articulated what many men seemed to be feeling during this period of transition: "In too many hospitals, mother and father are separated at the elevator door. She goes to the labor room and he to the waiting room. Though he wants to be with his wife — and she needs him as never before — his role is treated as a joke. One hospital even has a sign: 'Babies should be shown as infrequently as possible to fathers as it is a waste of nursing time.'"[122] Pollack's article, published in *Cosmopolitan*, joined many others in the pages of other popular magazines, including *Ladies' Home Journal*, *Woman's Home Companion*, and *Life*. They helped gain public acceptance of notions that men belonged with their wives when they labored and that the men were needed to help the women through these difficult hours. Women wrote many of the articles and joined a chorus of voices in the 1950s and 1960s pointing out the problems with separating parents-to-be. In a *Redbook* article a young mother remembering her labor experience wrote: "It was both ridiculous and cruel to keep my frantic husband pacing up and down the 'Daddies Room' hour after hour while I was lying miserably alone only a few yards away."[123]

Clearly, many men in the 1950s did not want to "sweat it out" in the waiting room while their wives suffered alone in the labor room. Peter Douglas, who gratefully recorded his wife's second delivery — at Grace–New Haven Hospital in 1950 using natural childbirth methods — recalled that he "did 'sweat it out' when our first little girl was born in 1947. My wife and I still do not like to recall that twenty-eight hours of physical pain for her, and mental pain for me. . . . I remember, all too clearly, my awful uncertainty . . . the sleepless endless hours of anxiety I spent in the hospital waiting room. Night gave way to day and day to night again before the baby came."[124] In contrast to this frustrating and alienating experience, the couple greatly appreciated being together for their next labor and delivery.

The changes came gradually and unevenly. A study of attitudes at the Sloane Hospital for Women in New York City in the early 1950s concluded that "some husbands want to be with their wives in the labor room and other husbands prefer to stay in the waiting room until their babies are born. They appreciate being able to make the decision themselves."[125] That last sentence is key: men were questioning hospital policies that did not allow them to decide for themselves the roles they would take during the births of their own children. There is no doubt that many men continued to prefer their separation from their laboring wives. Howard Johnson, whose wife delivered four babies in four different hospitals in the Midwest during the 1960s, wrote, "I never wanted to be in the delivery room. It never occurred to me. The procedure was, as I understood it, to just wait in the waiting room which I did."[126] A researcher in 1969 interviewed men about their preferences and found that half of them preferred not to be with their wives. The author quoted many of the men who wanted to stay in the waiting room. For example, "No, I wouldn't want to be with her during labor. I'd be frightened to death. I'm not the type. My stomach wouldn't take it. I stayed in the waiting room." And a second: "It's a woman's business, and I don't think she would want her husband there. I brought my wife to the hospital, and when the doctor told me it would take a while, I went to work. It helped to keep me from worrying."[127] A Chicago man who did not want to see any of his four children being born put it this way: "I couldn't think of anything less appealing than to watch my wife — the woman I love — in the middle of a messy business like childbirth."[128]

Yet the striking change of this period was that half of the expectant fathers wanted to be together with their wives at least during labor. Steven Barney, whose wife delivered at Madison General Hospital (now

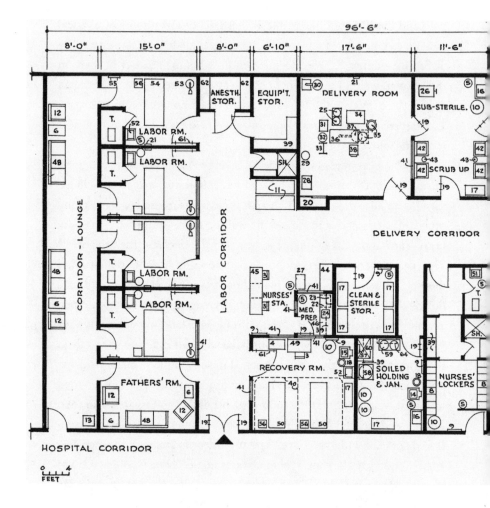

Meriter Hospital) in Madison, Wisconsin, in 1969, definitely wanted to
be with his wife in labor and delivery. He managed to accomplish this and
wrote about the experience in the local newspaper (he was on the paper's
editorial staff). He spent some time in the fathers' waiting room, nonetheless: "I had great expectations. Waiting rooms are full of such emotions, and all fathers share a common bond which makes them instant
allies."[129] This observation is an extremely important one. Men who sat
in waiting rooms, for a short time or for a long time, bonded with one another and shared an important life event and all the emotions connected
to it. Increasing numbers of men in these decades, empowered by their

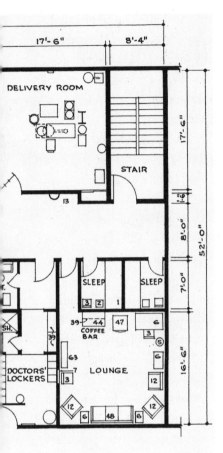

Floor plan model for a labor and delivery unit to handle 1,500 births a year. The fathers' room is within the unit and gives the men access to labor rooms as well as to a lounge-corridor. If hospitals could afford to construct such a unit, they would easily be able to allow the men to be with their wives during labor, although in this period most laymen still would not be permitted into the delivery rooms. John M. Jullien, *Planning the Labor-Delivery Unit in the General Hospital* (Washington, D.C.: U.S. Department of Health, Education and Welfare, Public Health Service publication no. 830-D-15, 1964).

waiting-room experiences with other men, voiced their willingness or even eagerness to join their laboring wives.

Despite the growing interest, many men who wanted to be with their wives were blocked by hospital restrictions based on architecture. Fathers' rooms in hospitals built before or renovated in the 1940s had been designed to be separate from the active obstetrics corridors. Men could not be easily incorporated into those spaces; they could not be allowed to roam the obstetric hallways because they might contaminate the area. Even as administrators developed some tolerance for allowing the men to be with their wives in the 1950s and 1960s, they felt forced to continue to bar their presence so that doctors and nurses could freely do their jobs without the women's health being endangered by the comings and goings of husbands. Hospitals had finally succeeded in bringing down postpartum infection rates, which had earlier been a prime cause of maternal mortality, and hospital administrators were loath to allow a practice they associated with possible infection transmission.

By the 1960s, and certainly thereafter, hospitals began to redesign the space of the old maternity suites and build new ones to allow "separate access to labor rooms" to "permit the husband to visit in the labor room without passing through the main corridor."[130] In such places, men had easy access to their wives' labor rooms without getting in the way of or endangering other patients. It took a long time—well into the 1980s and even beyond—for many hospitals to be able to build such flexible spaces.

Physicians practicing obstetrics in the middle of the twentieth century began to join the voices seeking more flexible hospital policies as they saw the benefits to the hospital staff and to themselves of having the men in the labor rooms supporting their wives. They, too, however, initially felt stymied. Dr. George Schaefer, for example, felt there was a role for fathers in labor, but his hospital did not allow it, and so he contented himself with advising "those husbands who want to wait it out [instead of going home] to bring their own books, magazines, crossword puzzles or even paper work from the office."[131] Robert Rutherford, another physician who early supported and worked hard to include husbands in labor so that they could provide psychological and physical supports, had to admit that if the laboring woman was unconscious, "the father is encouraged to stay in the Father's Room. . . . Neither [husband nor wife] has any desire to participate except passively."[132] But in those cases in which the woman was conscious, which happened more often as the natural childbirth movement grew in strength in this period, Rutherford believed men were necessary to successful experiences, and he tried to convince his colleagues to welcome them.

Most physicians in the 1950s and 1960s continued to insist that the men stay in their own spaces and not interfere with labor and delivery. In 1969, Earl Withycombe was a student at Massachusetts Institute of

Technology when his wife delivered their first baby at Boston Lying-In Hospital. "I had been told by staff that I would have to wait in the lobby and I would be notified when I could see Leslie," Withycombe wrote. "I understood, although the staff didn't tell me, that I would not be allowed into the delivery room." He sat in the lobby, accompanied by his mother-in-law and two friends. They played bridge as they waited. "At some point around midnight, a nurse came over to our game and told me to go stand by the elevator door." He did so: "The elevator doors opened and I saw Leslie lying on a gurney, with two young physicians standing at each end, both wearing masks and white coats. One of them was holding a swaddled newborn who was frowning. Leslie weakly grinned at me and said it was a girl." About fifteen seconds later, the elevator doors closed and "I was alone."[133] Withycombe's experience dramatically demonstrates why so many men began to view these separations from their wives as unacceptable.

The fathers' waiting rooms provided some positive experiences for the men who populated them in the middle of the twentieth century. Hospital practices varied significantly: some hospitals excluded other family members, others allowed it; some excluded laboring women, others allowed them entrance; some continued not to provide spaces for the men at all. Most hospitals, however, did designate specific rooms for the waiting husbands. The men found comfort in the company of others undergoing the same anxious ordeal, and they eagerly shared their stories and gave one another a needed boost. While most men did not try to grab their hatchets to storm the barricades of the labor rooms to join their wives, many in these years did find themselves increasingly curious about what the women were doing, concerned about their suffering, and eager to share the experience with the women they loved. The waiting rooms and the communal male experience they provided helped to prepare the way for the men to enter hospital labor rooms and ultimately to fight to get into delivery rooms. When that happened, the waiting rooms lost their initial purpose of keeping the fathers out of the way of labor and delivery and became instead places to which the men, and later whole families and groups of friends, could retreat for a brief respite from the intensity and pressure of being an essential part of labor and delivery.

3 * THE BEST BACKRUBBER

Fathers Move into Labor Rooms

Even as most men were confined in fathers' rooms in the 1940s and 1950s, some hospitals allowed a number of them to venture out of the waiting rooms for short visits to their wives during labor, and a few hospitals even let them stay through the long hours of labor, excluding them only when the woman went into the delivery room. The changes that allowed men to enter labor rooms came slowly and unevenly and demonstrate the heterogeneity of the hospital birth experience in the United States. The opportunity for men to be with their wives came first to those who could afford private labor rooms; it was related directly to socioeconomic class and privilege and also to race in this period of segregated hospitals. New medications that allowed women to be awake and pain-free during labor and the natural childbirth movement, which grew in the 1950s, joined to create social pressures pushing hospitals to let couples be together during labor.[1] The movement to bring fathers into labor rooms gained particular strength in the decade of the 1950s because it fit the period's pronatalist nuclear family emphasis: men's participation in labor could foster their involvement in the lives of their children.[2]

Dale Clark, who wrote in *Esquire* the vivid account of a fathers' waiting room quoted in the previous chapter, wanted all husbands to "grab hatchets" to break their way into their wives' labor rooms. He accomplished that goal for himself by ignoring the sign directing fathers to their own waiting room; instead he boldly accompanied his wife into the labor room, which he also described in memorable language:

> Now, at three o'clock in the morning, a single bulb glowed dimly in the labor room. Thousands of you who read this—fathers included—have never seen a labor room. This one was one of a series of small, narrow, utilitarian cells along a corridor to the delivery room. There was space in it for two narrow beds along the opposing walls, two low cabinets containing bedpans, a folding screen, and a single, small, straight-backed chair. One door opened from a toilet, shared with the adjoining cubicle. Above and outside the corridor door, a light would flash when Ruth pressed the push-button device attached to the head of her bed. It was a perfectly efficient and matter-of-fact—and terribly lonely—little cell. . . . A nurse came in with a tray of examining equipment. During each examination I was asked—for hygienic reasons, I suppose—to step into the corridor. . . . A man doesn't need to be a miracle worker to play his role to perfection. He merely needs to be there. Period. Instead of wearing out the carpet of the lounge on the floor below, he is simply required to pull up a chair to his wife's bedside.[3]

Clark's article was a public endorsement meant to encourage other men to do what he did and ignore the rules in order to be with their wives through the labor ordeal. It was probably a combination of good fortune that another woman did not occupy the second bed in his wife's labor room and his own brash assurance (or did he reveal that he would write up this experience in a popular magazine?) that let him get away with what most other men could not yet accomplish. During the 1950s, however, encouraged by their wives and the growing movement that Clark's essay represented, more and more men tried to do what he did and join their wives in labor.

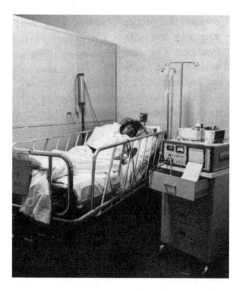

Woman in a labor room, confined to the bed with the bed rails up and connected to an IV. She is alone and unable to move about for the duration of her labor. Suzanne Arms, *Immaculate Deception* (Boston: Houghton Mifflin, 1975), 61. © Suzanne Arms.

Hospital Policies of Exclusion

In the face of emerging sentiment for men and women to share the labor experience, hospital policy changed slowly starting in the 1950s. Wesley Memorial Hospital, along with other Chicago hospitals, permitted fathers briefly to visit their wives in labor if they were in private rooms or serially if they were in semiprivate rooms. Men whose wives were in larger wards—those less privileged economically—did not see their wives at all: the cramped spaces and considerations for the privacy of other women precluded their presence.[4] Some hospitals allowed men brief visits to their wives' labor rooms during the day but not at night.[5] Other hospitals "send the father home when his wife is in labor and send him a telegram when his baby is born."[6] Many hospitals had different policies for each class of patient: "When the private patient is admitted to the hospital in labor her husband may stay with her. . . . The clinic patient is admitted directly to the labor unit where visitors have not thus far been allowed."[7] In contrast, in a small hospital in South Carolina, a man stayed with his wife throughout labor; he was sent to the waiting room only when his wife was moved into delivery.[8] Clearly, hospital policies and practices varied enormously. Most often, however, hospitals insisted that men wait outside the hospital maternity suites during most of their wives' labor and delivery.

Hospital policy keeping the men out of labor rooms had what many believed was very logical reasoning behind it. The exclusion policy developed as childbirth expanded in the hospital in the 1930s and 1940s (recall that half of American women delivered their babies in hospitals by 1938), when most women were sedated for much of the duration of labor, either routinely or by choice. Hospital staffs believed that if a woman was anesthetized, there was no need for her husband to be with her; he could do very little except get in the way. Dr. Joseph DeLee, in a widely used text he coauthored with Mabel Carmon, advised nurses that men may be admitted for short visits to their wives in labor, but it should be "as little as possible."[9]

Physicians who might have worried that the laymen, if allowed to stay in labor rooms, would challenge medical decisions or procedures need not—initially—have been concerned. Fathers-to-be, whether from the waiting room or the labor room, usually supported the period's routine medications and interventions. As one of them put it, "To hear the screams of a loved one in pain and know that you can do nothing about it is an excruciating torture. To pace the floor hours on end, distracted by anxiety, is a nightmare. . . . Imagine then the unspeakable relief of a vigil untouched by fear, a vigil during which you can watch your wife sleeping soundly, and know that she is not torn by pain or racked by terror."[10] Another new father wanted relief for the hard time his wife was having: "After 12 ½ hours my poor, beaten, bedraggled & beautiful wife finally went to the delivery room. Throughout the day my wife was in much pain. I kept trying to comfort her but of course to no avail. By her fourth hour of agony I was in tears and felt horrible because I couldn't help her. . . . Dr. Chung finally put her to sleep. I was terribly happy."[11] Once a man saw his wife in pain, often he was moved to support the use of medication to ease her difficulties, in the process demonstrating a faith that medical science could come to women's rescue.

In another example of how men might have contributed to rather than challenged common hospital procedures, a man related how he was integrated into his wife's 1949 long and agonizing labor experience. Because

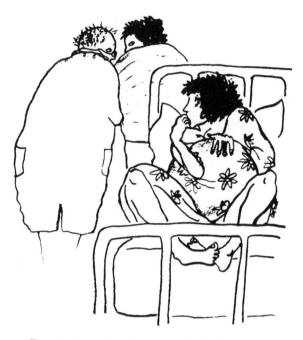

'The doctor and my husband decided between
them that I should have an epidural.'

Cartoon of laboring woman in bed while her physician and her husband confer behind
her back. Some women complained that this scenario left them out of decisions about
their own bodies. Sheila Kitzinger, *Rediscovering Birth* (New York: Atria, Simon and
Schuster, 2001), 124. Cartoon by Sue Gerber. Courtesy of Sue Gerber.

of a breech presentation, the physician was preparing for a possible cesarean section. The doctor decided not tell the woman about the com-
plication until later because, as her husband explained, "she worries too
much." But he did tell the husband, who remained with his wife through
much of the painful labor. The husband communicated his wife's need for
pain relief. "They finally gave her a shot & then let me quiet her down."[12]
In this example, the birthing woman was excluded from any contribu-
tion to decision making, about either the possible cesarean section or
the anesthetic, through the collusion of the physician and her husband,
which gave the man input into the pain relief decision. However, the language the man used, "they . . . let me," indicated that traditional hierarchies held and physicians made the decisions. Nonetheless, as men came

to join their wives in labor, doctors might sometimes include them in the discussions and practices that hid events from the birthing woman.[13]

Fathers who were admitted into labor rooms were not always involved in determining or even discussing potential procedures. At Genesee Hospital in Rochester, New York, for example, the obstetrician and the attending anesthesiologist together made the choice about anesthesia "for each individual patient according to the needs of the patient and the obstetrical situation."[14] One physician, while acknowledging that he might talk to the patient and her family about procedures, baldly stated, "The complaints of the patient and the annoyance of the family should be entirely ignored."[15] Indeed, the American College of Obstetricians and Gynecologists issued standards for obstetric practices in 1959 that noted that it was up to the medical staff to "assume responsibility for proper technic in all patient care."[16] Physician authority remained strong and generally accepted in this midcentury period, and the fathers usually did not dispute it.

Women's magazines in the 1940s and 1950s agreed that physicians should have ultimate authority. They typically advised their women readers: "You, your husband, and your family do not have experience enough to decide the 'best' method in your case. Let the doctor decide."[17] Many women agreed. One of them wrote: "I accepted everything that was being done. It never occurred to me to object. . . . I had great faith in my doctor and did not ever question his actions. I still feel kindly toward him."[18] Constance Ola, who had her first baby in 1950, wrote that she was "surprised by [the physician's] stance of authority," but by the time her second was born in 1952, she was more blasé about it: "Again 'authority' took over. . . . I was put to sleep."[19] Handbooks for fathers in this period similarly advised the men not to interfere with medical decisions. They should help their wives choose a physician and then "give him your full confidence and co-operation." Regarding anesthetics particularly, William Genne told his male readers to let their doctor know about any preferences but then: "Always abide by his decision. He knows what is best for your wife."[20] There was a general acceptance of medical authority because most people had a positive view of what medicine had to offer, in obstetrics as in other fields.

Most hospitals were slow to allow entry to the laymen. An obstetrical nurse practicing in Madison, Wisconsin, described a typical labor and delivery scene in the 1950s in her hospital, making obvious some of the reasons most hospitals did not want to include men in their practices:

> We gave drip ether. . . . There was another type that we gave . . . [in which] you strapped the instrument onto the patient's hand and you poured this blue liquid [trilene] . . . and they inhaled that and they couldn't get too much because then they would go to sleep and it would just drop off and if they needed more they would inhale more. . . . At that time you never called the doctor until the patient was ready to deliver. . . . The lady was in the labor room, we watched her progress until you thought she was complete [10 cm dilation] and that the fetus had progressed until you thought she was ready. . . . Generally after you decided that the patient was ready . . . you called the doctor and hoped that he got there on time. . . . But, the mothers were generally put to sleep.[21]

Given such practices, men would not have any role to play.

Most often cited as the main reason for hospital policies of exclusion was what hospitals perceived to be the need for routines and control in order to keep the maternity corridors and rooms free from any danger of outside infection. Postpartum infection was the single highest cause of maternal deaths in the period before the late 1940s, when the use of antibiotics brought the rates down. Since hospital maternity wards sometimes needed to be shut down because of high puerperal infection rates — and there were many examples of this in the 1930s — hospital staffs were always on the lookout for sources of infection.[22] They tried to isolate labor rooms completely, and even compulsively, by physically cutting off the corridor.[23] Husbands, especially if they came and went during the long hours of labor, were one culprit that was relatively easy to simply remove from the mix.

Trying to achieve thorough cleanliness, nurses actively sought to maintain what historian Sylvia Rinker has called "the rigors of scientific asepsis that defined the medical practice of obstetrics. . . . Physicians lent their authority, and nurses used it willingly to promote scientific birth restrictions. Asepsis rules required banning family and friends from the laboring rooms in the hospitals." Rinker went on to analyze the situation from the nurses' perspective: "Nurses willingly supported policies that separated a woman from her family on her admission to the hospital, stripped her of her clothes, shaved and purged her, and sometimes restrained her, all in the pursuit of asepsis. . . . The nurses who participated in such actions believed the scientific training they had received; they were convinced that such policies were justified to save mothers and infants from death. . . . Birth became an event not to be accepted and celebrated but to be managed and controlled."[24]

Birthing women did not necessarily understand this kind of motivation, and many of them resented the medical and nursing routines that forced their separation from their husbands. One woman wrote about her 1947 delivery at a New York hospital: "The labor went badly. Listening to the groans and screams of women already on the verge of delivery increased my own fears. Due to the insensitivity and impatience of a staff nurse who sat rocking in her chair next to my bed (I saw my husband only briefly and then was ordered to lie down) measuring my contractions with a large silver stop watch, the labor was longer and more painful than necessary. I would have preferred to be walking the halls with my husband."[25] Another woman wrote that hospital policy applied during her three labors in 1952, 1954, and 1956 in southern California included no walking in the labor room. "Women were supposed to lie quietly and wait for hourly checks."[26] It was fear about possible infections that led hospitals to insist on such careful procedures.

In Berlin Hospital in Waushara County, Wisconsin, more flexible policies in the 1950s accommodated birthing women's wishes to some extent. A woman was able to arrange to have her husband accompany her throughout labor, although the hospital barred him from the delivery room. For one woman who gave birth in the hospital in 1953, having her husband with her during labor was helpful as well as comforting; the person who recorded this woman's experience related: "She said that her husband was with her all of the time holding her hand and she stressed the importance of support of the husband. She said that after a hypo [injection] she was drowsy and would have forgotten her breathing, etc and he would sort of remind her of what to do."[27] Decisions made by other women delivering in the same hospital showed the variety of available opinions and options. One did not want her husband in the labor room. Another said the opposite: she couldn't have gone through labor without her husband. She "said that she took hold of the corners on his shirt collar and pulled when she had a pain and it just helped to have him there."[28] Hospitals in rural communities with fewer women in labor at any one time found it easier to be more responsive to women's varied wishes than did busier hospitals.

Hospital policies cannot be categorized easily, however, geographically or otherwise. In the New York City area, for example, Cornell University's New York Lying-In Hospital on the east side of Manhattan allowed men to accompany their wives through labor (and delivery) in the late 1950s. But when requested to do so in the 1960s, Hempstead Hospital on Long Island refused. The Reverend John Lawrence Ainsworth stayed with his wife during the birth of their first two children in the city in the late 1950s. The couple moved to Long Island and in 1962 wanted to repeat the experience of being together for both labor and delivery, but Hempstead, claiming it was health department policy, did not allow it. (North Shore Hospital in Manhasset, apparently, was the only Nassau County hospital to allow men in labor and delivery at that time.) Ainsworth contacted the department of health, which explained that individual hospitals established their own policies on this matter and most did not want to risk letting the men into the maternity ward:

> The reasons the hospitals have made this stand are several. As you may be aware, the problem of hospital-based infection is a serious one that has grown markedly in the past few years. To minimize any possible chance of infection on the maternity and nursery services, hospitals have established rigid controls; one of the most basic controls is the exclusion of all persons from these services except those actually giving medical or nursing care. . . . A second reason given for excluding husbands . . . is the severe nursing shortage. It is strongly felt by most hospital staffs that the presence of family members increases rather than decreases the nurses and physicians work espe-

cially if the labor and delivery are not completely uneventful. . . . I do not foresee an early solution to this problem.[29]

The health officer believed that "extensive education" would be needed before the entrance of husbands would be common, and she added that most hospitals were not "physically set up to be able to carry out such changes in policy."[30]

Architecture in rural and urban hospitals did indeed inhibit changes in this midcentury period. The administrator of Wautoma Community Hospital in Wisconsin, for example, "was quite concerned about the placement of the labor room adjacent to the delivery room." When considering changing hospital policy to allow men to be with their wives in labor, "he seemed rather reluctant to allow the fathers in the labor room since they have to pass the scrub sink where the doctors scrub."[31]

Hospitals made exceptions to their own rules when the men were physicians or physicians in training. One woman wrote of her two birth experiences in 1939 and 1941 at Israel Zion Hospital in New York: "Since my husband was a physician, he was with me during labor in the hospital cubicle."[32]

Women who labored alone in wards or multiple-bed labor rooms had the additional concerns of having to listen to other women in labor, similar to what my mother experienced in the 1930s. Marian Tompson said that when she delivered in 1950, she got to the hospital and was surprised "because all the women were drugged and they were screaming and yelling and moaning and I wasn't prepared for that."[33] Another woman described her 1951 two-day labor at Crouse-Irving Hospital in Syracuse, New York, in a four-bed labor room: "I was shaved, given an enema and prepared for the delivery room. . . . During that time many women came in, went through the whole process of labor and left to be delivered. I had to hear, and often when the curtains were open, see, the whole drama of each childbirth and must say, become more frightened by the moment."[34]

Marian Tompson corroborated Clark's description in *Esquire* of the stark labor room when she described the room in which she labored in Chicago in 1950: "It was the old wing of the hospital and very gloomy, dark halls, you know, and the labor room was—had big windows, but they were dirty! It was just like a pale ecru kind of wall. . . . It wasn't very comfortable. I think it created more anxiety than comfort in a woman going into that kind of a room." Tompson described the entirety of the hospital birth experience as emotionally sterile: "I felt that it could have been a broken leg or a[n] inverted toenail. . . . I was so excited! You know, I was going to have my baby, not one *person* acted excited—I mean, not one person said, 'Oh, isn't it wonderful that you're going to have your baby today.' . . . No empathy or understanding of the emotions that a woman was having."[35] Without their husbands, women strongly felt the institutional lack of sentiment.

The strictures on husbands carried through to other possible birthing partners as well. Women friends or relatives who might have accompanied birthing women to the hospital when their husbands were unavailable were not permitted into ward labor rooms. One woman wrote about her 1945 delivery at Beth David Hospital in New York:

At 3:30 PM my mother and sister and I left for the hospital. My husband was away at sea. . . . Finally, I was put to bed in the labor room. I had undressed and said good-by to my mother and sister. There were other women in the room in later stages of labor and nurses came and went and talked about "dilations"—I didn't know what that was. . . . After a while I became hungry and asked for something to eat. I was brought a dinner of spaghetti and I don't remember what else. I happen to like spaghetti and that seemed O.K. to me. Later, of course, I threw it up. They did not warn me that this might happen.[36]

The Wesley Hospital Fathers' Books add to our understanding of how the exclusionary policies worked. Some of the new fathers did not know what the hospital policy was, and they frequently asked whether they were permitted to enter the labor rooms. One man complained that his wife's doctor told him when they got to the hospital he couldn't see her "until after the baby is born."[37] Another confirmed this: "Can't even see your wife here."[38] But some men did visit their wives in labor regardless of stated visiting hours. Sometimes this was accomplished by personal permission. One father said: "They let me in to see Agnes and . . . [I] walked all over the ward with my wife."[39] Another related that the nurse admitted him to his wife's room, where she "allowed me to listen to the baby's heartbeat and it sounded just like my Elgin watch."[40] It was not possible to discern a pattern to the differences from the evidence in the fathers' books; probably economic considerations drove the policies, allowing for greater flexibility among paying patients in private rooms and less for poorer patients. Certainly women in private rooms would not bother other patients if their husbands were with them behind the closed door.

In contrast to the evidence of some degree of elasticity found at Wesley Hospital (and other private or university-run hospitals), Cook County Hospital, Chicago's biggest public hospital, offered no choice in the matter. A nurse who worked there claimed that the men "came as far as the front door with their wives [and then] were sent home and were not to be back until after the baby was born."[41] As historian Rosemary Stevens, the foremost scholar of American hospitals in this period, has noted, hospital growth in the fifteen years following World War II did not change the essential inequalities of earlier hospitals. Black and uninsured patients were more commonly found in municipal public hospitals where conditions were "often dreadful."[42] Policies of racial exclusion kept African American women out of most private hospitals in this period (Wesley was one of a few exceptions in Chicago); they had to deliver at Cook County Hospital, where space shortages forced most women to labor on stretchers in the hallways.[43] Even if black women had private insurance, staff physicians could find ways to, in the words of one scholar, "assure a remarkable degree of segregation of patients." David Barton Smith found that mid-twentieth-century Chicago physicians could "choose where to send each of their patients. They [were] reluctant to violate informal norms, for doing so could adversely affect their chances for reappointment."[44] Regardless of their capacity to pay for services, minority women, along with poor white women who also had little choice but to go to a crowded public hospital, were denied the kind of flexibility that might have allowed their husbands to accompany them through labor.

Many entries in the fathers' books reveal a definite variation in the application of the rules. Those men who pushed the issue, like Dale Clark did, might succeed in spending considerable time with their wives during labor.[45] Hospitals in small towns seemed more elastic in labor-room visiting policies than did many urban institutions. In Bell Plain, Iowa, for example, the maternity ward policy was "low key," and men were permitted to be with their wives in labor without any fuss. "They just stayed right in the room with us," one nurse explained.[46] In Moscow, Idaho, Sigurd T. Lokken was in and out of his wife's labor room in 1953, helping from time to time with back rubs and conversation. "She said that it meant a lot to her to have me nearby."[47]

Despite such exceptions, most hospitals, especially those with greater pressure of large numbers of patients and space constraints, continued in the 1940s and 1950s to insist that the men sit in waiting rooms or go home for the whole of their wives' labor and delivery. One man found the separation from his wife as she labored very difficult: "Now she is in advancing labor. The Doctor is supposed to be on his way. I'm trying to remain calm but I would rather be in the labor room with my wife . . . to help her with what little moral support I could give her. She is alone in the room—I should be with her."[48] He was unable to get the hospital to bend its rules, as was another man: "Haven't seen my darling wife yet. Read the magazines—ate my nails—am still awaiting. . . . Nurses say wife is in hard labor. . . . They won't let me see her, but say it should be some time this afternoon. . . . My dearest Ilene can't take too much pain."[49]

Occasionally a man revealed that, even if permitted to visit his wife in labor, he would choose not to stay. One man at Wesley Memorial Hospital watched his wife labor through contractions four minutes apart, "feeling them very hard, she was crying but tried to smile thru it. It sure takes a lot of Guts, and she sure has it. Brother that's more than I can take. I had to leave or I'd start bawling myself."[50] Variations in practices occurred sometimes because of institutional restrictions and sometimes because of men's own wishes.

Grantly Dick-Read and Natural Childbirth

Individual experiences of birthing women who felt they were not permitted to make the decision about the use of pain medication or the company of their husbands during their labors led them to seek other methods of delivery. Katherine Egan, for example, who delivered four babies during the 1930s and 1940s, said she was "forced to have anesthesia." During one of her labors, she said, an intern wanted to give her an anesthetic, and "I said I didn't want it, didn't need it, but they gave it to me anyway and against my protests." As a result, she described her birth experiences as "traumatic" and "a nightmare of impersonality," during which she felt a "helplessness to deal with events that bothered me most."[51] Helen Minton, too, did not get what she wanted during labor. She had had a twilight sleep (scopolamine and morphine) delivery in 1943, during which she felt "woozy, absolutely drowning in pain," and did not want to repeat that experience when pregnant again in 1948. She arranged ahead of time to have no pain medications unless she asked for them during labor, but her physician was at the opera when she was in labor in the hospital. She was strapped to the table and was in severe pain, so she asked the nurses for medication "and was told that my chart said, 'No Medicine.'"[52] Without her physician present, orders could not be changed. The husbands of these women, who were not with them during labor or delivery, could offer no help.

A study of maternal attitudes about labor and delivery in 1950 demonstrated that many women could not have a say in the procedures used during their births, especially the use of anesthesia. In responding to a questionnaire, women complained about "undesired anesthesia . . . forced upon the patient, unpleasant comments and scolding by attendants, a sensation of helplessness when strapped to the stirrups and delivery table."[53] Individual women reported that their wishes were stymied. One woman from Minneapolis said, "In the delivery room, they put a gas mask over my face, though I insisted I didn't need it. I tried to take it off, but my hands were tied. Everything that was wonderful was blotted out."[54] One of the main reasons women became attracted to less medicated delivery methods was their previous experience and perception of being forced into taking drugs they did not choose.

It was the combination of frustrations over not being able to make decisions about some particulars of childbearing practices, such as anesthesia, being strapped to the table, and the exclusion of laymen during labor, that led women and men to challenge medical decisions and authority more directly. Natural childbirth, when added to the growing dissatis-factions with hospital practices, led the way to the basic challenges that ultimately transformed childbirth in America's hospitals. Indeed, natural childbirth proved to be the strongest impetus behind attempts to change hospital policies about fathers-to-be in this midcentury period.

Dale Clark and his wife had read English physician Grantly Dick-Read's book *Childbirth without Fear*, which became widely publicized in the United States after the British physician's visit to the New York Mater-nity Center in 1947, and this had encouraged them to try to be together in labor. The Clarks had not received any formal training in his method, but they tried to follow on their own Dick-Read's prescriptions as described in his book. One of the reasons that Dick-Read's method caught on dur-ing the 1950s is that it fit so well with cultural patterns emphasizing the family and domesticity: Dick-Read believed that women's most important job was to bear children, and he wanted to make the experience more positive.[55]

Dick-Read taught that labor pain was brought about by tension, which was culturally produced from the fear and expectation women had that childbirth hurt and was a threat to their health. He thought that fear would lead women to tense their abdominal muscles, which would lead to holding back labor. If women could relax, he believed, their abdomi-nal muscles would relax, and labor could more naturally progress. Dick-Read called this the fear-tension-pain syndrome. He advocated relaxation techniques including positive visualization to ease women's fear and ten-sion and in particular deep breathing with the help of sympathetic birth attendants. His book also provided education in the basic anatomy and physiology of labor and delivery. His method became known as "natural childbirth" even though he did not disallow the use of medication to help the women who needed it. It was particularly attractive to women who did not feel comfortable with the hospital intervention routines common at the time. The term "natural childbirth" almost exclusively referred to Dick-Read's method during the 1940s and 1950s and then in the 1960s became applied indiscriminately to other alternative birth methods in-cluding those of Lamaze and Bradley.[56]

Dick-Read's method was the subject of numerous articles in popular magazines. During the 1940s, Bimbetta Coats happened to be in England for her labor and delivery, and Grantly Dick-Read himself attended her. She advertised her "glorious" experience in the pages of the *Reader's Digest*, read by more than one million Americans each month. "Dr. Read insists that no woman in labor be left alone for more than a few minutes during this first phase [the first stage of labor before full dilation]. He is in favor of the husband's being there until the actual delivery. . . . So there I lay in my pleasant room, my husband with me and Dr. Read coming to see me at frequent intervals." Coats liked her experience so much that she tried to replicate it when she was pregnant and back in the United States, but she was unable to convince her hospital to let her husband into the labor room. She managed as best she could alone to follow Dick-Read's precepts, and she advised American women, "If you are going to have a baby, and your doctor says you are normally formed, why not try Dr. Read's method? You will be rewarded with a joy and pride in yourself and in your child that you will never lose."[57]

According to physicians, most of the early Dick-Read births in the United States were initiated by the women themselves. One physician admitted in a letter to Dick-Read: "Women are reading your book . . . [and] are coming to their doctors and compelling them to get interested in natural childbirth. That is precisely how my interest was aroused."[58] In 1949 Angela Wyse and her husband "read a book by the English Dr. Grantly Dick Reed [sic]" even though "most doctors and hospitals were not yet recommending it," indicating that women throughout the United States learned of the method rather quickly. When Angela went into labor, the couple went to Lakeland Hospital near Elkhorn, Wisconsin, where they were able to be together during labor. She was attended in labor and delivery by Dr. Thomas Ambrose, the father of historian Stephen Ambrose, and a very accommodating nurse: "I still recall the pleasant feeling of pushing my feet into the rather ample stomach of the nurse in attendance."[59] By 1950, physicians at Yale University, Long Island College Medical School, Cornell Medical School, and the Johns Hopkins University Medical School found ways for their patients to deliver using Dick-Read's method and made arrangements for husbands to be with their wives during labor.[60]

Sigurd Lokken, who was able to be with his wife as she labored in 1953, grabbed their copy of the Dick-Read book as he ran out of the house to join her in the hospital.[61] Marian Tompson, who later became an activist in alternative childbirth methods, delivered her first child in 1950 in a Chicago hospital. She had read about Dick-Read's method and was eager to try it. Her physician, who usually anesthetized his patients, agreed to go along with her wishes. She was in a two-bed labor room, so her husband took turns visiting with the second woman's husband; it was hospital policy that he could not go with her into the delivery room. He waited outside, and at one point was sent home, and she "felt *totally* left alone. I mean the one person who really cared about me was gone."[62] At Methodist Hospital in Madison, Wisconsin, women wanting a natural childbirth influenced a change in hospital policy, which had excluded the men from the labor rooms. In 1952, the hospital and its medical staff "modified the former policy and now allow the husband to visit briefly with the patient during labor in the labor room for a maximum of five minutes at reasonable intervals." While five minutes would not have been enough time for women looking for support with their breathing and relaxation techniques, it constituted a foot in the door to change. At Methodist Hospital, women were permitted to visit their husbands in the fathers' room for longer periods of time.[63]

There are many stories of how individual obstetricians stepped into the breach of absent husbands and found ways to comfort the laboring women. Although physicians did not usually play a big role during labor and indeed some insisted on not being called to the maternity unit until the birthing woman was fully dilated and ready to deliver, a few seemed to greatly enjoy interacting with laboring women. One woman delivered her third child at St. Mary's Hospital in Passaic, New Jersey, and described a Dr. Palmeri, who roamed the labor floor singing the 1951 Hit Parade favorite "Hey there, You with the stars in your eyes." She fondly remembered the doctor making every laboring woman "feel that the 'stars' were shining brightest in *her* eyes. Dr. Palmeri was short, thin and wiry. He was Italian and had a thick crop of black curly hair, an olive complexion and wore a perpetual smile. In his hospital whites, he resembled a modern St. Francis of Assisi. Dr. Palmeri radiated warmth, cheer and self-assurance.

Fear and apprehension among expectant mothers diminished considerably in his presence."[64]

Along with the natural childbirth movement, new childbirth technology and medications were also associated with men being able to break down the barriers and be allowed into the labor rooms of American hospitals. When caudal anesthesia—the injection of a local anesthetic into a portion of the spinal canal called the caudal canal—became available and popular in the 1940s, some women were awake and virtually pain-free for their labors. Many hospitals altered their policy about excluding men if their wives received caudals and allowed husbands to be in the labor room. A woman who delivered in Passaic, New Jersey, in 1942 was among the first in her community to experience continuous caudal anesthesia. Her husband had arranged for a physician from Staten Island who knew about the method to come to Passaic to help his wife. Her experiences were publicized in the *Woman's Home Companion*, encouraging other women to try it. The birthing woman heard the moans of other women in labor, but she did not feel any pain. She drank coffee and relaxed with her husband and with the attending doctors who were there to learn more about this new method: "When I'd drained [the coffee] my husband lighted a cigarette and passed it over to me. I took it gratefully. . . . Meanwhile the doctors, my husband and I got into an argument about the European situation, each quoting his favorite news analyst. . . . After a while the tube from the supply bottle was attached to the needle in my back, and I was given a second injection of metycaine, later followed by a third. Then each of the doctors made an examination and decided it was time for me to go into the delivery room."[65] This kind of new medication that allowed the woman to be a conscious participant in events fostered changes and greater welcoming of fathers-to-be into labor rooms. One happy man wrote that his wife, having their second child, had a short labor, aided by "a coddle [sic] which really took care of the pain. . . . I am really grateful."[66] Alongside the increasing numbers of women who refused medication and wanted to be "awake and aware" for a "natural" labor and delivery, these methods helped hospital staffs understand that "sympathetic and continuous attention during actual labor must be maintained."[67]

Leading the way in establishing facilities for men to be with women who wanted to follow the Dick-Read method was Yale University's Grace–New Haven Hospital. As was the case with many hospitals, Yale's practice was influenced by the women who gave birth in the hospital. One such woman was Ethel Cates. After enduring a twenty-five-hour labor in a previous delivery, during which "the pain was agonizing, a beast that took over my body like two backhoes tearing out my insides," Ethel and her husband read Dick-Read's book and told their obstetrician they wanted to try the method for her second delivery in 1942. Her doctor, "though faintly skeptical, had gone along with my idea. I believe I was the first woman to suggest and use Natural Childbirth at Grace–New Haven."[68]

Under the oversight of Dr. Herbert Thoms, in 1947 the hospital began a demonstration program, following the urging of one patient well versed in Dick-Read's ways, which included allowing the husband to help during early labor: "The most important part of the program is the 'support' given during labor. This consists of aiding the patient to put into practice the relaxation and other techniques which she has learned previously. *No patient in active labor is left alone.* In the early part of labor the husband, a student nurse, or a medical student may be with the patient. At a later period, a nurse, a physician or both will be present."[69] Thoms became enthusiastic about the method and the results at Grace–New Haven when he realized that there was "increased safety to mother and child. Any program of obstetrical care in which the use of analgesics and anesthetics can be largely minimized or dispensed with will promote shorter labor, lessened bleeding, less necessity for new-born resuscitation, and fewer operative deliveries."[70] Thoms's experience led him to understand that husbands had an important role to play in natural childbirth: "We realized early that a large percentage of women wanted to have their husbands with them during labor," he wrote. "We set about making this possible." Furthermore, he believed that the man's participation would lead to a "more auspicious beginning of family life."[71] A woman who delivered in those early years using the Dick-Read method at Grace–New Haven with her husband at her side during labor remembered, "We joked about the fact that I didn't feel the slightest bit uncomfortable and my husband said, 'This is surely a wonderful way to have a baby,' and my doctor said, suddenly serious, 'Isn't it?'"[72]

Physicians in the Yale program carefully considered whether it was wise to have women making their own decisions. This thoughtful statement indicates some of the sensitivities evident at midcentury: "Formerly, we used to state to the patients that if they needed something, all they had to do was ask for it and they would receive it. We decided this was not a good procedure because it threw the responsibility back on the patient, at a time when the patient was relying on our care. We felt that we should assume the responsibility, not the patient. . . . Again in the delivery room we watch them closely, and we are the ones who suggest gas and do not leave it up to the patient to decide whether or not she should have some sort of anesthesia."[73] Physicians worried that they might be abrogating their own responsibility if they waited for birthing women or their husbands to voice their wishes.[74] Even when going along with couples who wanted to use natural childbirth, physicians believed they had ultimate responsibility.

Thoms noted that natural childbirth took more time and effort from doctors and nurses.[75] Although this concerned hospitals looking at the financial bottom line, many who delivered with the help of the Dick-Read method insisted that fathers' presence could actually ease the staffing situation. Mary Ann Grant, for example, wrote, "There is no hospital in the country today where a nurse can be spared to spend possible hours at or near the side of one patient. . . . The husband's presence actually releases a nurse to some great extent, in that most (if not all) of the mother-to-be's needs and wishes can be attended to by her husband, thus alleviating the need to summon a nurse from her other numerous duties." Another advantage, she noted, is that the father would know what was happening to his wife, "instead of sitting in the waiting room wondering and wondering."[76]

Those hospitals that used Dick-Read's method in its early years in the United States — generally university-based teaching hospitals — encouraged a nurse, a student, or the father-to-be to stay with the women throughout the labor. One physician wrote, "We usually keep the husband busy by letting him keep an accurate record of when a contraction begins and when it is over and how frequently the contractions come. . . . It is our intention to have the husbands participate in labor as much as possible."[77] At a New York hospital where the Dick-Read method was used in an experimental project in 1949 conducted by Carl T. Javert, a woman remembered that a nurse or a resident was always with her during labor so that she was not alone, but her husband was not allowed to be with her.[78]

The Dick-Read method as it was used at Yale's Grace–New Haven gained many advocates when it was splashed across the cover of *Life* magazine in 1950. The story followed the labor and delivery of Jean Barnes, the twenty-five-year-old wife of a life insurance salesman. In preparation for the coming event, both Jean and her husband attended prenatal classes. "The program also brought in that usually forgotten man, the father. Charles Barnes attended two lectures for fathers-to-be and, in the final weeks, went with his wife to confer with a pediatrician and a psychiatrist about child development, behavior, and needs." The story reported that including her husband this way gave Jean "greater security" and continued, "An important part of the security was the comforting knowledge that her husband, as well as a hospital nurse, would stay with her all through her labor until she was moved into the delivery room." Charles stayed with his wife during her entire eighteen-hour labor, including the times when Jean was sedated.[79]

Peter Douglas, a father-to-be, greatly appreciated being able to be with his wife during a Dick-Read delivery at Grace–New Haven:

> I was made to feel that I, too, was a participant in the great drama of childbirth. I was not separated from my wife until the very last stages of labor. This almost totally eliminated anxiety. I talked to her until a few moments before delivery, and I was able to see both her and the baby within an hour after birth. All the way along I knew what progress my wife was making. The sense of utter uselessness I'd had before was dispelled. I had no hesitation whatsoever in sitting with my wife in the labor room as long as I was permitted to do so. We talked freely and cheerfully until it was time for her to go to the

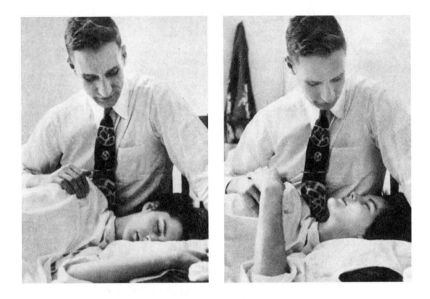

Three scenes from Jean Barnes's natural childbirth labor at Yale's Grace–
New Haven Hospital, during which her husband, Charles, watches as
she naps between contractions, comforts her, and waits while she rests. Charles
stayed with his wife the entire time of her labor and had some time for reflection.
Herbert Thoms, *Understanding Natural Childbirth: A Book for the Expectant
Mother* (New York: McGraw-Hill, 1950), 66. Photographs by David Linton.

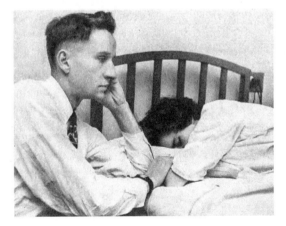

delivery room. I was able to minimize any discomfort my wife felt during contractions by rubbing her back as I had been shown by the nurse. . . . Since I could see her constantly and know that her discomfort was not great, I was freed from any sense of anxiety or fear.[80]

Some women, nonetheless, continued to feel that the best birth was the one that they could not feel or remember. One woman who tried the new methods in 1950 found her husband "useless" during labor and noted that "the birth attendants . . . all thought I was crazy to be doing this when most people were being knocked out. . . . The nurses were awful. They were used to people being anaesthetized and talked about me as though I wasn't there. They were totally impersonal."[81] Women and men continued to report negative experiences with traditional medicalized deliveries and also sometimes with their attempts with the newer, less medicated births. One woman who was sedated during her labor recalled: "My husband came in to see me during labor (then an unusual practice) and I disliked having him see me in such misery and looking so awful! He was loving and supportive."[82] As nurse Hazel Corbin realized, "There are mothers who want their husbands with them during labor, and there are mothers who do not want their husbands with them."[83]

The success of the Grace–New Haven demonstration of the Dick-Read method and women's and men's satisfaction with their birth experiences using the method continued to receive wide public attention. The physicians in charge of the program at Yale reported to fellow obstetricians in 1951 that after one thousand consecutive deliveries, they recommended the method, even though it might mean extra staff time: "We recognize that 'support' during active labor is the most important single factor in our program." Husbands could be relied upon for some of that support, but nursing staff was still essential.[84]

The issue of increased time and duties for nursing staff and the fact that most hospitals were not physically designed to accommodate men in labor rooms continued to pose problems even in those cases in which physicians were willing to support the new practices. Corbin admitted this in her remark: "Often this causes extreme difficulty because hospitals were not built or organized to accommodate the husbands during their wives' labor."[85] One hospital that allowed laboring women to be with their husbands had to keep the women "out of bed and out in the solarium with their husbands" because the hospital did not have "the space to provide for the isolation of each patient in a private labor room."[86] Many women did not have access to this kind of creative solution through the mid-1950s and continued to labor alone, with only sedation and the periodic checks from nursing staff to alleviate their anxieties.

There were a few physicians who visited the Yale program and came away unimpressed. A Dr. Steffen, speaking at a workshop in Wisconsin in 1953 following her visit to New Haven, said that (in the words of the recorder) "natural childbirth . . . may be all right for some people but not for her patients." The doctor felt that "the real trouble lies in the fact that the emotionally unstable woman is usually the one who goes all out for natural childbirth."[87]

Despite this kind of reaction almost demonizing natural childbirth, Dick-Read techniques gained in use and popularity around the country, especially among middle-class couples. Women read about it in their favorite magazines. A survey of seven women's magazines in this period identified growing interest in the subject of birth in *Redbook*, *Parents*, *Good Housekeeping*, *Ladies' Home Journal*, and *McCall's*, all widely read by white middle-class women.[88] The articles did not focus solely on the Dick-Read method, but as a result of increasing public notice, more and more women wanted to try to deliver their babies without medication. Many such women lived in communities where there were no doctors or nurses who had had experience with Dick-Read's relaxation techniques, but they nonetheless managed to accomplish Dick-Read-like deliveries without institutional support. Jan Ruby was one who did it this way, realizing that even without trained personnel, she was not alone. "There was my husband, sympathetic and convinced." She wrote in some detail about how they accomplished their goal in the absence of medical personnel trained in the method:

My husband was a wonderful help. He held my hand during the first stage contractions and warned me gently of any beginning tension in my fingers. His presence was a calm one and he was certain of success. That meant I couldn't let him down; and I didn't. He never squeezed my hand too tight nor did he talk to me except when I asked him to warn me of any signs of tension. His smile was enough. I knew he wasn't afraid for me because he realized I had the situation in control. . . . My husband had told them [the nurses] what I was doing when a contraction began and I went limp—and they cooperated by not talking to me at that time.[89]

A writer in *Better Homes and Gardens* focused particular attention on the husband: "For the first time, the husband has a real chance to help. Instead of being doomed to exclusion and frustration, to the pop-eyed, hand-wringing, corridor-walking role of the gags and jokes, he can now, in childbirth, as in other aspects of marriage, be a partner if he wishes to be." A man whose wife delivered at New Haven told the reporter, "Taking an active, informed part in labor is good for the soul—the husband's."[90]

One woman remembered that she did not like her labors in 1951 and 1952 when her husband was not permitted to be with her and she was "feeling very much alone having to lie there with my discomforts, only a nurse peeking in now and then and finding 'not yet.'" During one of her labors, she had to share a room with a woman who lost her baby, and that made her experience even more "unfortunate." She later wrote: "I do wish everyone in the northeastern U.S. then, and all over the country, could have had more options without being considered somewhat nutty. I feel sure that more fathers are happier now that it is more customary for them to have a larger role right from the start if they want it. . . . I would not want any prospective mother to feel as alone in her discomfort for even an hour or two as I did in Sept '51."[91]

Another woman publicized her delight with having her husband with her during labor. In a published "letter" to her childbirth instructor, she told how her husband timed her contractions in the labor room and "what a blessing it was to have my husband with me! . . . I didn't want him to hold my hand or touch me, but every few minutes I'd say 'Water,' or 'Draft—tuck in' or 'Bedpan' or 'Rub lower back,' . . . and he'd provide the requested relief—a godsend!"[92]

Those hospitals that continued to deny husbands entrance into labor rooms sometimes were able to incorporate nurses into more of a birth-partner role during the long hours of waiting with the birthing woman. Joan Ernst Wagner delivered her second baby (of eleven) in 1953 in Jonesboro, Arkansas, at St. Bernard's Hospital. Sister Florentine "sat with me herself and held my hand. She did not find it necessary to examine me at all, but just sat quietly beside me. . . . [She] took me to delivery room. . . . Lavern [husband, waiting outside] heard our baby girl's cry before the doctor arrived on the elevator. Sister had delivered her by herself."[93]

The best way to minimize the extra nursing time needed for women who were awake during labor, Thoms at Yale and others thought, was to train the expectant husbands in specifics about what they could do to help their wives. One frequent recommendation to fathers was to engage in vigorous back rubbing to ease the pressure.[94] The Yale staff believed that "husbands are the best back-rubbers in the world, bar none." As the *New York Times* reported, "By instinct, apparently, they know when their wives want a glass of water, the psychological moment to wash their faces or smooth their hair."[95]

Hazel Corbin was an early proponent of men attending their wives in labor. In an address to the Michigan Nursing Center Association in 1949, Corbin praised the Dick-Read method specifically, pointing out that before it was available a hospitalized woman "was even denied the solace of her husband's nearness during those hours of loneliness." She noted that Dick-Read's insistence that women in labor would relax more effectively with their husbands at their side had gained the men a role in the labor room.[96] By July 1950, a British surgeon and medical journal editor reported that "several American hospitals are experimenting along Dick Read lines. . . . They let young husbands stay with their wives until they go into the delivery room. . . . Devoted husbands are natural back-rubbers and feel much less like neglected spare parts hanging about dull waiting rooms."[97] One hospital that offered natural childbirth—on a voluntary basis—was Genesee Hospital in Rochester, New York. Noting the influence of the Dick-Read method and the Yale experience, an obstetrician reported that one year's experience demonstrated great public interest (29 percent of all deliveries) and commented on the ease with which men were incorporated into the labor-room experience. He thought the women were more satisfied, the duration of labor was reduced, and the babies were in better condition at birth.[98]

There was a huge emphasis on back-rubbing roles for men during labor during the 1950s. This practical suggestion gave men something specific to do: they could always try it if the situation seemed to be getting difficult.[99] But there was more than back rubbing to the growing interest in men attending their wives during labor. One obstetrician, for example, noted that prolonged labor "may be prevented by better personal care of the patient psychologically and emotionally." Another added that there was a lower rate of prolonged labors among private patients, implying that when women can have their husbands with them, labor can be shortened.[100] Birthing women felt support from their partners and coped better with their labors when the men were there. Not only did natural childbirth and men's participation begin to change the way women felt about their birth experiences in these midcentury years, but they also changed basic elements of what had been physician-directed and highly medicalized hospital deliveries and helped transform them into more consumer-directed and family-centered events.

Family Building

Accompanying their wives through labor was one concrete way men could increase their domestic function in the family, a subject of growing American cultural interest in the postwar period. As Elaine Tyler May has portrayed, the media in this period paid increasing attention to some domestic roles for men and to the importance of fathers playing an active role in children's upbringing. She noted a decade of movie and television interest in fatherhood as a "new badge of masculinity and meaning for the postwar man."[101] I Love Lucy addressed the situation of expectant fathers in 1953, as did the film Father's Little Dividend, starring Spencer Tracy and Elizabeth Taylor, released in 1951. Neither portrayed men accompanying their wives during labor, but Father's Little Dividend recognized the expectant father as a worrier.[102] Television and film portrayed an important family role for men.

Childbirth was an event and the labor room a place in which men could harness some of their anxieties about the world or their jobs and gain some control of their own family life. Nurse activist Hazel Corbin articulated this explicitly: "They are looking for security when they have their babies and they highly prize being together to share the great experience." She rued the separation of men and women during labor within this larger context and worked tirelessly to get hospitals to change their policies.[103] Addressing remarks to nurses, she wrote: "The hospitals which have permitted the husband to stay with his wife during labor . . . are finding that these procedures, unorthodox as they may seem, increase the emotional security of both husband and wife during this important event in their lives. . . . Doctors, nurses, and administrators are learning to adjust to the husband's active part in helping his wife relax in the labor room."[104] Vance Packard, too, speaking from the men's perspective, noted that previously "hospitals deprived the mother, in her moment of greatest need, of her main pillar of emotional support—her husband." In 1952, he celebrated the new childbirth methods on the grounds that "the step-by-step process of birth can be shared as a rich, family-welding experience."[105] Family togetherness could start in the labor room.

Religious hospitals, especially perhaps Catholic hospitals, seem to have played an important role in hastening the trend of men staying with their wives in labor. Although the data are not sufficiently complete to reveal the extent to which Catholic or other religious-based hospitals may have supported natural childbirth earlier or more enthusiastically than secular ones, their rhetoric of support for the family unit fits the family-friendly idea of keeping husband and wife together for this event. In 1950, an article in *Grail*, a Catholic magazine devoted to the idea "that God may be glorified in all things," lamented that young husbands are kept away from their wives when they were most needed. "During the hours of labor he sits helpless in the waiting room, weighted down by a very real sense of inadequacy. He is responsible for this baby. He should be by his wife. . . . He feels there must be some part in this for him. . . . He knows his wife needs him." The author continued, "In our Christian families the father is the head, he is the one who leads, supports, sustains. On this most important day his role does not change. . . . It is most necessary that on this day the parents be together. This is the day the mother most needs to know that her husband is by her side."[106] This theme of family building was very strong among those focusing on fathers' roles because of Christian teachings about men's responsibilities as head of the household. The same author pointed out that young men returning from war cannot be told that there is something that they cannot do. She continued that they needed to be able to carry out their domestic responsibility as husbands: "Now more than ever the mother needs him by her side to sustain, to encourage, to support her through this day of labor. . . . If under the stress of labor she forgets her part, there is no one who can help her back to her role better than her husband. If decisions are to be made she rests confident and secure in the knowledge that they can make them together. And as the head of the family the husband takes his responsibility gladly."[107]

A pamphlet published by Ave Maria Press and distributed through Catholic churches in the early 1950s quoted at length from a woman who had recently given birth. Her story put natural childbirth together with the Catholic emphasis on the man's role in the family: "I cannot over emphasize the role of my husband. I believe I would have broken down in some way if it hadn't been for him. He had read the parts of Dr. Read's book pertinent to his role and was reading it while I was in labor. He was calm throughout. He gave me hope and encouragement and helped me to relax and breathe properly. I felt lost whenever he left the room. . . . We both feel that this sharing of the childbirth experience is of very great importance to married life."[108]

The theme of building families was evident in secular as well as religious utterances. Including the father in order to strengthen family bonds and create meaningful experiences for both man and woman became a mantra at midcentury, and it was often associated with the Dick-Read technique. One author wrote, "The trained husband is the very best companion for a woman in labor. . . . The appreciation of these men at being included in the 'team' is beautiful to see. Going through labor together seems to made [sic] the whole affair more significant and satisfying to them both."[109] Mabel Fitzhugh wrote in the widely read magazine *My Baby*: "Unfortunately, there are still hospitals where the husband is not allowed to stay with his wife during the first stage of her labor. If people only knew what it might mean to parents, and perhaps to their children as well, to go through this most meaningful time together, working as a team, they would bring enough pressure to bear to make the practice universal. . . . His patient, calm understanding of what is happening to her is bound to produce a strong bond between them."[110] "Mrs. O. E." articulated the importance of having her husband with her during labor this way: "My husband and I shared the whole experience of pregnancy and labor together every step of the way. Somehow this has deepened our relationship and added to our sense of partnership."[111] In Seattle a man said, "It was the best thing we ever did together!" and a new mother exclaimed: "I felt we had . . . shared in a miracle."[112]

Interest in moving fathers into labor rooms in the decade of the 1950s to enhance family building succeeded in changing advice provided in obstetrics textbooks for nurses, one indication of the practice becoming more widely institutionalized. Whereas Joseph DeLee's textbook had advised including fathers as little as possible in the 1930s and 1940s, its new authors changed the rhetoric in the 1951 edition. Edward Davis and Mabel Carmon wrote: "Today we think of maternity as a family affair so the husband should be greeted and treated with the same courtesy as the expectant mother. He should be informed about the preparation that will be necessary for his wife, approximately how long these preparations will take, and then shown where he can wait." They advised that husbands can be helpful in timing contractions during labor if nurses are not available and if they have attended prenatal classes and "have an intelligent understanding of the progress of labor."[113] In the 1957 edition, Davis and Catherine Sheckler advised admitting the husband to the labor room immediately, and wrote: "The husband is more secure at the bedside of his wife when he is able to give encouragement and to offer physical support by way of back rubbing. It is very important for a woman in labor to have someone with her as much as possible in order to prevent loneliness. The nurse should recognize her great responsibility not only to care for the patient, but also to assist the husband in feeling a part of the experience. . . . The expectant father can be of great help to his wife provided the labor room staff makes him feel welcome." But, the authors cautioned, "when the nurse senses mounting anxiety in the husband, she can suggest that he go out to the fathers' waiting room for a cigarette. While his wife is attended by another nurse, she can talk with him, reviewing the patient's progress and offering the reassurance that enables him to resume his role at his wife's bedside with renewed confidence."[114]

This textbook and others like it for doctors and nurses put their advice in terms of the family's development, not just as a way to manage labor. "When he takes part in his wife's labor and feels involved in the birth of the baby, he is more likely to assume readily his role of parent and to derive a sense of fulfillment from it."[115] In Seattle, some physicians argued that "family centered" obstetrical care could strengthen "the moral fiber of their family unit." Letting the husband accompany his wife through labor was good for man and woman: "To the husband it results in an understanding of what the wife goes through, it increases respect and love for the wife. To the wife, having the husband present is a great comfort and gives her moral support."[116]

The Maternity Hospital in Minneapolis recognized the importance of allowing fathers to attend during labor. In 1953 a city newspaper published a story on changing practices. "The super-'scientific' techniques of not so long ago found no use for [the husband]; he was often treated as a sort of inconvenient accessory after the fact, and supercilious people in white shut him well away from the secret mysteries of birth," the reporter wrote. But now, in the Maternity Hospital "husbands are welcome. A man is beamed upon by the staff if he rubs his laboring wife's back."[117]

Many women who were alone in labor when they had their first baby and then had succeeding babies with their husband's help gushed about the transformation. Helen Glixon, for example, in order to see her husband during labor, had to visit him in the fathers' waiting room during her 1952 labor in Allentown, Pennsylvania, but in 1955 she labored at Columbia Presbyterian Hospital in New York City, where maternity policy had become more flexible. She wrote, "This time the entire experience was flawless—even to the extent that David was permitted to be with me in the labor room."[118]

In Clintonville, Wisconsin, the municipal hospital allowed the father to be in the labor room with his wife as long as he washed his hands and wore a "surgeon's gown." The hospital's reasoning fit the pattern becoming more common in the decade: "The father is an important member of the family and many of them want to give their wives the feeling of companionship, which only he can give."[119] An obstetrician told his colleagues that in such cases "the father [is] a member of the team. He must be made to feel welcome and important in his role. . . . [He] will often be most helpful in interpreting his wife's needs, and is most useful in a wife-supporting role, even though he but rubs her back, or fills her time with interesting and amusing projects and conversation."[120] Ideas about family togetherness promoted men's active role during labor.

A story in *Life* magazine in 1955 touted a combination of Dick-Read-method deep breathing and continuous caudal anesthesia and revealed that by mid-decade in Seattle women had considerable choices in their labors and deliveries. The story followed the birth experience of John and Mary Stouffer at Seattle's Virginia Mason Hospital. The reporter said that this hospital had allowed some husbands to accompany their wives in labor since 1949 because modern birth methods kept women conscious and wanting their husbands to "share the deep experience." Some physicians, the reported noted, "warn that the practice is unsanitary and that the sight of birth may upset fathers and harm marriages." But couples appreciated the experience together, and many came back to the hospital for succeeding deliveries. A photograph accompanying the story carried this caption: "IN THE LABOR ROOM John gives Mary lighted cigaret. He stayed with her during [her] nine-hour labor, reminding her to 'breathe deep, right down to your toes.'" When Mary received a caudal injection, John dozed next door.[121]

A California conference of health care providers and public health officials in 1955 revealed that significant differences of opinion on the matter of men's attendance at labor still existed. The majority of conference attendees agreed that "the husband should not be excluded from the labor room," but many believed that "better care can be given if the husband is not in the room." Those who thought the men should be allowed into labor rooms added the caveat "if they serve a useful purpose and propriety can be maintained." Dr. Edmund W. Overstreet from Stanford University observed, "There are hazards, other than infection, of the visitor in the labor room. . . . One hazard is the patient who puts on a 'show' for her husband, is uncooperative when he is present, and cooperative when

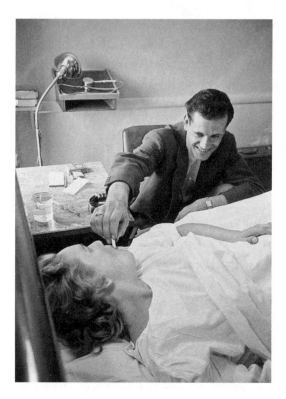

John and Mary Stouffer share time and a cigarette during labor at Virginia Mason Hospital, Seattle. "A Father Sees His Child Born," *Life*, June 13, 1955, 134. Photograph by Burton Glinn. Burton Glinn/ Magnum Photos.

he is not present." Chester L. Cooley, an obstetrician who practiced in San Francisco, agreed: "Certainly anyone who has been able to observe a large number of patients where no one is allowed, knows that the patient gets along better and has more confidence in her nurse; while where the husband is allowed, about every two minutes the husband comes out and grabs the nurse because he thinks the baby is coming."[122] Another constraint, many participants pointed out, related to hospital spaces. Many hospitals did not have private rooms for all patients in labor, and this physical fact limited fathers' participation. Despite these concerns, most conference participants agreed that many women in labor would benefit from the company of their spouses.

Around the country and increasing in availability and access, hospitals in the 1950s began changing their policies to allow men to accompany their wives in labor. Partners other than husbands were usually not (as far as I have been able to determine) included in these changes, and the rationale often stated was a traditional nuclear-family-centered one: sharing the experience could strengthen family bonds, connecting husband, wife, and child in a tighter union. (Some hospitals did allow "any other relative" of the woman's designation to attend if the husband was not available.)[123] By the mid-1950s, many couples, especially white, middle-class married couples and those with access to private rooms, could, if they so chose, experience labor together.

Pressures that led to men's initial steps out of waiting rooms and into labor rooms often came from the birthing women themselves and emanated frequently from those who wanted a less medicated natural childbirth. Togetherness in labor fit into a larger social pattern supporting and giving value to nuclear families, a trend that was particularly strong in the 1950s. Physicians such as Herbert Thoms at Yale, who came to believe in the efficacy and desirability of the Dick-Read method, supported the changes. Individual men—because they were impelled by their lonely, anxious time in hospital waiting rooms or convinced by their wives' needs—joined the movement and ultimately became its most ardent voices. The men wanted to be there to support their wives, and the women wanted the men's support. Both believed they could improve the childbirth experience and cement the family. Although initially these changes did not seem particularly radical, it was difficult for hospitals to accommodate the laymen, and the changes were achieved only slowly over time. Ultimately they did dramatically change childbirth practices. Men's initial forays into hospital labor rooms gave them more confidence and suggested specific roles to help their wives through the difficult hours. The changes accelerated in the 1950s, but not until later decades did men in labor rooms come to define the typical American hospital experience and significantly topple previous patterns of practice.

4 * HE WANTS TO KNOW

Prenatal Education for Fathers

Prenatal classes for pregnant women and their husbands — some developing as early as the 1930s but growing exponentially in the 1950s and 1960s — educated both parents for the experience of being together during labor. Hospitals frequently made these classes a prerequisite for the laymen to be permitted to pass through the doors from the public corridor of the fathers' waiting rooms into the labor corridor and, later, into delivery rooms. The classes opened new spaces in which the men could share experiences and feelings with one another as well as with their wives. In the classroom the male bonding that had occurred within the waiting rooms and through the fathers' books continued to sustain the men at the same time that the couples prepared themselves for a new level of intimacy and connection. Because most of the men who stayed with their wives in labor had gone through some prenatal education, we interrupt the labor-room narrative and turn in this chapter to the classes and how they developed.

Childbirth educators and hospitals offered the classes as a way to prepare first the expectant mothers and then the fathers-to-be for their roles during labor and delivery and also to teach tasks of infant feeding and bathing and encourage the men to be active in early childcare. Especially during the post–World War II years, the classes worked well within common cultural ideas about masculinity and men's role as head of the household and protector of the family. Educators taught basic knowledge and some practical skills, but they rarely, when including men in the classes, asked them to move very far from traditional gender roles. The classes were meant to expand men's domestic roles and connect them more closely to their families by engaging them actively in the birth processes and some infant care while still honoring their traditional role in the family. For the most part, prenatal educators discouraged challenges to hospital practices and did not intend to defy physician authority or confront medical hierarchies. Nonetheless, the classes empowered their men and women graduates to dispute hospital policies that excluded the men and act in ways that ultimately led to significant changes in labor and delivery routines across the country. They contributed, too, to a change in men's roles within their families.

In the early 1950s Vance Packard, a familiar Associated Press reporter and staff writer at *American Magazine* (and soon to be popular author of *The Hidden Persuaders*), helped to accelerate Americans' interest in prenatal classes. In the pages of *American Magazine*, Packard followed one couple, Ensign and Mrs. Bang, through their birth experience. He lauded the changes that allowed "a new method of training" that could lead couples to a satisfying and rewarding shared experience. Noting his own "frustrating and painful" time in the 1940s when he knew little about labor and delivery and had been "shunted into a darkened hospital waiting room," Packard celebrated that couples could now be prepared for the event and go through labor together:

> Ensign and Mrs. Bang's secret, we now know, was that together they had been rehearsing and preparing themselves carefully for this important event over a period of several months. . . . While the mother is training for parenthood, the father can be training too. . . . Until recent years we husbands were the forgotten men of pregnancy. This . . . deprived our wives of emotional support [and] it frustrated the

husband. . . . Ensign Bang went with his wife to the final sessions of her course covering the "rehearsal for childbirth." Together they saw demonstrated for them step by step just what would happen from the moment Mrs. Bang and the other members of the class felt the first twinge of contraction. Through a series of life-sized sculptures, they saw just how the baby would make its exit. And they learned, in a free-for-all discussion[,] just what they both could do to help the process along.[1]

Because Bang had attended the classes, the hospital and physician permitted him to remain at his wife's side during the whole of labor, during which, Packard noted, he "spent so many hours rubbing Mrs. Bang's back during her labor that he had a severe arm ache the next day!"[2] One vivid section of Packard's article retold a favorite story of the teacher of the class he had followed when researching the article: "Miss Janeway likes to tell her classes . . . of a couple who were sleeping curled up together. The wife's abdomen was against her husband's back. He woke up feeling a strange commotion behind him. But his wife continued sleeping. So he began watching the luminous dial of his wrist watch. When he established, after an hour of clocking, that contractions were coming regularly every 20 minutes and lasting about 30 seconds, he shook his wife and said: 'Wake up, honey, you're in labor.'"[3] Through these classes men learned to recognize the onset of labor, perhaps even before the laboring woman herself.

Early Classes

This new mid-twentieth-century era in pregnancy and childbirth, when the man could inform the woman of her own labor status instead of the other way around, began formally in New York City in the 1930s. Very few men were involved in prenatal classes in this early period; nonetheless, it is important to understand that a small number of pioneers set the stage for more men to become involved later on. Health expert and nurse Hazel Corbin, head of the Maternity Center Association of New York, worked to make the hospital birth experience more family friendly and encouraged men to take an active role in their wives' labor and delivery. The Maternity Center published a handbook for "pregnant mothers and expectant fathers" in 1932 and ran classes for the men, which were intended, in the words of historian Laura E. Ettinger, who has studied them most closely, to change men from being a "fifth wheel" during the months of pregnancy and during childbirth and instead "allow men to feel once again in charge of their families."[4]

Ettinger's study emphasized the traditional masculine roles encouraged in these early classes for fathers-to-be and also noted that the classes further reinforced a growing trend in the United States to rely on the physician expert to know what to do: "They encouraged men to push women to go to physicians during the prenatal, labor and delivery, and postpartum periods."[5] Corbin created a mock degree for the men who took the Maternity Center classes: "P.P."—Prepared Papa. The men who earned this "degree" had the responsibility to find good physicians for their wives and then pay particular attention to and obey the doctor's directions. They were taught to sit calmly in the waiting room and not worry as unprepared fathers might because their education helped them develop confidence in the doctor and hospital.[6] In those early years Corbin did not encourage the men to tear down barriers and try to be with their wives in the labor room. The Maternity Center classes were not radical in this sense. Nonetheless, these classes and others like them gave men and women information that they could not otherwise easily access, and this information along with their own experiences led men to seek significant changes in hospital procedures.

In Wisconsin, the state health department's Bureau of Maternal and Child Health instituted some prenatal education for women in the late 1930s. A public health nurse traveled the state and held informal discussion groups for mothers. The bureau stopped the service during the war, but restarted the classes in 1945.[7] The women appreciated the information provided by the nurse and requested that their husbands be included in some of the sessions.[8]

With a brief hiatus during World War II, hospitals in locations around the country began to advertise classes for expectant parents. In New Haven, a "Fathers' Council" was available to explain to men what to expect. In 1945 hospitals in Pittsburgh, Washington, D.C., and Los Angeles launched classes. In Flint, Michigan, classes began, and in Cleveland, Ohio, a "Men's Forum" educated fathers-to-be before the war and started up again after it. The Chicago Lying-In Hospital launched fathers' classes in 1949; in that year 154 men enrolled. In 1955, the hospital provided recognition to the men by presenting them with a wallet-size certificate.[9] Hospital maternity staffs noted that men returning from the war seemed particularly eager to participate. *Good Housekeeping*, which chronicled some of these postwar programs, noted that paternity had been "unhonored, unsung, even unrecognized" but that passing out cigars was no longer appealing as men's sole activity in birth practices.[10] Classes could help men break out of their customary disconnected role and participate more fully in the process. Classes run by the public health nurses in Wisconsin followed the Yale model.[11] The nurses made special efforts to attract the fathers to prenatal classes in rural parts of the state among ethnic Russians, Poles, Swedes, and Norwegians.[12] Men educated in such classes remained a minority of all new fathers-to-be.

Often nurses taught the women in prenatal classes and physicians taught the men. At a national 1950 conference of maternal and child health and hospital consultant nurses convened in Chicago, prenatal classes for fathers received much attention. One nurse noted there was wide interest among the men and that "it has been found that fathers' classes can be larger than mothers' classes." Nurses found that the men were eager to attend such classes and asked a lot of questions, unlike their wives, who were often quiet and "ashamed if they don't know everything." Some of the female nurses did not feel comfortable teaching the men even though they believed that, as one of them put it, "as a rule, physicians do not make good teachers for parents' classes as they are likely to stress pathology." The conference attendees reported a great deal of variety in classes around the country, but there seemed to be agreement that a good classroom teacher would be well trained: "She must be understanding and sympathetic, must have a sense of humor, must be enthusiastic and interested, must have a democratic approach and should not inject personal opinions."[13]

In San Luis Obispo, California, the local health department conducted prenatal classes in the postwar period, holding classes for women in the afternoons and classes for both parents in the evenings. The San Luis Obispo classes were modeled on the Fathers' Council in New Haven and included the use of lantern slides: "In the beginning the fathers were invited to those lectures given by physicians, but they now want to attend the ones given by the nurse. Their evident interest in the whole series shows that such a program should be planned to include them. The fathers have comprised fully 30 percent of the total attendance."[14]

The postwar curriculum in San Luis Obispo spanned ten classes: (1) anatomy and physiology of pregnancy (nurse); (2) hygiene of pregnancy (nurse); (3) nutrition (nurse); (4) labor and delivery (private physician); (5) layette and baby things (nurse); (6) aftercare of mother (nurse); (7) demonstration of baby bath (nurse); (8) care of the infant (health officer); (9) first year of life (health officer); (10) child from one to three years of age (health officer).[15] The classes included straightforward information, illustrated with diagrams, and some hands-on practice with a doll to learn how to take care of a baby. The Visiting Nurse Association in New York similarly began including fathers in the prenatal classes it led because "so many husbands wanted it." The classes taught that men should give their wives "sustaining affection" throughout the months of pregnancy and emphasized postdelivery work for the men, concluding that "baby care is best when it is given by both parents."[16] "Bringing up baby is Dad's job, too," agreed one graduate of the Maternity Center class in 1948, but, an observer noted, the men "want it clearly understood that they have no intention of taking Mother's place."[17]

At the Maternity Center classes for fathers in the 1940s, "students meet once a week, relax during the two-hour session in comfortable chairs in a spacious, attractive room." One lecturer, a physician and new father himself, noted that "men are much more interested in the scientific aspects of growth than women. They have so many questions to ask at the end of a talk that we sometimes have to turn out the lights in order to get them to leave."[18] Yale's Grace–New Haven Hospital offered two classes for the men alone and two more that they could attend with their wives: "The talks to husbands alone are concerned with pregnancy and labor, and are given by an obstetrician."[19] Herbert Thoms remembered that, soon after the demonstration childbirth program in the Dick-Read method began in New Haven, "it was sensed that expectant fathers as well as mothers were interested in learning more about the anticipated experience. As a result, evening classes for husbands and wives together were started."[20]

By the end of the 1940s, only 10 percent of the still small numbers of expectant parents who came to classes came because their physicians had recommended it. Some physicians might have feared that classes would lead parents to challenge medical decision-making authority, and indeed in that decade the recommendation for prenatal education included that "parents' classes should carefully outline the standards of good obstetric care so that expectant mothers and fathers are in a position to judge in a broad sort of way the medical, nursing and hospital care in their communities and thus be enabled to select that which will provide them with the highest standards of care."[21] Despite physicians' slow acceptance, prenatal classes were increasing. At a 1951 workshop on parent education, childbirth instructors provided advice about the fathers' education in such classes: "Be gentle and thorough in preparing the fathers for parenthood. . . . He wants to know . . . what is involved in labor and delivery, . . . so he won't be so frightened."[22] Women were pleased when their husbands attended classes.[23]

Nurses, too, came to find satisfaction in teaching both men and women in prenatal classes. One noted, "Some of my most satisfactory experiences have been when I could serve both the expectant mother and father. They seem to gain support from each other and the fathers are much less reluctant to ask questions. They also are more realistic about the practical aspects of planning for equipment needed and so on."[24] Other nurses continued to worry that men's presence in class would inhibit the women from speaking out. "Miss Millington said that she felt the presence of the fathers . . . stopped the group discussion."[25] Although practices differed around the country and men did not always have access to the classes, prenatal education thrived and was especially popular among white-collar parents-to-be.[26]

One important reason for the expansion of childbirth education was postwar funding policy for armed services personnel. The army agreed to pay for maternity care for female veterans and male veterans' wives only if

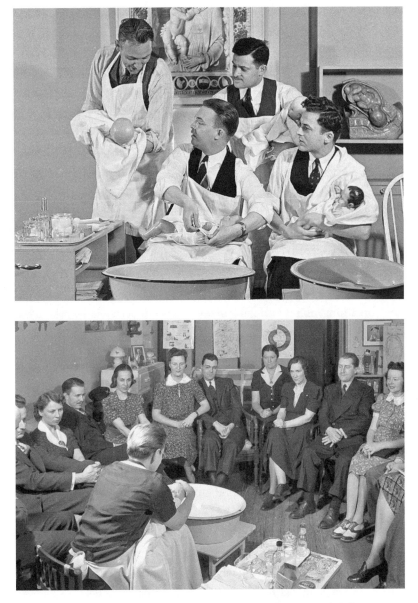

TOP Fathers-to-be learn how to bathe a baby as they practice with dolls in a prenatal class in a New York City suburb in the 1940s. © Lucien Aigner/CORBIS. BOTTOM Parents attend class together, watching the nurse demonstrate a baby's bath. Photograph by Percy Byron. Courtesy of Medical Center Archives of NewYork-Presbyterian/Weill Cornell.

the women delivered in the hospital. This policy encouraged people who might otherwise have continued to give birth at home to go instead into institutions. To the extent that prenatal classes were run by the hospitals or public health departments, and many of the earlier ones were, the women became exposed to this education. In such hospital-based classes, instruction often prepared women (and sometimes men) for the kind of obstetrical care they would receive in that hospital, rather than offering a more general course in available birth alternatives.[27] Most fathers-to-be, even if educated and middle class, remained relatively uninformed about what happened during labor and delivery until after midcentury.

Natural Childbirth Classes

The method championed by Grantly Dick-Read in the 1940s and 1950s to reduce the fear associated with childbirth — which included relaxation, deep breathing, and minimizing medications — played a large role in the emergence of new ideas and practices regarding men's presence in American hospital labor rooms. The Dick-Read teachings simultaneously were probably the single most important impetus leading to a proliferation of prenatal classes around the country at midcentury. As physicians learned of the method — especially from those involved in the Grace–New Haven Hospital demonstration project — they realized that their patients needed training to benefit most fully from the technique. Dr. Blackwell Sawyer, for example, who delivered babies in a small hospital in Lakewood, New Jersey, decided to give the method a try in his own practice after reading Dick-Read's book. Sawyer did not limit his prenatal education to the mothers: "Husbands have, in their anxiety, helped to instill terror in their wives. So when Sawyer patients come for prenatal instruction, they bring their husbands. And when the time comes for trundling wifey off to the hospital, the husband, anxietyless himself, adds to his wife's confidence."[28]

Hazel Corbin believed, too, that childbirth education often went hand in hand with interest in natural childbirth. She told a nurses' group that "the mother and father who learn together how naturally a baby is conceived, develops, and is born accept childbearing as a natural bodily function. To such informed parents it will seem common sense to expect their baby to be born by similarly natural processes."[29] And indeed, education in natural childbirth methods increased significantly after Dick-Read's visit to the United States in 1947.

Novelist Sloan Wilson (*The Man in the Gray Flannel Suit*) and his first wife had four children (one of whom died at birth) in the 1940s and 1950s. He wrote of these four deliveries: "On the advice of our suburban obstetricians, I had taken my wife to the hospital, paced the corridors in the time honored way, [and] accepted the news of birth with joy." But when his second wife got pregnant, his friends recommended natural childbirth, and Wilson cleared it ahead of time with his wife's doctor: "I didn't want to argue with my obstetrician in hospital corridors while my wife was in labor." The doctor agreed to let them try, although he did caution, "I just don't want you to think that childbirth is always as easy as natural childbirth enthusiasts sometimes paint it." With that caveat, Wilson and his wife attended classes and practiced Dick-Read relaxation techniques at home, and he was permitted to be with her during much of labor. But when his wife experienced a prolonged and difficult labor, Wilson left the labor room to the professional staff and concluded that "the abilities of a good doctor" were greatly appreciated. The classes had allowed the couple to be together for much of the time and helped them cope with the event and also kept Wilson's high regard for physicians intact.[30]

In many cases, women themselves first learned of Dick-Read methods, and in the absence of physicians able or willing to conduct classes in the techniques, they started their own. "Ann Onymous" described an informal society, of which she was a member, that started its own pre-natal classes. "We know that eventually the doctors will start their own pre-natal classes," she wrote, "but in the absence . . . we are doing what we can."[31] And British obstetrician Harvey Graham observed in 1950 that indeed Dick-Read classes were growing in America: "Several American hospitals are experimenting along Dick Read lines. They are also getting young fathers to attend the antenatal explanatory lectures." This, he pointed out, led the way for fathers to stay with their wives in labor.[32]

Writing in the popular *Better Homes and Gardens*, Lawrence Galton emphasized how much the Dick-Read method was changing the American birth experience. He began by describing a typical hospital experience at midcentury, which is worth reviewing in this context:

> Let's see what goes on in most hospitals today when a woman in active labor is admitted. After the customary examination and preparation for delivery, she's given a capsule of a barbiturate so she can relax and fall asleep while still in the early first stage. Later, as contractions become harder and more frequent and the cervix dilates increasingly, she may wake up, be given an injection of dermerol [sic], an analgesic, plus the amnesiac hyoscine, and she's off to sleep again. A few hours later, she'll wake up again because of the severity of contractions. Now, with the cervix fully dilated . . . [she] bear[s] down with abdominal muscles. Then, toward the end of the second stage, she gets an anesthetic, usually an inhalant like nitrous-oxide-and-oxygen, which puts her under until her baby is delivered.[33]

A nurse remembered, too, that in her hospital in the mid-1950s, women were "totally medicated during labor and delivery."[34] Another nurse confirmed that in the 1950s at University Hospital in Madison, Wisconsin, "from the time the patient started . . . dilating they were pretty well sedated . . . until the time of delivery and even after delivery because we were using nitrous in the delivery room."[35] Galton wrote how much Dick-Read techniques were altering this kind of medicated experience, using Grace–New Haven as his point of reference. "Expectant fathers . . . attend classes, learn the physical facts of labor and not only what to expect, but what they can do." Attending the classes allowed the men to stay with their wives during labor, during which they became active members of the birth team.[36] Their wives typically had fewer or smaller doses of analgesics and anesthetics and were awake to appreciate and endure the experience. As one woman told Galton, "It was a spiritual experience for me. I'm sure that those present and fully conscious in any birth room would admit that the presence of a Supreme Being is realized."[37] Dick-Read himself acknowledged that "childbirth is a demonstration of the incomparable genius of a Creative Force," but his method did not rest on religious belief, and, indeed, he strove to argue his perspective in secular scientific terms.[38] The prenatal classes paved the way for such enhanced birth experiences.

Natural childbirth remained controversial during the 1950s and 1960s, but even so, many physicians came to appreciate the Dick-Read method and later Lamaze techniques and saw that the father can be "an enormous help to his wife at many points" and that "he needs to learn the facts of parenthood right along with his wife."[39] The editor of the *American Journal of Obstetrics and Gynecology*, George W. Kosmak, noted a growing demand for parents' classes in 1952 when he encouraged his fellow obstetricians: "The doctors who have sent their patients to good classes have found that their mothers are better patients and that the husbands are more understanding and cooperative. There is also less fear and tension when labor begins and both mothers and fathers approach labor with a sense of balance and security."[40]

It is impossible to determine with any precision how many physicians and hospitals in American communities offered prenatal classes for prospective parents at midcentury or to know how many of those included the men. But it is clear that by the 1950s these classes had a loyal following around the country. An article first published in the widely read magazine *My Baby* noted: "The intense interest of fathers-to-be is one of the outstanding features of a preparatory class for mothers. They say, 'It all makes sense now,' after the meeting when they are shown the Birth Atlas and the mystery of the process is taken away. The men especially enjoy knowing how the muscles do the work. Their own responsibility as coach is explained, and their duties during labor are outlined."[41]

In this midcentury period, as prenatal classes were becoming widely available to middle-class parents, a great many men and women who were less privileged still had no access to such birth preparation or to natural childbirth. Louise Zabriskie, author of a popular nursing textbook, noted that classes and preparation for childbirth in general remained class-specific in the country during these years. Even in 1966, she thought that the "majority of women who come from the disadvantaged, low-income families" did not yet have access to prenatal education.[42]

Nurses and laywomen's organizations often stepped into the breach when hospitals or physicians did not provide classes. The Visiting Nurse Association of Brooklyn and the Queens Education for Childbirth Center in New York began their own weekly classes in 1956.[43] In Milwaukee a group of mothers who had read about the Dick-Read method and the experiences at Yale organized to provide natural childbirth opportunities and prenatal education for it in the city. They founded the Natural Childbirth Association of Milwaukee and held meetings twice a month, including the husbands.

> As a regular feature of each meeting, a mother related her experiences with natural childbirth. She would describe her thoughts and feelings during labor, the things which helped, and the periods that were most difficult. The comment repeated most frequently was that the hardest thing to endure during labor is the loneliness. Ideally the husband should be the one to provide moral support, but since husbands are not allowed to be with their wives in most Milwaukee hospitals, and frequently nurses cannot stay with a woman during her entire labor, we decided to try to provide a private duty nurse for those mothers who wished to have one.[44]

The Milwaukee group was innovative in two ways. First, its idea of hiring nurses to provide labor coaching for natural childbirth—as far as I can determine—was not systematically followed elsewhere in the country in the 1950s. Second, the parents who took the prenatal classes did more than educate themselves. They became activists in changing hospital procedures. This program led to expanded childbirth education classes, which in turn led Columbia Hospital and St. Michael Hospital to provide labor rooms where the woman trying the Dick-Read method could be separated from other laboring women and have her husband with her.[45]

With all this activity supporting natural childbirth and the rapid development of childbirth education classes in the 1950s, it is important to remember that the nation's hospitals and physicians were still much divided about the value of such experiences. Many women continued to want to labor and deliver with the help only of nurses and doctors and were happy for their husbands to go home or sit in the waiting room. Many physicians still had no experience in the natural childbirth methods and also remained skeptical that including husbands in prenatal classes or in the labor room had any value. Even in those instances in which doctors or hospitals provided opportunities for couples to pursue natural childbirth, "some patients preferred to be left with their obstetrician and nurse and had their husbands wait at home."[46] Nonetheless, the natural childbirth phenomenon spread, and with it spread prenatal education, which led to men's increased participation in their wives' labor.

In North Carolina, Asheville's two hospitals cooperated in developing an educational program for men and women that had been started by a nurse. Doctors originally had doubts about the necessity for the classes but became "unanimous in their enthusiasm." The fathers, too, appreciated the classes, and many of the ones who missed a class would make an effort to make it up later. Of the classes, one physician joked, "We know this plan is working. We've never lost a father yet."[47]

In 1957 Horace Harding Hospital in Queens, New York, started an eight-session course for both parents covering "physiology, development of the unborn baby, labor and care of the new baby, with special emphasis on exercises given in preparation for labor."[48] At another hospital, while women attended two classes during the day offered by a nurse, the physician presented two evening lectures attended by the couple together. The first of these "approached the psychological aspects of pregnancy and childbirth," and the second "emphasized the labor process and the hospital situation. . . . Things which the husband could do to support his wife during parturition were discussed."[49] By the end of the 1950s, the American College of Obstetricians and Gynecologists (ACOG) manual of standards for prenatal care included fathers' education and demonstrated widespread acceptance of the practice: "Fathers and Mothers Classes. A course of 4–6 one-hour conferences conducted by specially trained nurses and residents in large institutions under obstetric staff supervision has proved to be beneficial and popular. The purpose of such lectures is the dissemination of factual information and not the false promise of a discomfort-free pregnancy, labor, and delivery."[50] The standards did not have the force of law behind them, but they did influence many specialists. Despite its support of the basic concept of lay education, the ACOG revealed that it still had some ambivalence about drug-free methods with its use of the phrase "false promise," which seemed to be a negative taunt aimed at natural childbirth advocates.

Indeed, there was far from universal acceptance of natural childbirth methods or of prenatal education including husbands. A psychologist weighed in on the topic: "Because of the extreme detail in which the birth process should be learned, it is preferable that these classes be taught to mothers alone." In her estimation, men might be invited for "perhaps one or two sessions," but she did not go on to propose that such education could lead to a more active role in labor for the men.[51] Some hospitals held classes for mothers but excluded the men altogether: "We did not allow the husbands to attend any of the classes because we thought that our discussions could be more personal and intimate and with less embarrassment to the sensitive mothers if both sexes were not mixed."[52] Some programs, like the one at Mount Sinai Hospital's Klingenstein Maternity Pavilion in New York City, provided men's classes completely separate from the ones for women and emphasized formula preparation and baby bathing for them rather than information about labor and delivery.[53] The men-only classes provided opportunities for the expectant fathers to talk among themselves and get support for their activity.

Hospitals, health departments, and private organizations conducted increasing numbers of prenatal classes around the country. The *Ladies' Home Journal* publicized YWCA childbirth education classes in Seattle, Washington, in an article focused on the benefits of natural childbirth: the women "chatter about how interesting and how satisfying it was and how much they appreciated the presence and support of their husbands. Then men have plenty to say too—*they* did not pace the floor and chain smoke in the waiting room."[54]

A survey of fathers' participation in hospital childbirth and in prenatal classes around the country in 1973 provided the first national quantitative look at the practices and revealed significant regional variations. The study, sponsored by the International Childbirth Education Association (ICEA), along with a second one the organization conducted about men in delivery rooms, remains one of the few composite pictures of childbirth education and labor practices available for the period. The ICEA surveyed all hospitals listed in the 1972 edition of the American Hospital

Association Guide to hospitals that had maternity services. Asked if they offered prenatal classes, 53 percent of hospitals responded yes. Some of the women intending to deliver their babies in those hospitals might also have had access to privately sponsored classes. There were huge regional differences: in the East, 64 percent held classes; in the Midwest, 59 percent; in the West, 54 percent. In the South, however, only 28 percent of hospitals offered such education to their patients.[55] Since attendance at classes for the men opened the doors for them to be with their wives in labor, this survey provides important information about prenatal classes and also illuminates hospital maternity practices. Significant numbers of women and men in the United States did not yet have access to prenatal education and thus probably were not able to spend time together during the hours the woman labored in hospital-based childbirth. In the South, this characterized the large majority of couples.

Perhaps the best indicator of the popularity of prenatal natural childbirth classes comes from television shows, including one of the most popular in the 1970s and early 1980s, *Happy Days*. The show depicted the Cunningham family and especially teenage son Richie and his "greaser" friend Arthur Fonzarelli, known as the Fonz or Fonzie. The teenagers grew up, and Richie married and went off to the army, leaving his pregnant wife, Lori Beth. Lori Beth asked Fonzie to accompany her to prenatal classes (and later to the delivery room) in Richie's place. In the natural childbirth class, many wife-husband couples appear, including one African American couple, and most were excited to be sharing the experience. In contrast, Fonzie demonstrated his extreme discomfort. He wanted to be there in support of Lori Beth and for the sake of his friend, but when faced with what was actually going to be expected of him during labor and delivery, he balked:

NURSE-EDUCATOR: Now, as you know, natural childbirth is a way where the husband and wife, working as a team, use special breathing techniques to help in the birth of your baby. As you mothers and fathers, or coaches, will see in the delivery room.

FONZIE: Wait, wait, mayday, hold it! I don't know, first day [of class] and I don't want to overstep my bounds at all but I think you got

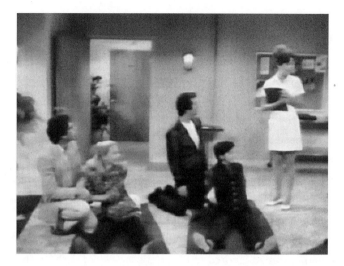

Fonzie attends natural childbirth class with Lori Beth, where he learns he is expected
to be with her all through labor and delivery. *Happy Days,* "Little Baby Cunningham,"
November 3, 1981. *Happy Days,* courtesy of CBS Paramount Network Television.

> that wrong there. When the fathers, or coaches, are in the
> *waiting room.*
>
> NURSE: No, the coaches are right there with the mother all
> throughout the labor and all throughout the delivery.
>
> FONZIE: Of the baby?!!
>
> NURSE: That's right.
>
> FONZIE (bends down to Lori Beth): Did you know about that?
>
> LORI BETH: Sure, Fonz, that's what natural childbirth is. Natural.
> What did you think it was?
>
> FONZIE: I thought it was natural childbirth. You're in the delivery
> room giving birth to the baby, I'm in the waiting room with a lot of
> other fathers and cigars. This is time-tested. I mean it worked for
> Adam and Eve, why fool around with it?

When the nurse-educator showed films of an actual birth to the class,
Fonzie, despite his efforts to stay cool, had to leave the room. Later, he
confided to a friend, "I didn't know I had to be *there.* I'm telling ya, this
natural childbirth thing is very unnatural."[56] Fonzie's discomfort gave a

humorous slant to the custom that had become, by the end of the 1970s, a common middle-class experience for fathers-to-be.

Responsible Fatherhood

Natural childbirth prenatal classes as well as those offered without promoting the drug-free methods often articulated that their main goals were to promote family togetherness and to define a role for the men that would help them develop their place as head of the family. As one writer put it: "Classes for fathers are springing up in many communities. . . . The men who attend are seriously concerned about their status in the family when the baby comes. . . . [The] father can regain his dignity in the family picture when a baby comes."[57] The classes were intended to make the men "fully able to relieve the doctor or nurses and assist their wife immeasurably in the labor room . . . working with her in this adventure rather than standing idly, nervously, and rejectedly by."[58]

Much of the impetus to greater inclusion of the men in prenatal classes came directly from the women and from their worries over being left alone during labor. One nurse wrote what she called a "bill of rights" for birthing women and declared the issues strongly. One of her provisions was the "right of every husband to be with his wife during labor." Author Mabel Fitzhugh believed that the men had to be trained in order to carry out a helping role for their laboring wives. Fitzhugh was most concerned that the birthing woman be able to have "her husband or someone with her who understands how to coach her during every contraction," and she left the door open for someone other than the woman's husband to be the helper. Yet the bill of rights itself mentioned only the husband's right to be there.[59] The inclusion of the husband spoke directly to a growing concern about the importance of shoring up the nuclear family. Men should be prepared to be there to help their wives through a difficult time, and in turn, their togetherness in labor would strengthen their future family life. In order to be together in labor, they needed to train together.

One obstetrician offered group counseling for expectant mothers and with the women probed some "attitudes of the husband during his wife's

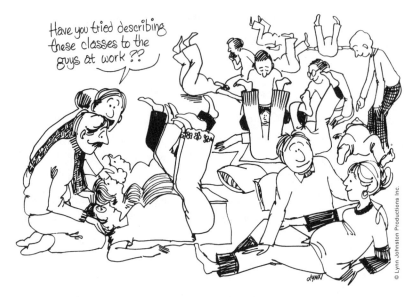

Cartoon of a natural childbirth class, illustrating how men bond in
mutual understanding in the classes. Lynn Johnston, *David,
We're Pregnant* (Minnetonka, Minn.: Meadowbrook Press, 1975), 62.
© Lynn Johnston Productions, Inc. Reprinted with permission.

pregnancy." This specialist pursued these questions "to help the women
understand that their husbands are also involved in their pregnancy and
childbirth, and to help them become better aware of the various feelings
men have toward pregnant wives and the meaning of parenthood to the
husband's way of life."[60]

Many writings about prenatal classes emphasized the connection
between the men's war experiences and responsible fatherhood. One
physician, for example, was happy to see that "young G.I. husbands are
proving to be earnest, interested, responsible fathers who take a develop-
mental attitude toward their children. . . . Classes for prospective fathers
are attended by many men whose babies represent a large investment of
time and interest even before they are born."[61] Encouragement to attend
classes often spread from prospective father to prospective father. Two
educators wrote that while some men were "rather shy about coming
to such a lecture [on prenatal care and delivery] . . . those who do come
. . . are very enthusiastic about the method." They overheard "husbands

talk[ing] to other men" about how helpful the classes were.[62] Prenatal classes provided one venue—along with the waiting room—where expectant fathers could meet and offer support to one another.

Articles in popular women's magazines helped to create a groundswell of interest in natural childbirth and in the prenatal classes that usually accompanied a hospital's adoption of the method. They emphasized preparing men for their future role as father. Dr. Milton Senn, for example, a physician practicing at Yale's Grace–New Haven Hospital, wrote in *Woman's Home Companion* how classes there helped men prepare: "They too will be instructed about pregnancy and childbirth so that a husband will know how he can best help his wife through this period. He will get some preparation too for his own important role as father of the family."[63] Many such articles highlighted how the classes could show the man how to provide help for his wife and prepare him for a fuller role in fatherhood after the baby arrived. This latter purpose, developing the man for his new role in the family, played heavily in a *Cosmopolitan* article. Author Jack Pollack wrote that the Medical Mission Sisters of Philadelphia practiced natural childbirth in their Santa Fe, New Mexico, hospital: "They prepare mothers and fathers for their roles in childbirth, thus establishing a sense of 'family' even before the child is born." Pollack quoted a new father, who summed up the meaning of natural childbirth and how much it worked to connect men to the pregnancy and childbirth experience when he wrote to the Maternity Center in New York. Identifying completely with his wife in the process (in a phrase that has since become quite common), he said, "We're pregnant."[64]

Birthing women experienced increased security when their husbands participated in classes and then during labor. One woman who attended classes with her husband at the Maternity Center in New York found that the classes were important for helping to create a "strong family unit, and the sharing of responsibility." In the 1953 article in which this woman's comment appeared, the author explained: "One of the most important factors in the sense of security this woman has developed has come from the knowledge that due to their training in natural childbirth, her husband will be allowed to be with her during most of the time she is in labor. His training has prepared him to take an active part at this crucial time, to offer support and comfort, to control the atmosphere around his wife during this critical period. . . . If both the parents had not received training the hospital would not allow them this experience."[65]

Prenatal education, although not available to all groups, spread throughout the nation by the 1950s. Nurse-midwife Alice Young Kohler, a Chinese American woman practicing in Hawaii, began classes modeled on the those of the Maternity Center and the American Red Cross class outlines that she "adapted to meet the specific needs and to fit into the cultural patterns of Hawaiian mothers." These classes did not necessarily explicitly connect to natural childbirth or family-centered maternity but had a more generalized parent education focus. Fathers wanted the education. Kohler opened the classes to the expectant fathers and found "the response was overwhelming—we had 54 registrations for this first evening class."[66]

The Chicago Lying-In Hospital, one of a few racially integrated institutions in that city, offered five two-hour classes in the evenings for fathers, black and white. *Ebony*—a magazine aimed at a middle-class African American audience—published a photo essay following John Moore, an electrical engineer, as he and fifty other prospective fathers "learned as much as any layman can about the physiology and psychology of childbearing and the techniques of child care." Moore, like so many other Chicago fathers of the same period, wanted a boy "so he can grow up to be a football player." The article did not reveal whether attending the prenatal classes gave Moore the ability to be with his wife during labor.[67]

Men played a leading role in encouraging greater participation from other men. William Genne, for example, wrote a popular handbook for fathers in which he addressed what he believed was one of men's greatest concerns. Genne explicitly argued that activities that traditionally were totally within women's sphere could be relevant and important for men. He insisted that the relaxation techniques associated with the Dick-Read method did not challenge men's masculinity and in fact would benefit the men as well as their expectant wives: "This is exactly the same kind of training the armed services used with pilots during the war. When they became tense after combat, physical therapists taught them exactly these same muscle exercises. Many husbands have been amazed at how it releases their own tensions and helps them to sleep better."[68] Genne urged the men to learn about their own hospital's policies regarding attendance during labor and to prepare themselves thoroughly for the experience: "A husband who has prepared himself to understand childbirth and to help his wife during labor is far different from the usual caricature of the waiting husband pacing the floor and strewing cigarettes all around." He exhorted his male readers, "Take advantages of the classes, conferences, and other educational services which many hospitals are now offering to wives and also to husbands in some cases."[69]

A story told by a nurse provides a concrete example of the need for men's prenatal education and some insight into what men knew and did not know about the labor and delivery process: "His wife just had her baby and he couldn't figure out why she wasn't through already, and I said, 'Well, you know,' I said, 'You know she had to have, the doctor had to do an episiotomy. He had to cut her bottom between the rectum and the vagina to make room for the baby. So she wouldn't tear.' And big tears streamed down his face. 'They cut my wife!' . . . He should know what's going on. . . . I can remember him crying just as plain as day."[70] Prenatal education, including information about the episiotomy, a common procedure in hospital obstetrics at that time, would have helped the situation and eased the man's concerns.

Prenatal education in the 1960s expanded rapidly—along with the women's movement, which championed women's control of the experience, and the growth of childbirth education organizations that emphasized family-friendly maternity care. Increasing numbers of young parents actively sought out hospitals where the father-to-be could be included in labor and physicians who were friendly to the idea. "Attendance at the lectures," wrote one obstetrician, "gave the husband a chance to enter more actively into the part of becoming a parent, since they enabled him to coach his wife in doing the exercises as well as to help her to carry out other instructions." They helped to calm his fears "just at the time that his wife needed someone who was not extremely apprehensive. The floor-pacing father is no longer a part of the labor-room scene."[71] The International Childbirth Education Association fostered this "family-centered childbirth" and worked to promote prenatal education that would lead to men's active participation in labor.

By the 1960s the Dick-Read method was no longer the only impetus to including men in prenatal education and subsequently in the labor room. An article in the popular magazine *Redbook* in 1962 noted that couples planning their births were now "thinking for themselves" and working out with their physicians "sensible childbirth procedures," picking and choosing more eclectically.[72] Indeed, by that time, there were more available techniques from which to pick. French physician Fernand Lamaze, who brought Pavlovian ideas into childbirth with a method called psychoprophylaxis, was growing in popularity in the United States. His method claimed to block pain sensations to the brain by creating countersignals in the form of conditioned reflexes, initiated by a program of breathing techniques and abdominal massage. Lamaze offered childbirth without pain, in contrast to Dick-Read's childbirth without fear. Lamaze required shallow chest breathing to allow the uterus room to do its work; Dick-Read emphasized deep abdominal breathing leading to complete relaxation and easing of tension. Both advised prenatal education for women and the men who helped them. Robert Bradley, an American obstetrician, entered the scene in 1965, promoting education for the father and explicitly stressing the importance of preparing him to be an active labor "coach." Bradley, author of *Husband-Coached Childbirth*, had first been drawn to natural childbirth through Dick-Read's work, but he altered the methods with an emphasis on trying to increase the father's role in childbirth. Bradley's ideas were very important to those interested in including laymen in the labor and delivery process. Together these methods provided alternatives, and childbirth education, associated now with a more generic "natural childbirth" notion, took more diverse forms.[73]

A 1962 edition of a widely used nursing text noted, "Many hospitals still do not allow a husband to accompany his wife to the obstetric floor, but it is the profound hope of the authors that more and more will come to realize the benefits to be gained from such a routine by all concerned." The text prescribed "classes for expectant fathers," where the men could learn infant care and also what to expect during labor and specifics of breathing exercises.[74] Novelist Sloan Wilson recalled what he had learned in his natural childbirth classes: "We husbands were told to tell our wives to relax, becoming quite sharp about it when we saw them stiffening their arms and legs."[75]

Women were initially more interested in and engaged with natural childbirth methods than were their husbands, and numerous stories relate how the pregnant woman often had to put pressure on her husband to attend classes. In one slightly humorous account of men's attitudes about such classes, a new father named Hal Higdon wrote about his experience when it came time for him to attend them:

> I balked and teased and said I wouldn't go. So, naturally (I was beginning to hate the sound of that word) one night my wife trundled me off to the hospital and into a large classroom, where about twenty or thirty other men were already seated. We all looked as though we would rather have been any place than where we were. . . . Soon we were instructed in the secrets of parenthood—changing diapers, mixing formulas and other such challenges. We were told, as our wives had been, how to recognize three signs of approaching labor . . . [and then had] a demonstration period.[76]

When the couple toured the hospital during one of their joint classes, the man noted that "all the essentials are on one floor—labor rooms, delivery rooms and the fathers' room—the latter graced by a man sitting nervously behind a growing pile of cigaret butts." But because he and his wife had taken the classes, Higdon stayed with her throughout labor, although he was not permitted to enter the delivery room.[77]

A woman wrote about her experiences: "My husband was firmly opposed to the idea of attending classes. . . . In over three years of marriage I had never seen Len so adamant, and this time nothing short of tears could compel him. So . . . I cried." The woman did not recommend this kind of pressure to others, however, since her husband never fully engaged and did not help her practice her breathing during pregnancy and also was not very much help in the labor room.[78] Sandra Eiseman, who in 1967–68, along with Carol Fowler, started the Childbirth Education Association in Madison, Wisconsin, and offered Lamaze-oriented prenatal training, noted that very often the pregnant woman would be the one to initiate men's attendance at the classes.[79]

Once the partners came to class — however reluctantly — they usually admitted they felt empowered to participate in an event that they came to see as meaningful to them. A nurse-midwife who worked to implement family-centered care realized that "pregnancy is a crisis period for the husband, and unlike his wife, he receives little outside support for the demands made upon him." Her advice seemed to be to try to bring dad in but not to exert too much pressure on him.[80] In a study of men's attitudes toward the classes they did attend, the researcher found that men "became less anxious after attending birth preparation classes," even if they attended only at their wives' suggestion.[81] Jim Fox, who took prenatal classes along with his wife at Sunrise Hospital in Las Vegas, "had to be begged, prodded, bribed or threatened to go to a class on childbirth. 'I thought it would be a bunch of women sitting around having coffee and gossiping.'" But he found the Bradley method, which he learned at these classes, extremely helpful, and he happily became "an integral part of the birth."[82]

As more men became educated, they accompanied their wives during labor, and many began to push to be able to follow the process through delivery. T. J. Blasing and his wife, Carolyn, were both interested in prenatal education so they could be together in labor and delivery. They learned from their friend, who had just attended the delivery of his child, that they could accomplish this only if they took the prenatal classes, so they signed up immediately. In 1969, their class had about fifteen women and four or five of their husbands. The following year when they signed up for repeat classes, about "half of the women had husbands who attended classes regularly and were planning to be in the delivery room." In 1974 they did it again, and Blasing noted, "By this time, it was quite routine for fathers to watch the delivery."[83]

Many male doctors became receptive to prenatal education and to the presence of men in the labor room because they perceived easy communication with the fathers. One physician made very explicit his reasons for supporting the practice: "A properly trained expectant father can be an ally to the doctor," he wrote his fellow physicians, adding that the husband "can be given advice and guidance not only for the benefit of his wife and himself but also to make the physician's task easier." One of the ways he could be a useful "ally" was that the man would more rationally understand the doctor's "verbal instructions."[84] Such perceived male bonding and easy communication—in a period when the vast majority of obstetricians were men—flourished also among the men attending prenatal classes. Irwin Chabon, author of one of the most popular texts championing Lamaze techniques in the 1960s, wrote about the men: "They sorely need the education offered in order to assume their proper role. When they are in the company of many men in the same situation, sharing the same hopes and fears, trials and tribulations, much, if not all, of their anxiety is alleviated. Group education makes the husbands more sophisticated helpmeets to their wives."[85] The shared space of the class-room acted as the shared waiting room had earlier: it provided space for the men to talk to one another and gave them increased confidence to move into the labor rooms and play a helping role.

A California physician told a story about the benefits of prenatal classes in terms of husband-wife sharing: "I recently delivered a nurse of her third baby. She had a somewhat immature husband who was rather aloof until he went through the classes with her and really changed his attitude. He was very supportive during labor and was very excited about the delivery which in turn made his wife feel happy with her husband's participation." The physician reported that he saw many such situations and concluded, "I have no doubt a shared experience greatly strengthens the marital bond."[86] Having gone through the classes together, the men could support one another and also support their wives more meaning-fully.

The classes worked to prepare both parents for the experiences, and one man glowed with praise: "It allowed us both to be part of a generation that could experience and share the pain and joy of our child together. It was a unique experience." In Westchester, New York, one childbirth edu-cation center opened in 1978 with the explicit purpose of "advancing the role of the father in the birthing process."[87]

Television audiences of *The Mary Tyler Moore Show* in 1976 saw an epi-sode about these new trends in fathers' participation. News anchor Ted

Baxter featured in his wife Georgette's birth experiences. Ted voiced fear about childbirth, and yet, trying to please his wife, he attended prenatal classes with her. He came to the office bragging about them and showing off his stopwatch, which he would use to time her contractions. As the episode developed, however, the watch malfunctioned, and Ted fell apart during Georgette's labor. Mary and Lou Grant took over and delivered the baby in Mary's apartment. Ted felt like a coward for leaving Georgette at such a critical time, but he drew a laugh when he said, "This is the most frightening moment of my life. Why isn't Georgette here when I need her?"[88] The show demonstrated that prenatal education had reached prime time.

As Lamaze classes spread around the country, natural childbirth gained adherents outside middle-class America. By 1967, the Bay Area Chapter of the American Society for Psychoprophylaxis in Obstetrics (ASPO) announced that "the Lamaze method in the Bay area is no longer available to only the middle-class patient." The organization held classes at the Fairmont Hospital clinics, the University of California Hospital clinic, and the Salvation Army Home, as well as at the Berkeley Night School.[89] The *Chicago Tribune* ran a series of articles about childbirth and fathering in 1972, advocating men's participation in childbirth and rearing as "a contemporary style of masculinity." Joan Beck, author of the series, encouraged men of all socioeconomic classes to actively participate in family-centered childbirth programs by accompanying their wives to their prenatal checkups, attending prenatal education classes, and being there to support them in labor.[90] This kind of newspaper attention spread knowledge about prenatal education widely and brought a greater variety of couples to the idea of wanting to try to work together in labor.

While it is not possible to know whether the classes aimed at a broader population changed the curriculum itself to connect explicitly to the varying needs of the greater variety of class, ethnic, or racial groups, it is evident that prenatal classes changed their emphasis in the 1970s. They looked much less at baby care, layettes, formula preparation, and breast-feeding and more at birthing techniques of labor and delivery. Women's modesty no longer determined class activity. Advice became: "Exercise classes on body mechanics, relaxation, and breathing control should be

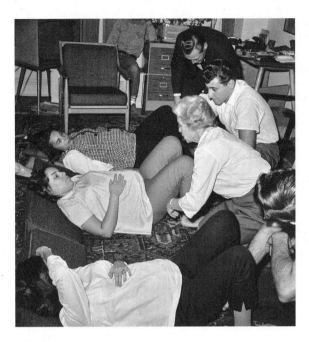

Natural childbirth class, 1964. The men are down on the floor helping their wives with the prenatal exercises as the instructor demonstrates what to do. © Bettman/ CORBIS.

practiced with the husband by his wife's side coaching just as he will during labor."[91] Many classes were associated with a specific method, such as Dick-Read or Lamaze, and others made it clear that, as a Planned Parenthood class in California put it, although associated with Lamaze, "the course . . . differs from 'natural childbirth.'"[92] Some educators stressed the importance of physicians and nurses meeting individually with the fathers who intended to accompany their wives so they could evaluate each other and the staff could assess how the man would fit into hospital routines.[93]

Some classes separated men and women in the 1970s, not because of modesty but because educators realized the men would benefit from talking to one another. Men who had recently been through the experience of labor and delivery often ran these discussions. "The men seem to need reassurance that what they have learned in the past weeks of class will all fit into place as labor progresses and that they will not be hesitant to start active coaching. . . . Probably the greatest benefit of this fathers' group discussion is for the fathers to be able to talk to an experienced father who in essence says, 'I've been through the experience, it

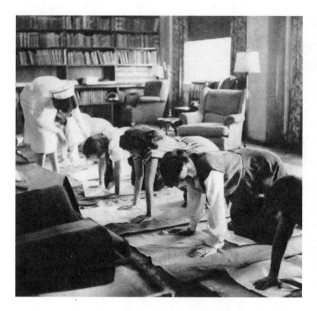

A prenatal class without the fathers; the women are practicing pelvic rocking, a position to help them tolerate labor contractions. Herbert Thoms, *Understanding Natural Childbirth: A Book for Expectant Mothers* (New York: McGraw-Hill, 1950), 34. Photograph by David Linton.

was great, and you can do it too.'"[94] The masculine group cohesion thus encouraged increased interest among novice fathers-to-be and gave them gender-specific support that allowed them to enter labor and delivery with more confidence. Male bonding had moved from the waiting rooms to the classrooms, where it similarly worked to embolden the fathers-to-be to more active roles in labor and delivery.

Indeed, studies at the time found that a woman's perception of pain was not necessarily affected by having attended prenatal classes with her husband but that "taking 'prepared' or 'natural' childbirth classes was correlated with seeing labor as a more positive experience" for both men and women. A study by Shirley Tighe Frank found that "men who took [prenatal] exercise classes perceived the labor as a more positive experience than men who did not take the classes."[95] Another study similarly concluded that "formal childbirth education prepares a father for labor, gives specific role cues for an effective performance of his role, and therefore, makes his role in childbirth congruent with the strength and competency characteristic of his husband role."[96] Men who were encouraged to play a responsible fatherhood role found that it could start in the prenatal classroom.

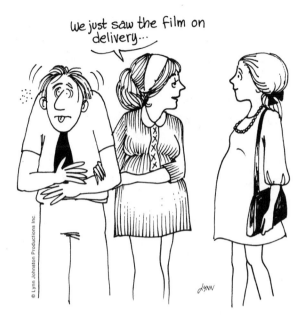

Cartoon of a couple leaving a natural childbirth class where they saw a film on delivery, upsetting the father-to-be. Lynn Johnston, *David, We're Pregnant* (Minnetonka, Minn.: Meadowbrook Press, 1975), 63. © Lynn Johnston Productions, Inc. Reprinted with permission.

Many prenatal classes included films of labor and delivery. Although they were to desensitize men and women to what was ahead, some men reacted strongly to the explicit scenes, as Fonzie did on television. Branko Terzic, for example, wrote that when his wife, Judy, was pregnant in 1980, they went to the classes together. Terzic said he was "ok" about the classes but might have "preferred to pace outside of the delivery room," except that his wife wanted him with her. During the classes, they saw a film of labor and delivery: "As the baby started to emerge there was a rush of blood the likes of which can only be seen in modern horror films. Apparently this was too much for my sensitive soul as I remember keeling over out of my chair onto the floor of the classroom."[97] Similarly, Sloan Wilson reported seeing a film in the classes he attended: "We saw a French movie in color of a woman giving birth to a child without drugs. . . . Although I had seen combat during the war, the gush of blood and other fluids which accompanied the birth of the child shocked me, and I wondered more than ever if I was going to be a great rock of stability while my wife burst forth with life."[98] Other men found the films enlightening in helping them to anticipate what was ahead. In one class, fathers appreciated the films and slides that showed the father-to-be "exactly what is expected of him in his role through childbirth."[99]

Two educational films from the 1970s provide a sense of what fathers and mothers visually experienced in class. *The Story of Eric*, which was released in 1973 by the ASPO, was a thirty-five-minute film that followed the pregnancy and birth of Wendy Johnson in California. Wendy, who narrates the film, was a teacher (shown in that role) who was looking forward to a Lamaze delivery. Her husband, Rich, was at first reluctant to get involved in the birth, but the classes committed him to participating in the process. In the film, we see the couple in class and follow Wendy to see her doctor, who is very supportive of the Lamaze method. The couple practice at home, and Wendy opines that they drew together more closely during this prenatal period than at any other time in their relationship. When Wendy begins labor, Rich listens to the heartbeat and times her contractions. He rubs her back. Her doctor considers a cesarean section as labor proceeds slowly. After fourteen hours, Wendy finally makes good progress, and Rich remains solidly in support. She is wheeled into the delivery room as Rich gets dressed in sterile gown; he later admits he was nervous but helps her throughout. At the end of the film, Wendy shows the baby to the camera and remarks, here is "our son Eric, brought into the world by our combined strength."[100] Prenatal classes were intended to further this kind of family togetherness.

A 1976 film focused more directly on the father. *Through a Father's Eyes* features four different fathers: two young white men, one young African American man, and the last a middle-aged white man. The film visually depicts the father's role during labor and delivery, sometimes including cutting the umbilical cord. The births all take place in the hospital but show different scenarios, including a delivery room and a combined labor-delivery birth room, use of pain medications and natural delivery, and physician and midwife attendants. Before going to the hospital, one dad says, "Sometimes I wonder if the actual thing does occur, would I be ready for it, or would I be doing the right things? Would I be making her

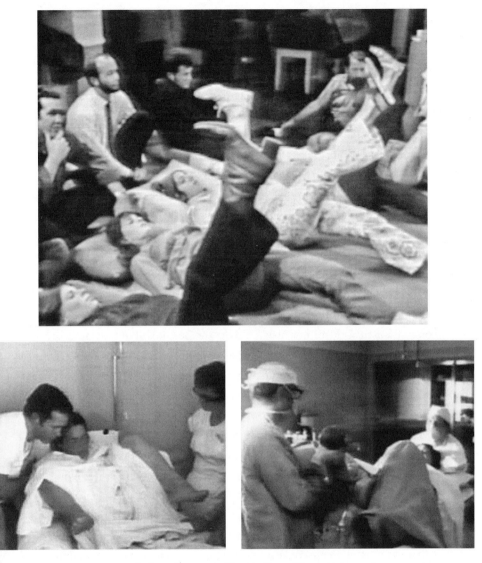

Still photographs from the Lamaze film *The Story of Eric*, which was shown in natural childbirth classes around the country in 1973. Women practice in prenatal class with the help of their husbands; a husband supports his wife as she pushes the baby out; and together they watch as the physician lifts the baby for them to see following delivery. Courtesy of Lamaze International.

feel good in so many ways? Now she told me, all I have to do is be there, which made me feel better." Another father said after the delivery, "I got the chance to see my son's shock of dark hair, right there, and that was incredible. I started crying. Then I realized, we made it. A star is born!"[101]

Men and women in prenatal classes across the country watched films such as these. The films provided information and visual familiarity that the men could carry with them and use as preparation for the roles they themselves might play in their own labor and delivery experiences. They were—literally—a dramatic introduction to what lay ahead.

Prenatal teachers came to understand that the experience in the classroom could have an effect on how the men saw their role as parent and ultimately on the whole family unit and the larger society. Some childbirth educators addressed the need for "better preparation for the problems confronting an involved father in modern American society." They called for health care professionals, sociologists, and journalists to take up more deeply and more seriously the meaning of fathers' participation in childbirth. One author insisted that "the best possible time and place to work out resolutions to the social pressures an involved father will confront is during the pregnancy, with the help of trained instructors in a classroom setting."[102] Many believed that if men trained for childbirth and attended their wives in labor, they would be better parents for the experience and bond more closely with their children.

As classes proliferated, they took on men's and women's needs for serious attention to the changes in their lives wrought by impending parenthood. Classes became more than practical instruction and included more introspective topics for discussion. What was the meaning of family-centered maternity care? One author writing to nurses believed that "true" family-centered care meant that "both parents are encouraged to attend prenatal classes . . . [where they can] focus on changes both the husband and wife are experiencing and the feelings these changes generate in them." If close examination by the men led them to not want to participate directly in labor, those feelings should be stated and addressed by the couple and respected by the nursing staff.[103] A different author wrote about the many "crises" couples faced during pregnancy, including what method to choose for labor and delivery and whether the father would stay with the birthing woman when she labored or delivered. She wrote, "Suppose his wife wants him to, and he doesn't? Suppose he wants to be there, but the expectant mother says no?" She worried that "some of the emotional crises faced by the expectant father are associated with his fears about being pushed, literally and figuratively, into the delivery room where he is afraid he cannot cope." She believed that the "evangelical zeal" of some childbirth educators put too much pressure on the men particularly and advised that teachers allow many opportunities in prenatal classes for the men to voice their fears.[104]

In Bedford County, Pennsylvania, mental health workers explicitly sought to improve parenting behavior in classes they organized. Labor and delivery formed a relatively small part of their concerns, but they found that the event of childbirth caused much anxiety among prospective parents. Classes significantly reduced these anxieties, and women reported satisfaction at seeing their husbands involved in sharing the experience. Men appreciated learning the facts of birth as well as the chance to support their wives throughout the event. As a result of the classes, a Lamaze group started a complementary prenatal class, and the local hospital began allowing fathers who graduated from the course to attend in labor and ultimately in delivery.[105]

A survey of the feelings and meanings behind men's experiences with their pregnant and laboring wives in 1976 concluded that many fathers had a positive attitude toward childbirth following their education. One father told the researcher, "I found that as I participated in more activities surrounding the birth, I became more and more excited about the life developing inside my wife. I went to the hospital and clinic a few times, we are taking Lamaze classes, and these have all made me feel more a part of what is happening, not just a spectator."[106]

Many men seemed to undergo a transformation between the beginning of a course of study and its end. One childbirth educator recalled that one of the men in her class sat through the early sessions "with crossed arms and a very sour expression on his face." She thought he was there only because his wife wanted him to be there. "By the end of class, though, he was a different man. He's going to be one of the greatest supporters of Lamaze."[107]

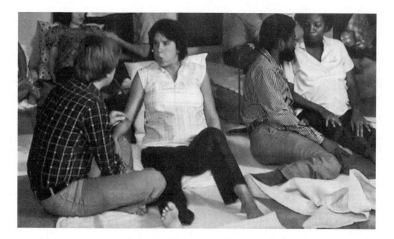

Couples in natural childbirth class, practicing their breathing together.
Leah Yarrow, "Fathers Who Deliver," *Parents Magazine*, June 1981, 66.
Photograph by J. T. Miller. © J. T. Miller.

Men attending Lamaze prenatal classes in Chicago in the 1970s revealed that they were "highly involved in the experience of becoming
parents. There was a sense that their lives would change as a result of
becoming fathers, but they seemed unsure about what those changes
would be." The expectant fathers reported that they experienced "a wide
variety of physical reactions . . . due to the emotional strain of the period."
Most important, "they had a sense that, like their wives, they too were
experiencing an important development in their lives." They did not see
themselves as secondary to their wives or their role only as helpers but
viewed their participation as "central to [their] experience as an expectant father."[108]

In the 1970s the prenatal classes helped to create the setting and the
cadre of men who worked hard to increase fathers' participation by staying with their wives when they moved from the labor room into the delivery room. In the 1980s, a prenatal session in New York was "typical
of increasing initiatives in the medical profession and among parents
themselves to become more supportive of expectant fathers. The notion
that fathers-to-be might suffer an emotional upheaval similar to that of
their wives, and even some of the same physical symptoms, is no longer
dismissed as a crude joke."[109] Educators saw fathers as necessary partici-

pants, and hospitals and physicians took them more seriously. Not only did fathers believe that childbirth was a "mountain top experience for them," but they also wanted to have "an equal say in what happens to them."[110] Birthing women might have initiated the men's participation in prenatal education, but the classroom experience—and certainly the labor room experience—provided men with definite ideas about their own roles in childbirth.

Most of the activity related to providing support for women in labor and the prenatal education that led to such support spoke only of including the birthing women's husbands. There were many individual instances in which women could be accompanied in class and supported in the labor room by their mothers, other female relatives, or female partners. But not until the 1970s did the phrase "or a supportive person of the woman's choice" become included in the literature, and even then it remained unusual.[111] There was by the 1970s a growing cultural acceptance of the married couple being able to share the birth experience together but little acknowledgment that women might have other people in their lives, including other relatives or perhaps lesbian lovers or men to whom they were not married, or friends with whom they might want to share these intimate and meaningful moments.

5 * PEACEFUL AND CONFIDENT

Mothers and Fathers in Labor Rooms

With more and more fathers present in hospital labor rooms during the middle years of the twentieth century, couples spent more time alone together during labor than ever before. During the period of home births, men had traditionally waited outside the birthing room. Increasing medicalization of childbirth in the hospital also separated birthing women from their husbands, as it did when men waited in fathers' rooms. But by the 1960s and 1970s large numbers of men, initially most of them white upper and middle class, found ways to get into labor rooms to be with their wives, especially after taking prenatal classes together. Because husbands were usually the only ones allowed into their wives' hospital labor rooms, these rooms became spaces for a new togetherness and intimate sharing. This chapter explores men's continuing struggles from the late 1950s through the 1970s to find their place in hospital labor rooms and looks more closely at what the women and men did once they were able to be together. Expanding their roles of masculine domesticity, men found that sharing their wives' labor involved them more closely in family life.[1] Their positive experiences in the labor room led them to want to increase even further their participation in childbirth.

Despite the growing acceptance of men in hospital labor rooms, their presence in maternity corridors remained not only controversial but sometimes physically impossible in many hospitals in the late 1950s, the 1960s, and even into the 1970s. Many hospitals could not accommodate the men without intruding on other parents; this was especially true in multibed labor wards and even in semiprivate labor rooms. The practice of men spending time with their laboring wives was easiest for all concerned if the family could afford the extra expense of a private labor room. Thus, togetherness in labor revealed significant class differences throughout these decades. Owing to the segregation policies of many hospitals during this period, however, it revealed race differences as well, and at first shared labor was the privilege only of middle- or upper-class white families.

Most hospitals in the South and many elsewhere admitted African American birthing women, if they admitted them at all, to separate, and often inferiorly equipped, wards until federal law and the threat of funds withdrawal required them to integrate. The 1946 Hill-Burton Act, which funded most midcentury hospital building and expansions, required that hospitals applying for the funds not discriminate on the basis of race, but it included an exception clause if separate but equal accommodations were provided. Between 1946 and 1963, federal grants totaling almost $37 million were made to racially segregated medical facilities.[2] Only in the decade following the 1964 Civil Rights Act did hospitals desegregate, some of them only after a fight in the courts. One hospital in Columbia, South Carolina, did not integrate its maternity wards until 1969, and then, says historian E. H. Beardsley, "largely because declining births made having two wards redundant. Before putting white women in once all-black quarters, however, the black section was remodeled and refurbished." In 1966, when Medicare threatened to withhold funds to Rex Hospital in Raleigh, North Carolina, the hospital admitted its first black maternity patient.[3] In the North, too, many hospitals remained segregated in the midcentury period. In Detroit, for example, where fewer than 1 percent of births took place out of hospitals in 1954, forty-two hospitals reported births. Of these only twenty-eight reported more than two per year to African American mothers. Ten hospitals in the city did not admit African American patients at all.[4]

Gradually, through increasing use of private rooms paid for by birthing couples, hospitals began to accommodate those who wanted to be together during labor. In Milwaukee, the parent group that organized to bring the Dick-Read method into labor practices in local hospitals (and which hired private duty nurses to help a woman when her husband was not allowed in the maternity suite) succeeded in bringing changes to two hospitals in the city before 1960. "Slowly the hospitals are making changes to incorporate the practice of the natural childbirth theory. . . . Physical changes in the hospital itself [are beginning to occur] — for example providing private labor rooms so . . . [a woman's] husband could be with her at a time when she needs emotional support."[5] Columbia Hospital in Milwaukee "provided a special room for mothers who have prepared for natural childbirth. It is apart from other labor rooms so the mother has a quiet atmosphere that is more conducive to relaxation. Her husband may also be with her during her entire labor." Similarly, St. Michael Hospital in the same city, a smaller institution, "has permitted husbands who desire to be with their wives during labor to do so."[6] The Chicago Lying-In Hospital allowed David Roberts to be with his wife during labor in 1962. He wrote about the experience: "I felt so close to my wife and shared the labor with her up until the birth was about to occur. Then they rushed her off to the delivery room and I was left in the waiting room by myself."[7] Those couples able to pay for the private rooms were increasingly able to accomplish their goal of being together through labor.

Yet the issue remained contentious throughout the period. The editors of the *Ladies' Home Journal*, in whose pages many of the popular debates about obstetrical practices played out, concluded in 1960: "Labor-room practices are coming in for the heaviest criticism of all. . . . The inertia of many hospital administrations and medical staffs, plus the expense of redesigning labor rooms, makes it often 'routine' for husbands to be barred."[8] There were many hospitals around the country in which it was impossible to find the spaces for men to be accommodated into labor rooms, and practices varied enormously. Hospital architecture posed one of the biggest obstacles to change and to men sharing the experience of labor with their wives.

Hospital administrators began to feel pressure to alter the geography of the hospital as more and more paying patients sought shared labor-room experiences. A study of 645 women in Boulder, Colorado, in the 1970s revealed how deeply ideas about husbands and wives sharing labor had penetrated American culture and birthing practices. Roberta Scaer and Diana Korte surveyed what women wanted so that a proposed new maternity wing of the town's Community Hospital might be constructed in response. The authors found that "the most important concerns of respondents are . . . keeping the family together and receiving the support of the hospital staff." The researchers interviewed a random sample of women whose births were announced in the local newspaper, a group of women who had enrolled in La Leche League (a breast-feeding support group), and a group of women who had enrolled in classes taught by local childbirth instructors. Between 98 and 100 percent of the interviewees wanted the option to include the fathers in the labor-room experience. Interestingly, the women did not have as strong feelings about friends or other relatives sharing the experience: only 42 percent of the random-sample women said they would appreciate the choice about whether to have friends and relatives in the labor room.[9]

The Committee on Maternal Alternatives in Baltimore conducted a survey of its own fashioned on the Boulder study. The participants included the 1,354 residents of Baltimore who used a commercial diaper service in the months December 1978 and January 1979. When asked whether the baby's father should be in the labor room, 99.5 percent agreed (91.3 percent strongly agreed). Eighty-one percent of respondents said that in fact they had had the father in the labor room with them during their last labor. The women who wanted but were not permitted to have their husbands with them were those whose husbands had not taken prenatal education classes. One of them said, "The only change would be that my husband could be with me during labor even if he doesn't attend a child-birth class—just for comforting purpose (I was scared and lonely during labor)."[10]

The arrangement of hospital spaces affected men's ability to be with their wives during labor. Some birth stories revealed how close and yet how far labor rooms were from fathers' waiting rooms and how hard it often was to traverse the short distance. The geography of labor and delivery could be potent. Robert Goldfarb, who marched through the doors into his wife's private labor room, described the physical layout of their hospital maternity unit and revealed much about hospital spaces: "We passed [another woman's] husband as we walked in, and though they were separated by only a swinging door and a short strip of corridor they were completely apart. I had the feeling that he might be picturing her as sleeping comfortably under anesthesia or else chatting before the strong pains started. She was doing neither and no matter what she felt he might be doing—dozing, drinking coffee—he was standing alone in an empty room."[11] Only a swinging door and short corridor stood between a man in the waiting room and a woman in a labor room, and yet it was impossible to close the gap between them.

The labor-room spaces themselves often could not accommodate the men. What Dale Clark had described as a "cell" seemed to be just that, a very small room big enough just for a bed. One woman wrote that she was "locked up in a room the size of our linen closet. The walls were lined with ominous looking rubber and the bed was high and narrow and impossible to get into without a goodly boost from behind."[12] A woman would labor alone in a private but sometimes very small room or she would find herself in a labor ward, separated from other laboring women only by a curtain. Many hospitals could not alter these spaces quickly even if they had wanted to and, if they responded at all, adapted spaces only for those who could pay for them. Policy thus was determined often for economic reasons.

Describing what hospitals should aim for in maternity unit construction, one author wrote, "Labor rooms are at best single rooms adequately soundproofed and isolated for privacy. One popular arrangement locates them between the maternity beds and the delivery rooms with corridor doors arranged so the father can be with the mother in the labor room without having to enter the delivery suite."[13] Yet one physician who wished the men could be with their wives wrote, "Most husbands must be prepared to endure a lonely period of waiting, since many hospitals do not have facilities making it possible for them to be in the labor room."[14] The rooms that did accommodate the men often were cold, stark places, sparsely furnished with bed and chair; yet inside these spaces, no matter how small or austere, couples frequently found great comfort and intimacy with each other as they went through the long hours together.

Natural Childbirth Impetus

Fathers' participation in labor, although not the exclusive province of natural childbirth advocates, received its strongest support from proponents of unmedicated birth. Marjorie Karmel's 1959 book *Thank You, Dr. Lamaze* added significant impetus to the changes already occurring in American hospitals, most of which had been based on the Dick-Read method.[15] Karmel was an American woman who had delivered her first baby in France attended by obstetrician Fernand Lamaze. She enjoyed her Lamaze birth experience so much that she tried to convince other Americans it was worthy of adopting. In her much cited and widely read book, Karmel described her Paris delivery:

> Dr. Lamaze called the signals . . . and I performed automatically.
> . . . From the moment I began to push, the atmosphere of the delivery room underwent a radical transformation. Where previously everyone had spoken in soft and moderate tones in deference to my state of concentration, now there was a wild encouraging cheering section, dedicated to spurring me on. I felt like a football star, headed for a touchdown. My fans on the sidelines. Dr. Lamaze. Mme Cohen, the midwife, the nurse, all exhorted me, "POUSSEZ! [PUSH] POUSSEZ! POUSSEZ! CONTINUEZ! CONTINUEZ! CONTINUEZ! EN-CORE! ENCORE!" . . . Each time a contraction began and I started to push again, the cheering section burst forth. It was fantastically exhilarating.[16]

The satisfaction and the feeling of triumph that Karmel experienced with her Lamaze delivery struck a chord with American women, and during the 1960s the method caught on quickly, especially among women who could afford the extra costs of a private room in the hospital. Two weeks after her book's publication, Karmel called Elisabeth Bing, a Dick-Read-method childbirth educator, and said, "Since my book has been out I've been overwhelmed with demands from women asking where they can learn the method." Karmel convinced Bing to learn and then teach the Lamaze method, and others quickly followed suit.[17] In Madison, Wisconsin, for example, Lamaze childbirth education classes—and consequent practice of the method—began in 1967.[18]

More and more couples looked for hospitals where a man could be with his wife in labor, specifically seeking what came to be called "family-centered childbirth." Two national organizations, both started in 1960 and led by laypeople—including fathers—and physicians, played key roles in this movement. One was the American Society for Psychoprophylaxis in Obstetrics (ASPO), since renamed Lamaze International, founded by Marjorie Karmel and Elisabeth Bing.[19] The ASPO was first a physician-only organization (Karmel and Bing did not vote) but quickly developed three divisions, for physicians, parents, and professional educators. Elly Rakowitz, an early activist, recalled that the physician members were brave to support the movement in those early years when many of their colleagues thought natural childbirth was a fad that would soon disappear and that nonmedical people had no business interfering with medical practice. The three groups of participants mirrored the supporters of natural childbirth and father participation throughout the country.[20]

The ASPO in these early years made a conscious decision to work within the system, in Rakowitz's words, "by conservatively moving toward reform in maternity care [rather than taking] radical stands by aggressively demanding acceptance of its beliefs." The founders believed that the Lamaze movement was concerned with women's rights in the specific area of obstetrics practices, but they sought to effect change in gradual stages, trying to "crack . . . open" the doors rather than bringing in the hatchets.[21]

"At first," Rakowitz remembered, "no one wanted to take the responsibility of allowing fathers to be present in labor rooms. Doctors would say it was up to the hospitals; hospitals would pass the buck back to the doctors; patients were never quite sure where the final decision lay." Permission for men to be in the labor rooms, when it came, was always prefaced by "*if* the obstetrical floor isn't busy, and *if* there is no laboring woman in the other bed in the room, and *if* prenatal classes had been attended . . . *if* they didn't behave, if, if, if . . . they'd be asked to leave." The ASPO helped parents' voices be heard.[22]

The second important voice for natural childbirth and fathers' participation in "family-centered" maternity services was the International Childbirth Education Association (ICEA). The organization's philosophy included a statement that the "father's waiting room lacks medical reason and denies couples their rightful joy in sharing this unique family experience."[23] The ICEA was founded by Hazel Corbin, head of the Maternity Center Association of New York, who convened a conference of childbirth educator representatives from around the country. Its first national meeting was held in Milwaukee. The group consisted primarily of lay educators and parents, but it also included physician members. It did not directly challenge physicians' authority and worked within a notion of hospitalized childbirth; at the same time it championed providing parents with information they needed to make informed choices about childbirth practices. It actively sought to include fathers in hospital labor rooms.[24]

An educational film released in 1960 demonstrated what ideal family-centered maternity looked like. It depicted a family-centered maternity service at St. Mary's Hospital in Evansville, Indiana. When the hospital's maternity service did not attract the number of patients expected after its opening in 1956, it started a family-centered program that became very popular. The film showed "Mrs. Smith" arriving at the hospital and being directed immediately to a labor room. "Her husband accompanies her. Admitting details are handled by him either in the admitting office or in the labor room after Mrs. Smith has settled down. During labor Mrs. Smith is never left alone. Mr. Smith is permitted to stay with his wife throughout labor, and if by chance it is necessary for him to leave, a nurse or aide will replace him." A pamphlet about the program in Evansville noted, "There is a chair in the labor room which can be converted into a bed so that, if Mrs. Smith remains in labor for some time, her husband may remain with her. If he wishes, he may spend the entire day and night."[25] Wide showing of the film indicated national interest.

Giving a sense of how common shared labor was by 1961, the *New York Times* reported that at Mt. Sinai Hospital (where Elisabeth Bing taught her Dick-Read and then Lamaze classes) "nearly half of . . . [the] expectant fathers remain with their wives during labor." Most of the ones who do, the supervisor of the maternity unit said, "are a tremendous help."[26] Although the Mt. Sinai numbers also indicate that either many couples did not choose to be together or that the hospital's facilities were not adequate to accommodate all the couples who wanted to be together in labor, they clearly reveal that more and more couples wanted shared labor. Yet practices around the country still varied, as some hospitals began permitting couples to be together in labor rooms and others continued to refuse the privilege. Doctors Hospital in New York City did not permit fathers to leave the waiting rooms in this period; other hospitals allowed them in labor rooms for short periods, and many opened their doors more completely.[27]

Deborah Tanzer, a psychologist whose work influenced many birth attendants, assembled many birth stories in her 1967 Ph.D. dissertation investigating natural childbirth. She was herself a proponent of the method. The women she interviewed revealed how much the presence of their husband during labor meant to them. One said, "My husband was always there, every time I looked up. . . . It was such a comfort to have him there. He'd let me sleep between contractions, and tried to wake me up when they'd come. I cannot *possibly* conceive of a woman going through labor and not . . . having a husband there." A second one related, "By this time I was *really* in a state, and I think I would've gone nuts or something if John hadn't taken control of the situation. He did his best to calm me, and we started timing the contractions. And within an hour we had the situation in control, and I started applying what I had learned. But I really feel it was because of my husband, that I couldn't've done it alone."[28] Tanzer concluded from her study that "the husband's presence in labor can serve an important function not performable by anyone else in our modern society."[29] Another psychologist noted that men and women exchanged traditional gendered roles during labor and they needed to be psychologically prepared for that. He wrote, "The husband who remains with his wife in labor assumes some aspects of the female role (giver of comfort), while the wife, who is doing hard physical work, assumes the masculine role. This healthy merging of male-female roles should be encouraged since the father's participation helps to lessen his guilt."[30]

Psychologist Shirley Zussman attributed most of the interest in husbands' participation to the natural childbirth movement. She interviewed forty couples, twenty of whom had been together during labor and twenty not. She said that "for those husbands who chose to be present during their wives' labor, there was almost unanimous agreement that it was a gratifying experience." One man admitted that he was "taken aback" when his wife suggested to him that he stay with her but that he actually liked being there: "It was better than being bored waiting downstairs. I felt involved, part of it. I like the sense of action." A second man said, "I felt it wasn't as bad as I thought it would be. I had imagined a labor room as a place where women scream and writhe in pain. Actually it was routine — calm, no trauma. I felt good that I had agreed to be there because I knew it made my wife feel better." Another man admitted that he agreed to be there only because his wife wanted it, but he, too, concluded, "The whole thing turned out to be very satisfactory. Things went extremely well. . . . I felt in control." Zussman concluded, "For the group of husbands who chose to be present the experience was essentially positive. Some enjoyed the sense of involvement, being on the scene where something was happening, the sense of sharing a vital experience."[31] The more experience in labor men had, the more they found it satisfying and spoke positively about it.

A "Lamaze Father" publicized his positive experiences in the pages of the popular magazine *American Baby*. When his wife was in labor, he wrote, "I was excited with anticipation but felt none of what I thought would be that first baby 'father's panic' that is so much a part of our cultural folklore." He said he had been welcomed at the hospital and was glad, when he passed the fathers' waiting room, that he would not "be spending the next few hours pacing the floor, separated from my wife." Instead, Ron Goodman wrote, "I was right beside her, timing the contractions, holding her hand, and giving her support. Judy kept saying how glad she was to have me there. . . . I was necessary, I was helping."[32] Women came to rely on their husbands' support during labor.

Alone Together

Since women had described being alone during labor as the worst part of the hospital experience, it is not surprising that when couples could be together in labor by the late 1950s, they greatly appreciated it. Actress Julie Harris described her labor and delivery in *McCall's* in 1956, and her experience (which also demonstrated how difficult it still could be for men to stay with their wives in labor) confirmed how meaningful the time together could be for the couple. In her case, the hospital staff seemed willing to show some flexibility for the star, but even she faced skepticism and pressure. Harris took the New York Visiting Nurses' course for expectant mothers, and she and her husband, Manning, read Dick-Read's book and did the relaxation exercises together during her pregnancy. Harris described events to Betty Friedan:

> Manning stayed in my room and timed my pains for a while. Then he left to have breakfast while the nurse got me ready. . . . Manning came back. . . . I felt proud that I was relaxing so well. Manning would hold my hand and smile at me and not interrupt till the contraction was over. . . . He's been preparing for this birthing, too. It made me feel peaceful and confident, somehow, just his sitting there and not being anxious, and the feeling of his hand. . . . The nurse kept fussing: "Your husband shouldn't be here." Then the supervisor came. "If my husband leaves, I leave," I said. "He's not in anyone's way. Can't you see that he's helping me?" The supervisor said: "Yes, I see; he is helping you," and let him stay. . . . The next nurse kept trying to give me pills for the pain. "No!" I had to interrupt my breathing to insist I didn't need anything. . . . All I wanted was Manning's hand to keep me patient. The excitement mounting within me stayed a calm excitement, not all the nervous panic I'd always felt before going on stage. The feeling of Manning's hand grew more and more important.[33]

Harris articulated how much her husband helped her cope with her contractions and identified what many believed to be the most important

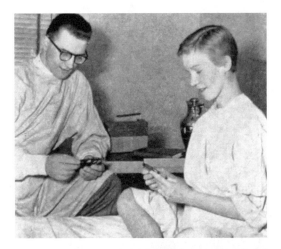

LEFT Couple playing cards together during labor. M. Edward Davis and Catherine Sheckler, *DeLee's Obstetrics for Nurses*, 16th ed. (Philadelphia: Saunders, 1957), 222. © Elsevier. BELOW Couple together during labor; the father-to-be reads while his wife naps. M. Edward Davis and Catherine Sheckler, *DeLee's Obstetrics for Nurses*, 16th ed. (Philadelphia: Saunders, 1957), 222. © Elsevier.

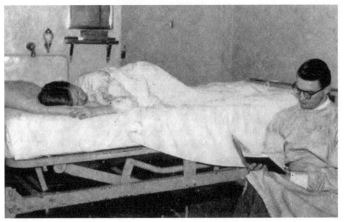

role for a husband during labor: helping his wife relax and stay on top of her pain by providing comfort and moral support. He was not required to do anything specific—just being there and holding his wife's hand could suffice.[34]

Medical literature increasingly emphasized the emotional comfort husbands could provide for their wives, and some gave detailed advice about how to divert the woman's attention away from her pain, as in this statement about labor management: "When labor actually begins . . . he is given a cap, gown, and mask and invited into the labor room. . . . For

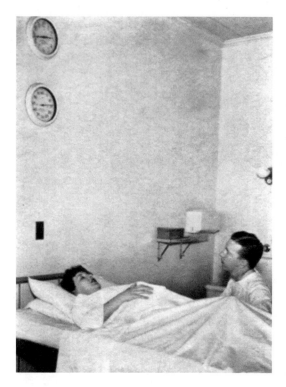

Couple together during labor as the man times his wife's contractions using the wall clocks. M. Edward Davis and Catherine Sheckler, *DeLee's Obstetrics for Nurses*, 15th ed. (Philadelphia: Saunders, 1951), 262. © Elsevier.

diversion, the husband many times reads to or plays cards with his wife, or they may listen together to their favorite radio program."[35] Indeed, many couples reported such activity to pass the time.

William Genne, who in the 1950s wrote a popular handbook for fathers-to-be — whom he called "AEF," the Army of Expectant Fathers — advised the men to inform themselves as fully as possible to get ready for a strenuous labor, as if for a sporting event. "We are on this team. We need to understand what the game is all about, where the goal is, and how to play our part."[36] Genne did not endorse any specific method of birthing (although he included a section on relaxation breathing in the manual) and advised men that their wives would probably be sedated. He added, "An increasing number of hospitals allow the husband to remain with his wife during the first stage of labor. This is a great help to both of you because it may take six to eight hours, sometimes more, for the cervix to become completely dilated. These hospitals find that the wife who has had the helpful presence and comfort of an informed and understanding husband during these hours is usually a much calmer and more co-operative patient for her physician."[37] This language, which admits to preferring the man's presence to his absence in the labor room, is not revolutionary in any other sense. Rather, the manual provided practical advice within the context of complete acceptance of physician and hospital authority. "When the baby is lower in the pelvis, the pressure may cause discomfort in the lower part of the back. There is a bony prominence on the backbone below the waist. If the husband will slip his hand under his wife, so that the heel of his hand is under this bony prominence, she will often feel more comfortable. The husband does not need to press, the weight of the wife's body on his hand is pressure enough." Genne continued, "Always be guided by your wife's comfort. If she likes it, all right. If she does not, try something else, or just allow her to rest as comfortably as possible. Merely your presence can be a big help to her and give her a sense of calmness and security which is very beneficial."[38] Backrubs had taken the place of boiling water for men's most important role, but just being there was significant in itself.

Genne's book and other advice articles and manuals gave men courage to enter into the world of women's labor. They also provided knowledge about the anatomy and physiology of labor and very specific ways men could participate and help their wives. This knowledge in turn helped make the men braver in challenging their exclusion from labor rooms at the same time that it strengthened their faith in medical practices. This kind of writing put the expectant father clearly in his role as head of the household:

A husband who has prepared himself to understand childbirth and to help his wife during labor is far different from the usual caricature of the waiting husband pacing the floor and strewing cigarettes all around. His calm and confident presence during the first stage of labor can bring reassurance and power to his wife. Of course labor is hard work. It is a tremendous effort. But it need not be a nightmare of an unknown horror for either husband or wife. The couple who have prepared themselves physically, mentally, and spiritually can face with confidence the unfolding drama of birth, the climax of which will bring into the world the baby, making their love for each other incarnate.[39]

Sometimes the men who sat with their wives in labor felt extremely stressed by seeing their wives in pain, a reaction that itself indicated the couple's emotional closeness. "It is not a pleasant thing to watch your wife suffer," wrote Peter Browne. "I wished I could take some of the pain for her, but there was nothing I could do except hold her hand and ruffle her hair encouragingly now and again." He graphically observed, "Every gasp tore at me; I could feel sweat running down my neck."[40] It is not surprising that men who watched their wives suffer sometimes supported the use of medication that would relieve their pain.

A big impetus pushing hospitals and physicians to be friendlier to fathers-to-be entering labor rooms came from a two-part exposé of "cruelty in maternity wards" in the *Ladies' Home Journal* in May and December 1958. A significant proportion of the articles dealt with the complaint that "women undergoing labor are left alone for long periods of time. . . . The husband is excluded from the labor room at the time when the wife needs him most."[41] A woman from Waseca, Minnesota, wrote to the *Ladies' Home Journal*, "I was left all alone most of the time although I begged to have my husband with me. They would not allow him in."[42] Ninety percent of the hundreds of women who wrote to the *Journal* pleaded, "Let us have our husbands with us."[43] The editors concluded that allowing the husbands into the labor rooms "will give the mother the support and reassurance of a loving presence. It will provide her with the small comforts that mean so much, yet without taxing the hospital staff. Someone to hold her hand or rub her back; to wipe the perspiration away or bring the cooling drink. *We earnestly urge the medical profession to review the rule which bars the husband from his wife's side.*"[44] The magazine editors believed that the majority of American hospitals still kept fathers confined in the waiting room.[45]

In contrast to the numerous accounts the *Ladies' Home Journal* provided of women who were not permitted to be with their husbands during their labor, the magazine also published a happy account of a couple allowed to be together in labor. Muriel and Robert Goldfarb shared the experience and described it as "one of the most tender moments in the family's life." After attending classes, they went through labor together in a private room. Bob said, "From the beginning it was different for me. No longer was I shut outside."[46]

Many men and women eagerly shared their birth stories in the pages of American magazines in these midcentury years. One new father, who had been through natural childbirth training with his pregnant wife, told what happened during his wife's labor: "I brought along a good book, sat by my wife's bed and read choice passages to her, held her hand when she wanted me to, gave her back-rubs, wiped her face with cool cloths and just talked. The twelve hours of labor sped by without the tension that increases pain. As my wife says, 'It's easier to be calm and relaxed when someone is there who acts that way.'"[47] When they entered hospital labor rooms, men found tasks for themselves, reading, timing contractions, rubbing their wives' backs, talking, and providing reassurance.

By 1959, the standards set by the American College of Obstetricians and Gynecologists (ACOG) accepted a role in labor for the husbands: "Someone should be in constant attendance [during labor]. The husband or a relative may stay with the patient during labor, providing their presence is desired . . . their influence is constructive, if adequate physical facilities are available."[48] A popular obstetric textbook in 1966 looked even more favorably on laymen in labor rooms: "Of all the devices for the psychologic support of the patient during labor, the most important one is the physical presence of another human being. . . . The husband can be invaluable for this duty."[49] Despite such support for the practice, many physicians and birthing couples called attention to "inflexible, assembly-line obstetrics" that still existed in many hospitals and that took "precedence over the mother's emotional needs."[50]

Inside the shared labor rooms, couples found ascetic and undecorated surroundings. When writing about the experience, they emphasized the intimate time together rather than the starkness. "Happy the fathers," wrote the Ladies' Home Journal, "[who are] allowed to lend the emotional support of their presence, if they wish, at this tremendous family event."[51] The parents of "Jeremy" wrote to Elisabeth Bing describing his

Couple together during labor as the nurse instructs the father-to-be about rubbing and supporting his wife's back. M. Edward Davis and Catherine Sheckler, *DeLee's Obstetrics for Nurses*, 16th ed. (Philadelphia: Saunders, 1957), 224. © Elsevier.

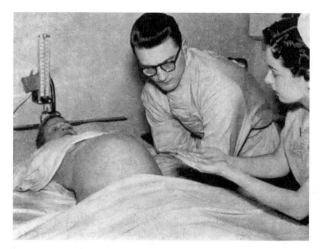

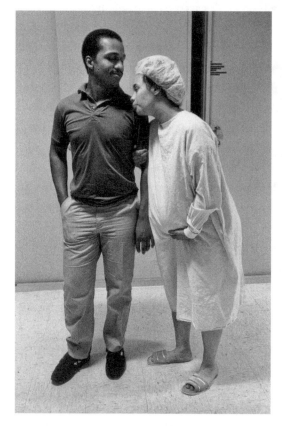

Couple together during a natural childbirth labor during the 1970s as they pace the hospital corridors instead of being confined to bed, pausing when she has a contraction. © Suzanne Arms.

birth. Sharon wrote that they arrived at the hospital at 2 PM; a hospital staff member told her husband to go to the waiting room, but he said "no, he was going to be with me, and no one made any further protest." In labor, Gerry wore a white coat, and "Gerry and I sat around and joked and chatted. I did some slow breathing while he timed the contractions." As labor progressed, "Gerry . . . was very busy popping lollipops in and out of my mouth, wiping my brow, timing the contractions, keeping an eye on my relaxation and calling out the time of the contraction." Gerry was more aware of his surroundings. He felt overheated and kept shedding clothes. He looked around him: "The labor room had all the charm of a labor union meeting hall: Harsh lighting, flaking walls, dreary institutional colors." He nonetheless acknowledged, "It felt great to be there." He noticed, "The only disturbing thing was the weeping and shouting we heard from other women on the floor." Once settled in, and with labor progressing, Gerry later remembered, "We were both elated. There was a sense of being absolutely alone together, a sort of true sexual intimacy."[52] In the same vein, in Dodgeville, Wisconsin, Paul Messling fell asleep in bed with his wife during her labor, to the consternation of the nurses. "I said this was how we got pregnant and I wasn't getting out of bed."[53] The rooms, no matter how austere, fostered intimacy.

Women sometimes could not predict what they might want from their husbands during labor. Trina B. had a baby in 1969 in a Madison, Wisconsin, hospital. She had a thirty-six-hour labor with her husband in the labor room for much of the time. She said, "We settled into this room. Labor had started. I was having contractions and E. kept trying to read to me [which they had decided earlier] and I finally told him, 'Please be quiet.'"[54] Similarly, Anita D. limited what her husband could do during her 1975 labor experience in a New York City hospital: "My husband was massaging my feet. That was so important. I didn't want him touching me anyplace else but he massaged my feet all the way through the whole time and that was really very important."[55] Ronnie Rae R. labored in 1969 with her husband's company and advised others, no matter the particulars: "Share the moment with [your] husband. Be really close with everything, every step."[56] A woman from Marietta, Georgia, put these sentiments very succinctly: "I would rather have my husband with me than any specialist. A loving husband's hand in yours is by far the best sedative in the world."[57]

The 1970s witnessed real changes in men's participation in labor in American hospitals as most hospitals came to accept men's presence in the labor rooms. Merle Gross and her lawyer husband, Barry, helped to lead the way in Chicago. The couple's very public descriptions of their activities during labor illustrated how couples coped during the hours together. Merle told a reporter, "During labor I was really working hard and was getting very sleepy. . . . I was constantly saying thank you to Barry for all the little things he was doing for me. I teased him about missing his calling—he looked so medical in his scrub suit, with his beard hanging out underneath the mask. The strongest memory I have is of my husband's super masculine behavior. Gentleness in men I always find very touching because they are so big and clumsy."[58] This appealing account encouraged others to try the shared experience.

There are common threads running through the labor-room stories in the 1970s as men learned the many ways they could help their wives through increasingly strong labor contractions. Jerry Martin told of his wife's labor in California: "I held her hand and talked to her. I told her that it was the peak and would be over before I counted to twenty and it was. I kept wringing out the washcloth and keeping it cool on her forehead and face."[59] In Chicago, a man who was permitted to be with his laboring wife only briefly said, "I can't show Tina I'm all nervous because she looks to me for security. You know how it is, we have to be big heroes at times like this."[60] Men might have expanded their family activities when they helped their wives during labor, but they did not travel far from the traditional masculine role.

A 1972 labor story provided more details:

My husband joined me in the labor room and timed my contractions which continued to be irregular. He encouraged me to concentrate on the focal point [a common natural childbirth recommendation]—a king of hearts card clipped to his front pocket. I was very drowsy [she had accepted a sedative] when my cervix had dilated to seven cm. My husband kept me alert by talking with me, wiping my forehead with a cool cloth and holding my hand. . . . It was such a comfort to have my husband with me. Unfortunately when I reached ten cm, the doctor was not yet at the hospital. With a strong urge to push, I waited one hour for him. . . . This was the time I most needed my husband's encouragement. He was wonderful and reassuring.[61]

One observer noted that "whether it's curiosity or a sincere desire to participate in the birth miracle, [the fathers-to-be] conscientiously take childbirth courses and know as much about breathing techniques and contractions as their wives. The men are tremendous towers of strength during the long hours of waiting." One couple prepared very practically, as the husband related: "Carol prepared a couple of sandwiches and some fruit so that I wouldn't have to leave her. And frankly, I was afraid to. . . . So I sat, and grunted, and read a mystery, and talked, and every so often a nurse would come in to check Carol and I would have to leave the room. But, you know, for the life of me, I'm not sure if I ever ate that lunch."[62] Ruth Forbes opined that "during the actual labor he can be a tower of strength encouraging her, keeping up her morale, reminding her what to do if she forgets, acting as a link between her and the medical staff. He is not just there as an observer, but as a participant, helping at all stages so that the couple can give birth together, and can share the delight and joy."[63] These examples of expectant fathers trying to be heroes for their wives and a woman in labor making her husband a sandwich demonstrate that incorporating men into labor maintained conventional gender expectations.

Birthing couples came to appreciate and highly value togetherness during labor. One study conducted during the 1970s revealed that 92 percent of women whose husbands were with them found their presence "beneficial" in raising morale and improving physical comfort. Most of the studies of men's participation in their wives' labor during the 1970s concluded that a husband offered "unequalled ability to support his wife during the particular stresses" of labor and that "it is the father whose presence preserves her personality intact. For this role, he alone is best qualified."[64]

Actor Donald Sutherland joyfully wrote about his experience with his wife in labor: "The only pitfall of working together was laughing, which, when it occurred during the contraction, caused Francine her only discomfort throughout the birth."[65] A study of thirty middle-income couples who had attended childbirth education classes found that most of them reported that they worked well together in labor. "Men timed contractions, breathed along with their wives to help them stay 'on top' of contractions, massaged backs, brought ice chips and juice, translated and transmitted requests from their wives to doctors and nurses, gave constant caring attention and encouragement, and were consistent reminders to their wives when labor was most difficult that the women were not alone and that labor would end." The study found no negative effects of the experience on the men and no women who complained of their husband's interference or overinvolvement.[66]

During the 1970s, men's involvement in labor expanded well beyond its early (white) participants. Increasing racial integration of hospitals meant that more African Americans had access to previously white-only hospitals and wards, many of which were more flexible in labor practices than the less equipped black hospitals. Even so, hospitals found informal ways to keep black and white patients apart. At the University of Chicago Lying-In Hospital in the mid-1960s, the maternity service contained East and West units, which in effect divided patients along racial lines.[67] Although hospitals integrated at different paces through the 1960s and 1970s and indeed over the rest of the century continued to find ways to discriminate, many middle-class black couples were able to find ways to be together in hospital labor rooms.[68]

In the 1970s *Essence* followed two couples' birth experiences, demonstrating that being together in labor had crossed previous racial barriers for middle-class couples. In the first story, African Americans Charlotte and Ozell Bonds related their "initiation into parenthood," with Charlotte emphasizing how important Ozell's presence during labor was for her:

Finally . . . Ozell appeared in the doorway. He paused momentarily as if to reassure himself that he really wanted to be there before coming over to the side of the bed. As soon as he asked me how I was doing, I forgot about all my trivial complaints and began to tell him about

the funnier things that had happened. . . . I jerkily shifted from one
breathing level to the next, trying to stay ahead. Ozell began coaching me and I was soon able to adjust. . . . Although he looked like he
was ready to drop, Ozell never stopped wiping my forehead, spoon-
feeding me ice and doing other things to help me relax. . . . Ozell
stood behind me while pressing an ice pack against my spine. Two or
three times, his hand moved during the peaks of contractions causing
pain to ripple through my body. "Can't you keep it still," I snapped. It
wasn't just the movement that bothered me. No. He was so hung up
watching that machine [monitor] that I didn't think he was paying
me any attention. . . . I only wanted Ozell to stay close to me. Feeling
his strength as he squeezed my arms and shoulders reassured me I
could make it.[69]

Ozell, meanwhile, had learned from the physician that the baby's heartbeat was irregular, and he understood that it was his job to keep that information from Charlotte while at the same time helping her cope with
discomfort from her contractions and from the monitor that was tracking
her labor. "I was sure that Charlotte didn't know that a problem existed
and I was equally sure that there was no need for her to know at that
time." He knew that he watched the monitor too much because of his
knowledge, and he took frequent breaks for a cigarette in the fathers'
waiting room to regain his strength and composure.[70] It is impossible to
know how often men carried knowledge that their wives did not have
that added to their stresses during labor. Physicians consulting with husbands — man to man — and not informing the birthing women of potential problems might have been common and might also have partially
explained physicians' willingness to incorporate the men into the labor
process.

Another *Essence* article similarly encouraged men to accompany their
wives through labor. A woman who was company coordinator for the
Minority Business Enterprise program at Pacific Telephone Company
in San Francisco wrote about her own experiences. Patricia Patterson
explained that she and her husband, Jimmy, decided on natural childbirth and enrolled in classes together. When she started labor, she wrote,

"Jimmy grabbed some magazines (he was going to read at a time like this?) and I took my bag and put it with the baby's things. It was unreal. . . . Off we went, relatively calm, unlike the movies where the husband goes speeding off with his wife moaning and groaning." To help her concentrate during contractions, she brought to the hospital a twelve-inch statue of a Masai warrior to use as her focal point. After being prepped, Patterson was taken to a small private labor room. "Jimmy, with all our paraphernalia, was escorted in and given instructions on how to call the nurse. There we were. The room was dimly lit, and in the far corner was a shelf where we placed our warrior—who caused a lot of conversation." Patterson continued, "It was about 5:30 AM, and we had begun using some of the slower breathing exercises. Jimmy would feel the tightness of my stomach when the contractions started and signal for me to begin my breathing. This went on for a while with a gradual increase in the intensity and the duration of each contraction." The darkened room was intimate as the two worked together.

> I remembered to relax in between and Jimmy helped me by timing the contractions and breathing with me. . . . I found it increasingly hard to concentrate on my statue, and Jimmy had to remind me constantly. Jimmy took short rests every now and then, but the magazines he'd brought along were put aside as the contractions got rougher and closer together. There seemed to be no relief. . . . Jimmy was busy wiping my brow, giving me ice chips and wiping my mouth. . . . Jimmy spurred me on.[71]

By the 1970s, a majority of American men and women were finding it relatively easy to be together during labor. An ICEA survey of hospital practices in 1973 revealed some regional variations in the practice, but it also showed how widespread the policy changes were: In the East, 87 percent of hospitals allowed the fathers to be in the labor rooms. In the Midwest, the shared experience was allowed in 97 percent of hospitals, comparable to the 98 percent in the West. The South lagged somewhat behind, but there, too, a significant majority of hospitals, 73 percent, permitted the practice. The national average was 86 percent.[72] It is important to note that at the same time in the South only 28 percent of hospitals offered prenatal classes to parents-to-be and thus did not necessarily tie the men's presence to the education.[73]

Sharing labor together led many to wax eloquent about how meaningful the experience was for the men and for the relationship. One woman described laboring at home with her husband's help in 1974 and finally deciding to go to the hospital: "We stopped and bought donuts for the nurses. I remember how close I felt to my husband when we arrived at, I think it was the emergency entrance. . . . My husband [said] 'We're here to have our baby.'" When the same woman delivered again in 1977, she recalled, "Here I am in labor and things were getting intense. It was so wonderful having my husband with me. . . . I have such memories of closeness, it was almost like making love in a way. It was a really intimate experience."[74] It was the closeness that spurred on many couples and enhanced their relationship.

Health Professionals Respond

Many physicians at midcentury remained adamantly against laymen entering the maternity corridors, whether the couple wanted natural childbirth or regional anesthesia. The president of one of the major national organizations of obstetricians, Dr. Brian Best, said in his annual address in 1958, "I have often suspected that the woman in labor instinctively prefers the minimum of curious spectators, and I have always doubted the wisdom, or as some today would have us believe, the necessity of the husband's presence during labor." He went on, "To the husbands I say there is no romance in watching their wives labor." Best believed birth was "woman's (and all females') supreme moment, when she accomplishes independently a feat not permitted the male, and during which he is powerless to help or hinder."[75] Her independence was not, presumably, total: there was still an important role for the obstetrician.

An article in *Redbook* described for a lay audience the still common midcentury medical objections to husbands having any input in medical decision making:

Some obstetricians view their own personal roles as similar to that of a ship's captain on the bridge, directly responsible for the safety of mother and baby. They alone, they point out, are fitted by training and experience to deliver babies safely. They plan the delivery, direct the hospital staff, make the decisions and perform the critical maneuvers. If the mother appears to be in pain, they nod to the anesthesiologist and pain relief is provided. If something else is needed, they say a word to the nurse. If the birth is proceeding slowly, they may speed it up with forceps.[76]

It was this idea of total medical authority that led some physicians to try to keep husbands out of labor rooms even in the 1970s so as not to "be watched at every turn. . . . [The physician] can have better control of the situation."[77] A physician observer agreed in his interpretation about why some physicians were still reluctant to give the layman a significant place: "The role which a physician occupies in relationship to patients . . . is that of the absolute monarch, and it is a position the average physician does not like to abdicate."[78]

Redbook further elaborated by quoting an obstetrician who had never let a husband near his laboring wife: "A husband wouldn't want to be present unless he's a sadist who enjoys watching his wife suffer. And a wife wouldn't want her husband there unless she's a sadist and wants to show him how much suffering he is responsible for."[79] In a similar vein, Dr. Robert H. Stewart wrote, "It is not fear in a woman who desires her husband to be present during labor and delivery, but only basic sadistic instincts in which she forces him to realize what he has done to her body, and the suffering and tearing of her tissues which she can endure, and thus prove that hers is the superior sex." Of a husband who might want to be with his wife at such a time, he asked, "Is it possible that he is masochistic in this desire?"[80] In the face of statements like these, some couples must have paused before requesting the "privilege" from their physicians.

Physicians sometimes equated husbands' presence with natural childbirth and dismissed both together. In 1974, American Medical News staged a debate about natural childbirth in its pages that revealed some of the divisions among medical practitioners. Against the practice altogether was Robert H. Barter, a professor at George Washington University in Washington, D.C. Barter said that *Newsweek* had quoted him as having said, "Natural childbirth is great if one is going to have her baby in a rice paddy." Claiming not to have changed his mind "one iota," Barter went on to say: "Failure to use epidural anesthesia, when it is available, to make childbearing a painless process is not only ridiculous but foolhardy, for both mother and baby do better under carefully controlled conditions of delivery. . . . In conclusion, *it is high time that obstetricians themselves rid our specialty of these non-medical, non-professional persons, who have been allowed to make inroads into the science and art of obstetric care.*" Barter concluded, "Permissive obstetric practice, with the help from all of the do-gooders and cultists, would like to take us back to the Dark Ages of obstetrics."[81]

Supporting natural childbirth and fathers' participation in labor in the debate was John B. Franklin, a professor at Thomas Jefferson University in Philadelphia. Franklin's answer to Barter portrayed natural childbirth as part of a family-friendly practice and not at all threatening to physicians or to health: "It is my belief that the expectation that all labors are natural events provides a setting in which a woman and her husband can accept responsibility for themselves in labor, a fact that aids the physician, reduces his accountability, and makes . . . intervention an event that is readily accepted because it is only done for fetal well-being and not for physician convenience."[82]

Letters to the editor following this exchange overwhelmingly supported increased participation of both parents in childbirth and demonstrate that physicians as a group were accommodating to the changes. Dr. Daniel J. Buckley Jr. of Decatur, Illinois, wrote, "It is appalling that a professor in a medical school could have such a narrow, closed mind [as Barter]." Dr. William G. Gerber from San Francisco found Barter's message "an elegant portrayal of the type of arrogant, misinformed stance that makes militancy seem necessary to women and other groups interested in dialogue with the medical profession." Dr. Peter A. Goodwin of Isle of Palms, South Carolina, wrote, "I feel pity for him, for his students, and for many of his patients." And Dr. W. Scott Taylor of Albuquerque,

New Mexico, concluded from Barter's remarks, "I feel it is high time we physicians begin to pay more attention to the wants and needs of our consumer patients."[83]

Indeed, the tide had turned by the 1970s, and medical opinion was generally accepting of men in the labor room. One physician wrote that initially he had "considered the husband in the labor room a nuisance" but changed his mind. "It was not long until we realized the benefits of having the husband play a supporting role to his wife during labor. We have been using, in most instances, less analgesia and anesthesia. . . . When the husband is playing the proper supportive role, the wife in labor does not require the depth of analgesia that is required when he is not interested or is not present during labor."[84] As this physician pointed out, there were medical reasons as well as social ones for including the men.

Physicians — some with trepidation, others more eagerly — played a significant role in paving the way for natural childbirth and for laymen's presence in labor rooms during the 1960s and 1970s. The term "natural childbirth" in the 1960s came to encompass the methods of physicians Grantly Dick-Read, Fernand Lamaze, and Robert Bradley. Bradley likened a father's participation as a member of the birth team to nineteenth-century physicians' realization that they needed to wash their hands before doing vaginal examinations, both, he thought, excellent ideas that had been too long ignored by the medical profession. "History has shown physicians to be, characteristically, overly cautious followers rather than daring leaders," he concluded.[85] But Bradley, Dick-Read, and Lamaze did lead the way to many of the changes during these years. Many who championed their natural childbirth ideas in hospitals across America, fueled in large part by Herbert Thoms at Yale, were physicians. Perhaps the doctors yielded more easily to pressure from their patients in part because they did not spend the long hours during labor that nurses did. Perhaps they understood the issue from their own perspectives as fathers.

While some physicians worried that a woman would fuss more in labor with her husband present as she tried to put on a "show" of how much she was suffering, others observed that women were much calmer with their husbands present. Some women indicated that they did not want their husbands in the labor room because they believed "they can be braver without them."[86] Others appreciated their husband's "presence and cool hand."[87] Indeed, trying to generalize is fruitless, since there were so many different opinions and practices across the country, and locally couples may not have been able to find the kinds of experiences they sought. But the trends are clear, and in the 1960s increasing numbers of middle-class couples experienced labor together, and the numbers of hospitals allowing this togetherness grew exponentially. By the 1970s, men were common sights in hospital labor rooms.

A clinical professor at the University of California who practiced at French Hospital in San Francisco in the 1960s fully supported husbands in labor rooms. He evoked a gender bond between male physicians and the laymen and because of it believed that men could be good allies. In his hospital, he wrote, "during labor the husband is allowed to stay with his wife. He is very good company for her and will willingly attend to all manner of little chores, thus relieving the nurse who is concerned with other patients too. . . . Completely untrained husbands are astute students, and if simply told what to watch for, will report to the nurse any abrupt change in their wife's pattern."[88] Any understanding between the fathers-to-be and male physicians obviously decreased as more women entered the practice of obstetrics, but by the time women reached a significant number in the specialty, the presence of men in the labor room was already established.[89]

Since they were the ones spending the most time with laboring women, nurses held the burden of having to adjust to very different patterns of care as men became incorporated into hospital routines. When women were sedated or anesthetized during labor, nurses' role was careful observation; when laboring women had their husbands with them, nurses had to find ways to welcome the man and help him support his wife "in the way that seems best to both of them."[90]

In hospitals that allowed the husbands to visit with their wives in labor, the nurses were instructed to tell the husband to leave each time the woman was being examined. One obstetrical nurse told the story of her own childbirth when her husband "just felt that here was this important experience and he was the one that was being told to leave all the time." He went to the fathers' waiting room during these times but was not pleased by his repeated banishments.[91] Similarly, Sloan Wilson did not like the policy: "While the doctor examined my wife, I was told to go and stand in the corner, because my presence apparently embarrassed the nurses or somebody. Standing there with my face to the wall like a bad boy, I felt the tension rising within me almost to the breaking point."[92] While some men were mobilized into action to expand their roles by such adverse experiences, the nurses bore the brunt of the extra work involved in adding the men to the list of people to whom they had to pay attention. Personnel shortages in the 1960s made hospitals claim that husbands could help by taking some of the routine care of the laboring woman from the nurses, and in some cases it worked this way. But overworked nurses did not always feel the relief.[93]

Taking care of the father became a common addition to labor-room nursing duties. One author advised: "As labor progresses the father, too, may fatigue, become flustered, or lose his self-confidence and require the nurse's assistance or reminders in performing his role." The nurse should remember also that "the father needs to take care of his personal needs" and may need to leave the room occasionally. She should cover for him during these absences.[94] Most men appreciated helpful gestures such as being brought coffee and juice.[95]

Sometimes nurses were caught directly between physicians and the birthing couples. Carolyn Splett, an obstetrical nurse beginning in the 1960s, related that each doctor kept a 5×7 card with specific instructions for the nurse, who had to remember the different preferences of each physician. When hospital policy allowed fathers in the labor rooms, situations could sometimes arise that were very difficult. Splett related, "I can remember some conversations where every time there was an exam done, then the nurse would say to the father, 'You have to leave now because we are going to give an exam.' And the father would say, 'It's okay. I can stay here.' And then there would be this power play with the nurses [who] would [say], 'The rules are that you have to leave.'" She remembered that the doctors would give a hard time to nurses who cooperated with prepared childbirth, "saying that we were going to be wide open for a lawsuit because we were letting these people make decisions for themselves."[96]

Later Splett moved to Missoula, Montana, where things were very different. She said, "The biggest hurdle we had in Missoula was getting fathers involved. And . . . I took more guff and more criticism from the nurses who did not want [fathers] than I did from the doctors who by this time said it was ok."[97]

Nurse Hazel Corbin actively supported men's entry into labor rooms. She realized, "No one is more petrified . . . than the woman alone in labor. If ever a woman needs her husband's moral support and assurance it is then." A birthing woman should not look on her husband as someone who pays the bill and hands out cigars. "How much more wonderful for her to have someone she can really talk to and lean on, someone who understands this fundamental thing that is happening to her."[98] Sister Colette in Kenosha, Wisconsin, agreed: "His presence not only gives his wife emotional support, but he can actually help her . . . to make 'the most' of her labor contractions by reminding her when to breathe and when to relax. He frequently can tell when a 'contraction' is beginning by placing his hand on his wife's abdomen before she is aware of this occurrence. He can also 'time' the length and frequency of the contraction in the absence of the nursing staff."[99]

As Splett had noticed, some obstetric nurses had a negative early response to Lamaze methods. Bonnie Miller remembered that her initial reaction to Lamaze in 1958 was that she thought the women who wanted it were "freaks." She said that the nurses in her hospital (in Madison, Wisconsin) were "very concerned because I think . . . the husband . . . got involved in trying to limit the wife's pain medication and we really did believe that if a patient was in pain they ought to be able to have something for that."[100] Letting the men observe their wives in labor led some men to demand more pain relief medications for their wives, and in the Lamaze cases it might have led them to demand less.

Over time, most nurses came to appreciate the men's presence. One concluded from her experiences with men accompanying their wives in labor that "it is a very good thing and creates few problems." She praised the men, saying, "Most husbands are so unobtrusive and yet so helpful that afterwards we forget all about them. Patient and untiring, they sit with their wives throughout labor, . . . run errands and demand no attention for themselves, and their actions go largely unsung."[101] Another nurse agreed, "If she wants much sustained back-rubbing, there is nothing like a strong, patient husband to do the job."[102] Nursing historian Sarah Williams found that although it took time for many nurses to accept the inclusion of husbands, ultimately they became strong advocates.[103]

Men Respond, Some with Ambivalence

Despite the growing numbers of women who wanted their husbands with them for the help and support they could offer and the growing numbers of men who wanted to share the labor experience with their wives, there still were men and women in the 1960s and 1970s who did not think labor was a time when the parents-to-be had to be or even should be together. One woman admitted that during labor she thought of her mother and what she had been through to bring her into the world, and she wished her friend who had delivered her own baby just six weeks earlier could be with her. Her husband, she thought, "was in the way. He didn't know how to rub in any of the right places." She was glad when the doctor suggested that her husband leave: "Actually I wanted to do this alone. . . . I was alone, like a mother cat, on my own, this was my thing, and I felt like scratching the eyes out of anyone who got in my way. It was very primitive."[104]

During the 1970s, some men, too, voiced doubts and began to buckle under the pressure to do things exactly right and to be that idyllic, gentle yet masculine "tower of strength." A nurse put her finger on a key issue in 1971:

> Unfortunately, in some instances where the husband is allowed to be with his wife in labor, he is often expected to give her *full* support during the experience, and is, indeed, made to feel guilty if he finds he cannot do so. I have heard proponents of the psychoprophylactic program in preparation for childbirth put this kind of pressure on the father-to-be, and that can be as harmful as if he were not allowed to participate. . . . The emotionally involved husband *cannot* and *should*

not be expected to take over the total conduct of labor. He, himself, is in need of support at this time so that he may give support to his wife.[105]

Indeed, a study released the same year found that 34 percent of husbands were "upset by some aspects of labor," including witnessing their wives' pain and feeling helpless to do anything for her.[106] Another study found that men who spent some time with their wives in labor often came away feeling "generally apologetic and disappointed." Many expressed anger toward the staff, claiming the doctors did not follow through on plans agreed on ahead of time or that the doctor was too strict and not sufficiently encouraging.[107]

Increasing numbers of studies focused on the psychological aspects of the experience, and researchers worried especially about men's reactions. One study reported the story of an obstetrician who separated the couple because the man was suffering "much more anguish than his wife." The researcher related: "A wife asked her husband during labor what he was thinking. 'I'm feeling guilty,' he replied. 'You're having this pain and there is nothing I can do.'"[108]

A 1977 study followed forty-five first-time fathers and found that most had participated in their wives' labor. Eighty-nine percent of the men "were in the labor room during the entire labor except for short 10–15 minute intervals." Jo Manion, the author of the study, found that 19.5 percent supported their wives minimally, 39 percent moderately, and 41.5 percent offered optimal support during labor.[109] This variation points to an issue that may be impossible to quantify for the nation as a whole but gives a good indication of the approximate variations in men's and women's labor experiences. We cannot assume that once men entered labor rooms they all behaved similarly or felt the same way about their experiences.

A popular fathers' handbook of this period advised men: "Don't let anyone decide for you if you should be in the labor room. . . . You are not a heartless coward if you choose not to be in the labor room, nor a devoted hero if you do." Yet the message in the book remained mixed. Author George Schaefer admitted that some physicians believe that the father's "proper place is in the hospital waiting room, or even better, at work or in a nearby movie or coffee shop," and yet he continued the discussion of whether men should be in labor rooms by emphasizing the role men could play. The laboring woman, he wrote, "is mighty lonely. Her husband can give her the companionship she needs, especially when the doctor and the nurse have to leave temporarily." He told a story of a couple who were not together in labor for their first child, in which the woman was "very tense and consequently her pain was so severe that she demanded a degree of anesthesia that could have endangered the baby." During her second labor, however, the woman's husband was with her, and it "went smoothly. The mother was so relaxed that she did not require even the lightest anesthesia. To prove that it was the father's presence that was making the difference, the doctor would occasionally ask him to leave, whereupon the wife would become terribly tense and restless and complain of severe pain."[110]

Schaefer's message that the men should never stand in the way of physicians' medical judgment was unambiguous. He told expectant fathers never to interfere "in any way with the doctor or his assistants. . . . Remember that you chose your doctor because you had a great deal of confidence in him. Don't lose that confidence now." He told the story of a man completely convinced that natural childbirth methods were preferable in all circumstances. The man berated his wife when she wanted an analgesic, "telling her that she was a disappointment and that her cowardliness was endangering his baby." When the obstetrician determined that he had to deliver the baby by cesarean section, "the husband refused to sign the necessary permission form." Whatever "inner need the husband had," Schaefer did not approve.[111]

Alongside euphoric descriptions of experiences men and women had together during labor could be found a few that were considerably less positive. In 1975, Nirvana K. delivered her second baby in California. She had wanted an unmedicated childbirth but in the end had accepted an epidural. She recalled, "I told my husband, 'Now I really want to do this the whole way.' Because I didn't know if we were going to have a third. I really wanted to do this the whole way, 'Could you help me through it?' And he, like most men, it was very difficult for him to watch me in pain. And he did think, 'what are you trying to prove?' And I'd say, 'I'm not trying to prove anything, I want it. I don't want it. I want it. I don't want it.'"[112]

Many fathers-to-be used the words "we" and "they" in describing events, stressing the togetherness of the couple and sometimes an oppositional relationship with the physician. One father said, "I was involved and could see everything that was going on. They weren't going to get anything past us. We were a team." Another wrote about his anger and frustrations: "We told the doctor that we didn't want any drugs. . . . Then when Cynthia was complaining of fatigue, he gave her a paracervical block. It seemed to stop labor for a little while and really stopped her urge to push. This made me angry. . . . Also, I think that the most important male present should be the father. . . . The husband shouldn't be made to feel like an intruding appendage." Another man said he felt like the medical people made him feel like an "innocent bystander" and he could not do very much to help control events.[113]

Television sets sometimes intruded into the couple's ability to share the labor experience fully; they also sometimes helped the man bond with the male physician. If the laboring woman wanted her husband's support and he was instead watching television — most frequently sports events, which men sometimes watched with the doctor — labor might not be seen as a time of intimate togetherness. As one man who was watching football during his wife's labor in 1974 said in defense of his activity, "I was *there*! I was *there*." He saw his role mainly to protect his wife from possible unwanted outside intrusions, and watching television did not hinder him from that role.[114]

Men who shared labor with their wives in the 1970s found being in the labor room rewarding yet challenging. One described what he did: "Whenever a pain had a peak in the middle, my biggest function was to maintain back pressure and support. . . . The ripples were strong enough so that I felt like I could correlate those ripplings with the peaking and the subsiding of her pain."[115] Many, though, described their difficulties more than their accomplishments during the labor process. One said, "At one point it seemed like labor would go on forever. I couldn't understand why it was happening so slowly."[116] Because he did not always understand what was happening, another man related, "Sometimes during labor I was frustrated and angry."[117]

American Baby responded to this sense of unease among some men who accompanied their wives into labor rooms. Sally Langendoen advised men about what to do if their wives panicked and lost control. Using traditional roles for men, she thought the most important message was to "render himself the authority" and take command of the situation. She presented stories of couples who used her technique successfully. In one, Tony gave the man's perspective:

> When I got into the labor area after Linda was admitted, I heard someone screaming. It was a shock to find out it was Linda. I thought she would be able to deal with it after taking the course. The first thing I did was put my hands on her cheeks and my face up close to hers, and then I started going through the breathing with her because she was completely out of control. She responded to me. It took a lot of time because she would get control for a short while, and then another contraction would come that was more than the others, and then she would lose it and I would have to go through the same thing all over again.[118]

Brenda told the woman's side of another couple's story:

> I got panicky, but not so much panicky as I wanted to give up. Carlos felt I should keep working, and he was right. He got me back on track. He stood right in front of me, and he had to stand in front of me in every direction because I was flailing all over the place at that point. He ran from side to side and made sure he did the breathing ten times as heavily as I was doing it, and he made sure I didn't look at anything but him. We had to work for half an hour that way. I responded to him.[119]

These dramatic illustrations provide a glimpse into the pressures that men may have felt when they contemplated their role in the labor room. They might be called upon to respond at a highly intense level. Thus, women's need for their husbands' support becomes clear, but so too do the men's worries and some of their voiced frustrations and disappointments or even anger. A man may be prepared to notice tension in his wife and how to help her breathing techniques, but calming her at the level of such panic may be beyond his capabilities. In response, nurses were taught to try to help the situation and provide some "inner" support measures, such as "allow him to discuss his concerns and feelings. Identify and support his changes as he moves through labor. . . . Praise him. Allow him to separate easily from the woman if he wants to escape. Respect his decision regarding involvement."[120] Labor could present difficult situations.

By the 1980s, men's participation in labor had become routine in American hospitals. The major obstetrics textbook supported Dick-Read, Lamaze, and Bradley methods as effective and recommended "the presence of an involved, supportive father."[121] With experience, obstetrical nurses more easily integrated the men into the labor-room practices. One nurse surveyed men and women delivering at Magee-Women's Hospital in Pittsburgh and found, "Supportive nursing care contributed to this positive emotional climate, and required assessing the unique needs of not only the patient but, at times, her husband. . . . Nursing care and support was provided directly or indirectly as needed." In a specific example, Judith Maloni wrote, "The nurse might suggest to the husband that his wife could use more encouragement or that her mouth was dry and maybe she would like some ice chips. In this manner, rather than replacing the husband when his assistance was not fully meeting his wife's needs, nurses worked to increase his effectiveness and help the expectant parents maintain control of their birthing experience."[122] Sometimes extra nurses were necessary during labor and delivery because of the father. In one such case in Milwaukee, Branko Terzic had fainted while watching a birth film during a prenatal class, so during his wife's labor and delivery the hospital provided an extra nurse in case he had the same reaction again; Terzic did not faint for the actual occasion.[123] The men found their supporting role most satisfying when the hospital staff was able to help them with information and some practical advice along the way. Their needs as well as their perceptions of their wives' needs were changing hospital practices.

A 1981 study that explicitly examined nurses' and fathers' support of laboring women found that "fathers were five times as likely to touch their wives as were nurses to touch their patients," illustrating that a close marital relationship may have aided labor. Looking at the experiences of forty women, the researchers concluded that "well over one-half of the support the women received came from their husbands." After the experience, the mothers remembered and commented on their husbands' support as most helpful. The men just had to be present to be perceived as helpful and supportive and to have reduced anxiety.[124]

Fathers-to-be often spoke of their main function in labor as being supportive of their wives and helping out in ways that she would identify. But many also had their own reasons for attending labor. A 1982 revision of the *Fathering* handbook included a new section categorizing seven kinds of fathers' responses, and they help us to understand some of the dynamics at work in this period. Authors Celeste Phillips and Joseph Anzalone used interviews, observations, and questionnaires over a five-year period to collect men's emotional responses to their labor participation. One group likened the birth experience to an athletic event and talked about playing a "good game" and "working as a team." A second group was proud when their worst fears did not materialize. A third group voiced heightened respect for women for having undergone such a difficult job. Another group of men felt that they had lived through a profound experience that made them feel more complete as a husband or father. A fifth group emphasized their connection to their wives and used the word "we" to describe events: "We did it . . . and then we had contractions . . . when we went into labor . . . now we are one." Some men described the new insights they gained by participating in this basic experience. The last group Phillips and Anzalone identified was composed of those men who spoke about their engrossment in the process and in their children and the "profound experience" of birth.[125] As men became more accustomed to labor participation, their responses became more nuanced and more connected to themselves rather than just to their wives.

The fathers-to-be were helped along in the 1980s by childbirth classes that included teachings about men's participation more directly. For example, fathers were sometimes separated from their wives during prenatal classes and attended special "coaching" sessions. One such class was taught by a man who had recently attended his wife's delivery; this teacher utilized a special "script" that included "an analogy between a labor coach and a football coach" and "how to deal with the wife's discouragement." This course also addressed the men's feelings and the difficult situations they might face: "The main point I want to stress is that there may be several times during the labor and delivery that you may be conflicted about what to do. It is tough being a labor coach. . . . There are always things about which you'll be uncertain. You'll have to make decisions that make you feel very uncomfortable at times."[126]

Philip Taubman, a new father, found natural childbirth and his role in it nothing short of "traumatic." He told the *New York Times* in 1984, "It is never easy to watch someone you love suffer. . . . Try telling your wife that, ultimately, despite efforts to keep her mind off the labor, the only thing you can do to relieve the worst pain she's ever experienced is to coach her on breathing fast and wipe her brow periodically with a wet washcloth. I was also frightened. It was the lack of control. . . . Every instinct is to take action, to do something to protect and help my wife, [but I] was stymied by the principle that her suffering was necessary."[127]

Although it was often rewarding to play an active role and be a positive support in their wives' labor, it was not easy for some men to do so. Nurse Pam L., reflecting on her own deliveries in the 1980s and her experiences of being with laboring women since, said, "I think that sometimes dads feel to[o] sorry for the women. I've seen a few labors that have not gone well because the woman has had an epidural and a lot of the reason was because the husband wasn't being supportive. 'Oh, just get an epidural.' 'Oh, the poor dear, she is in to[o] much pain, oh the poor dear.' That was literally the words the guy was using. He was making her feel weak, like a little girl, instead of strong." Pam believed that good labor support was crucial and could "make or break a labor." Men needed to be taught so they could better help their wives.[128]

These stories illustrate that men's experiences in labor rooms were not always positive, although frequently the positive aspects were most emphasized in public. Social and individual expectations grew so strong in the 1970s and into the 1980s that men felt they no longer had the choice of waiting outside. Their experiences chewing their fingernails and not knowing what was happening as they sat in the waiting rooms had not been positive, except in the sharing of their experiences with other men undergoing the same emotions. Their experiences in the labor rooms with their wives, while often warm and intimate, also held some negative aspects. Most men voiced their enthusiasm about being able to help their wives and be an active participant in the important family event, although some of them admitted their role was fraught. As men publicly shared their experiences with one another and as increasing numbers of handbooks and manuals appeared to help them think through their possible roles, men continued to work to influence (and to their minds, improve) policies and procedures in American hospitals. In their very ambivalences, men who accompanied their wives through labor helped to identify the ways hospitals, doctors, and nurses could better accommodate the men and women who labored together. The changes they wrought did not necessarily move in a linear direction of increasing the successful participation of the men or improving women's labor experiences, but they did reflect the men's changing interests and increasing involvement in the childbirth process.

6 * SIDE BY SIDE

Men Move into Delivery Rooms

Even as hospitals opened the labor-room doors to men, allowing them to be with their wives for the long hours of the first stage of labor, the same hospitals insisted that the men go back to the stork clubs to await the birth of their babies. The delivery-room exclusion policies began to be resisted, though, especially by advocates of natural childbirth and those men who had been with their wives during labor. Debates about whether to permit fathers into delivery rooms grew heated during these mid-century years. From the 1940s to 1970 the question was argued in medical meetings and aired in the press and popular magazines. State and local legislatures passed laws and ordinances about it. One husband was said to have chained himself to his wife to ensure his presence throughout, claiming, "I love her and she needs me."[1] Despite the pressure from an increasing number of couples who wanted to be together when their baby entered the world, hospitals were slow to change their policies that excluded the men from delivery rooms. Practices varied widely around the country, by individual physician and hospital as well as by region, class, and race of the birthing woman. Among other issues, hospitals worried about keeping infection out of what they considered to be an operating room and saddling the nurses with the additional responsibility of watching the men and tending to them if they fainted. This chapter pursues the story through the decade of the 1960s, the years when the men, especially relatively privileged men, began to move into delivery rooms.

The Pioneers, 1940s and 1950s

In the 1940s most women did not have and did not expect to have their husbands with them during delivery. Hospital policies and board of health regulations typically barred fathers from delivery rooms primarily because of the fear of infections they might bring from the outside but also because of worries about lawsuits if something went wrong. The Chicago Board of Health, for example, forbade fathers from entering any surgical suite or delivery room, a policy it did not change until 1967, when the state of Illinois left the delivery-room decision to individual hospitals. Even for natural childbirth men were not welcomed. Joan Gerver, who participated in obstetrician Carl Javert's "experiment" in unmedicated natural childbirth at New York Hospital in 1949, wrote, "Husbands were not included in the training or allowed in labor or delivery rooms. It never occurred to us that my husband should be in the delivery room. Nobody's husband was. One's expectations are influenced by the childbirth customs of the time and place."[2]

A woman who had a frank breech vaginal delivery (in which the butt rather than the head presents first, making vaginal delivery more difficult), with a long painful labor, provided one reason why women did not expect the company of their husbands. She wrote, "A few days later my mother told me she had never seen a man cry as Bernard had cried during the birth. I was glad he was kept out of the room."[3] Another woman, who delivered her baby at the Scranton State Hospital in 1943, wrote, "I would not have wanted my husband in the room, I really felt that the nurses in the room were really efficient and helpful."[4] Other women were more conflicted on the issue. Moya Sullivan wrote about her 1945 delivery at Beth David Hospital in New York: "I think if my mother or my husband had been in the delivery room, I would have felt happier. But by the same token, they could not have taken away the pain and seeing me in pain would have caused them much distress."[5]

Many women in the 1950s still felt that they did not want their husbands with them. Mildred Cherry, for example, picked for her attendant a woman physician who spoke her native Yiddish, and she had a happy experience at Brooklyn Jewish Hospital. She wrote, "I would have liked my husband to be with me in the labor room, but I'm not sure I would have wanted him in the delivery room. Perhaps that's because I knew it wasn't possible and therefore didn't consider it."[6] Many birthing women did not include their husbands when they planned their deliveries. Despite her sister being a nurse who worked at the Chicago Maternity Center and coming from a family of nurses, one woman wrote, "It never occurred to either me or my doctor or my husband that our daughters' father should be present at the births."[7]

But during the decade of the 1940s and increasingly in the 1950s some couples did begin to think about being together for delivery, and men started to figure out ways to accomplish this. Fame might have helped a few individual men stay with their wives. Aviator Charles A. Lindbergh noted in his diary that he attended his wife's 1942 delivery. He arrived at the hospital after she had already been taken into the delivery room: "Put on cap and gown and extra-thick mask, as I have a cold and didn't want to take any chance of giving it to Anne. . . . Dr. Pratt showed himself to be a highly skillful obstetrician, with an extremely efficient staff. He uses his hands with great dexterity and creates confidence in anyone who watches him work."[8] Even his mild illness did not prevent Lindbergh's presence.[9]

Although Lindbergh's experience was uncharacteristic, there were already in the 1940s a few individual physicians and hospitals that welcomed fathers. A story from 1945 shows that practices in American hospitals varied significantly even before natural childbirth had its impact. A nurse from Texas, Joanna Long, wrote that she had worked in a large hospital where "it was the strict rule of the hospital that the husband did not see the wife from the time she entered the labor-room until she had delivered and returned to her own room on one of the other floors." But when Long took a different job in a small twenty-bed hospital, also in Texas, the maternity ward of which had just one labor room and one delivery room, the practice was very different: "From the time the young couple entered the front door of the hospital, the husband was privileged to stay with his wife. . . . These two were exciting characters in a thrilling story building up to a terrific climax. . . . The young father wept happy tears unashamedly as he kissed [his wife]." From these experiences Long concluded: "When I think of the comparison of the two methods, the biggest argument in favor of the father's presence in the delivery room is that he should not be cheated of one of the greatest emotional experiences in his life."[10] A physician at the St. Croix Valley Memorial Hospital in Wisconsin during the 1950s "believed that the father should attend the birth in the delivery room," the two stories demonstrating that rural hospitals may have been more flexible than urban ones in these years.[11] Further sustaining the idea of rural flexibility was a conversation among the women in a prenatal class in Wisconsin in 1952. The women all agreed it would be "nice" to have their husbands with them, and Mrs. S. related that "her uncle was with her aunt in a little hospital. They dressed him like a doctor and he stayed with her."[12]

As early as 1946 at Virginia Mason Hospital in Seattle, at least one physician routinely allowed the husbands of women getting continuous caudal anesthesia to accompany their wives throughout labor and delivery. Robert Rutherford, the obstetrician who initiated the program, surveyed physicians in his hospital about letting the men stay with their wives through delivery and found that "little interest was demonstrated except to raise a number of reasonable questions regarding legal responsibility, infection hazard, and the doubtful motivation of any husband who wanted to be with his wife during this strictly feminine act."[13] Despite his colleagues' worries, Rutherford began the program, and about half of the women who received caudal anesthesia chose to have their husbands with them throughout labor and delivery. He provided printed information for the men and included them in prenatal education and on hospital tours. Rutherford admitted there were some disadvantages: "The doctor must be able to work before an attentive audience — namely the patient and her husband." But, he assured his colleagues, the physician was not deemphasized by the husband's presence; rather, "the physician emerges not as a technician but as an expert teacher who is starting a young couple off on that exciting next phase in marriage—parenthood." The advantages far outweighed the disadvantages, Rutherford thought.[14]

Flexibility and individual variation about men's presence in the delivery room in the 1940s and 1950s might have been greater than any study of general policies would allow us to know. At the University of Kansas hospital in 1949, Gail Ravitts endured an eighteen-hour labor. "My husband was with me the entire time. . . . My husband had talked his way into the delivery room—a practise [sic] not common in those days. His father had been a country doctor, and he had assisted in home births, and convinced the attending physician that he would not faint, and if he did, he'd be glad to lie in a heap in the corner."[15] A 1949 delivery in Michigan provided another example of how individual men found ways to be with their wives during delivery. Joseph MacLeod and his wife had read Dick-Read's *Childbirth without Fear*, and he was committed to helping her through both labor and delivery. "When the final time came," MacLeod wrote, "we entered the delivery room [and] the MD said to me, 'Where are you going?' I told him that I was considered part of the act. He responded . . . 'we cannot take care of you when the action starts. Well, suit up and stand over there in the corner. When I think you are all right, I'll signal you to come over here. If you are not all right, do not utter a word, just slump down in the corner and stay there.'" MacLeod passed the test and witnessed the delivery: "The results were compassionate and awesome."[16]

Even husbands who were physicians were not routinely included during delivery in these years. One woman wrote, "Since my husband was a physician, he was with me during labor in the hospital cubicle, but [he had to step] out of the delivery room at times of births. That was the programming of those dark ages!"[17] Some hospitals allowed physician-fathers into delivery rooms, in accordance with the letter of the law, if not its intent: "We would like to have some of our husbands watch their wives [in] delivery, but this is impractical due to hospital rules. Occasionally this is done if the husband happens to be a doctor, as hospital rules permit only doctors and nurses to be in surgery and the delivery room."[18] Because they fit technically within the rules, physician-fathers might have had slightly easier access to delivery rooms.[19]

The increasing popularity of natural childbirth—Dick-Read in the 1940s and 1950s and Lamaze and Bradley in the 1960s—and the family-friendly rhetoric that accompanied it, especially among paying middle-class Americans, pressured hospitals to allow fathers into delivery rooms. Following Dick-Read's 1947 visit to the United States, Herbert Thoms and other obstetricians at Yale's Grace–New Haven Hospital began what became a renowned program adopting the British physician's natural childbirth methods. At first, new dads stayed outside during delivery and met their newborns at the delivery-room door.[20] Peter Douglas, one such father, was happy to have shared labor with his wife, but he could not join her for the delivery: "I was able to see both her and the baby within an hour after birth." Douglas continued, "The eventual goal of the natural childbirth proponents is to have the father present throughout the birth process. I, for one, feel that this would serve to strengthen even further the bond between parents which is the inevitable result of living through the miracle of childbirth together."[21] A woman recounted another, some-what later variation at Yale: "Instead of standing next to me in the actual [delivery] room, he was in a TV/video room immediately behind my head and had access to all kinds of machinery to take pictures so we have pictures from ALL angles. (He could talk to me from a microphone in 'his' room.)"[22]

A Mr. Owen attended his wife's labor at Yale in 1947 and got so emo-tionally involved that he "became intensely anxious to follow through by being present at the delivery." Then, he wrote: "When I was finally and officially barred from the delivery room, I was quite frankly furious. For the next twenty-five minutes I thought of nothing else, forgetting com-pletely that my son was being born, and I should be happy." Owen felt that the policy of exclusion was "not the best way to start father-child relationships."[23]

Women attending prenatal classes sometimes learned why men were excluded. One nurse-educator told her class in 1955 that "surgical technic was more important than having a father in the delivery room. . . . You don't know if your husband is there or not." One of the women challenged her and said "she would know. She would want to know her husband was beside her." But the teacher had the final word: "It was not safe," she said, referring to the worry about infection.[24]

The best-known example of promoting fathers' participation in the early years came from physician Robert Bradley, the "father of fathers," whose book *Husband-Coached Childbirth*, published in the 1960s, actively encouraged men to demand to follow their wives into delivery and to play an active role throughout labor and delivery. Bradley started including fathers in delivery in his own practice in 1947, basing his thinking on Dick-Read's writing and his own experience. "At this stage of my medical career, no husband, to my knowledge, had ever been allowed in that forbidding no man's land known as the delivery room," Bradley remembered. One event made him want to change that pattern: after a particularly exuberant natural delivery, Bradley walked from the "joyful scene" at delivery to the waiting room to tell the new father the happy news. He was shocked to see "the frightened, anxious, distraught face of the man whose love and affection had been shared with this woman to produce this child. It struck me like a sledgehammer. What on earth was this lovely woman kissing me for? Why was I the object of her gratitude . . . while her young lover sat uselessly in the waiting room, fearful and anxious over his sweetheart's safety, eagerly wishing to see the outcome of his love for her, the baby, yet deprived by isolation from the most meaningful emotional experience of their lives together?"[25] But even Bradley thought that the decision about fathers in delivery should not be automatic or legislated by general hospital policy but rather be "at the medical discretion of the individual doctors."[26]

Through the decade of the 1950s, as the Dick-Read method became more popular, increasing numbers of couples wanted to have a family-friendly experience during which they would share the whole of the birth experience together. But they continued to face strong medical and institutional resistance. Mary Rogers, an obstetrical nurse, remembered that the physicians believed "the father was in the way, you know, or he's going to faint. . . . They'd say the delivery room is too small or it'd take another person to watch the father." In those cases in which the father wheedled his way into the room, Rogers said, some physicians felt the fathers had to leave. "But I don't remember hearing of anybody falling or hitting their head on the radiator or the kinds of liabilities that they were concerned about."[27] The International and Fourth American Congress on Obstetrics and Gynecology, meeting in New York City in 1950, supported the idea of men being present at delivery, although the presence of laymen in delivery rooms remained rare and contentious in American hospitals.[28]

Delivery Rooms and Policies of Exclusion

Delivery rooms in mid-twentieth-century hospitals were sterile, cold spaces, but, unlike the bare labor rooms, they were filled with equipment. The delivery room looked to one woman "like a curiosity shop." She continued, "I'd never been in a state before to notice all the strange pieces of apparatus there. [This was her third baby.] But now I was curious about them and asked questions."[29] Delivery rooms typically contained the rubber-sheeted delivery table, which could be broken in the middle, with stirrups and handles to allow for a lithotomy position (with the woman flat on her back and her legs in stirrups) and with a headpiece that could be lowered if necessary. Alongside the table would be artificial and emergency lighting, including a spotlight, an incubator, mirrors, an oxygen supply, a heating lamp, and an instrument table on which might be rubber gloves, basins, various kinds of forceps, scissors, retractors, needles, catheters, aspirators, dilators, syringes, gauze, and blood transfusion apparatus. By the 1970s, monitors might be tracing fetal and maternal heart rates. The rooms smelled of disinfectants, and the lighting presented an otherworldly glow. Delivery rooms were equipped as operating rooms, prepared for a possible emergency cesarean section, and as infant care units, ready with a heated crib and resuscitators. Often the rooms were quite large, so that medical personnel could move about easily and medical students, interns, and residents might be able to observe. Doctors and nurses were garbed in gowns, caps, and masks. The spaces were meant to provide a germ-free environment. Especially in well-funded hospitals, the rooms could be imposing monuments to modern medicine.[30] The spaces themselves could be intimidating to the laymen who might enter them, making them feel the power of medical science.

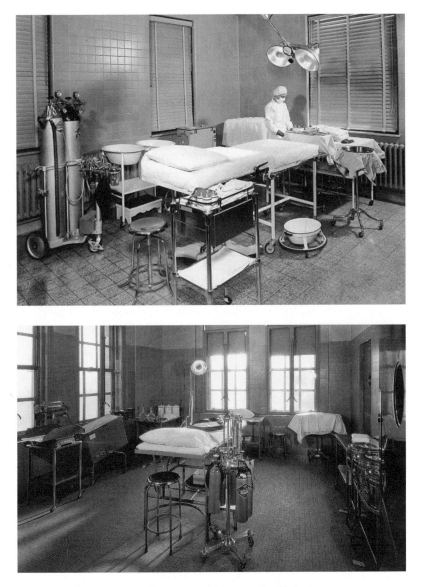

TOP Delivery room at Abbott Hospital, Minneapolis. While the room may not appear to twenty-first-century eyes to be filled with fancy equipment, in the twentieth century it seemed intimidating to laypeople. Note the oxygen tanks and the overhead lights. Nestler & Grover, Minnesota Historical Society. BOTTOM Shiny and bright delivery room at New York Hospital, Cornell Medical Center. Courtesy of Medical Center Archives of NewYork-Presbyterian/Weill Cornell.

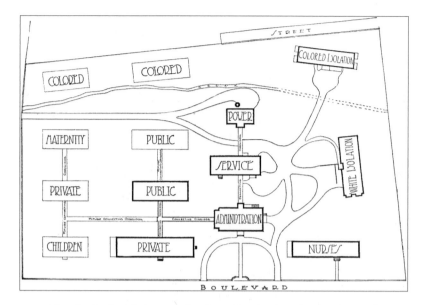

Plot plan for St. Luke's Hospital, Jacksonville, Florida, indicating the racial segregation in the hospital. Edward F. Stevens, *The American Hospital of the Twentieth Century* (New York: F. W. Dodge, 1928), 21.

Racial segregation in many midcentury hospitals meant that black and white women would deliver in separate delivery rooms, which complicated architectural decisions. "Where the service is large enough, separate delivery rooms can be allocated. . . . An ideal arrangement, if it should prove not too expensive, would be to have an auxiliary delivery room for each class of patients on the same floor with the patients' quarters."[31] The plot plan for St. Luke's Hospital in Jacksonville, Florida, provided three wards for "colored" patients, all separated from the rest of the hospital.[32] In segregated hospitals, the most fully equipped delivery rooms were reserved for the white patients. African American parents in segregated institutions rarely, if ever, had the choice of laboring or delivering together.

One of the reasons hospitals excluded the laymen from delivery rooms, in addition to legal and infection considerations, was that the men's presence could interfere with the privacy of other patients. Glass windows and common corridor space did make it likely that the fathers would encounter or be able to see other patients. Even in those cases in which hospitals and physicians were sympathetic to adding the men, not all facilities permitted it. At Kaiser-Walnut Creek in the San Francisco Bay Area, a nurse wrote that labor rooms presented no difficulty because they were private, but the two delivery rooms in her hospital were across from each other and glassed in: "If a woman is delivering in one, the next woman's husband would not be allowed in, to protect the first woman's modesty."[33] Apparently no one thought to put up curtains.[34] Physical facilities remained one of the most stubborn barriers to fathers' participation.

As hospitals remodeled in this midcentury period, they provided more private and safer access to labor and delivery rooms. But since even hospitals with the most rigid policies of exclusion occasionally allowed physician-fathers into their wives' delivery rooms and a few physicians—like Rutherford in Seattle—included individual laymen as they saw fit, it is clear that it was not just the physical spaces and see-through windows that made hospitals pause before including the men. Class and race considerations were also prominent factors guiding hospital policy.

In those cases in which the fathers-to-be were admitted, they, too, were decked out in surgical scrub suits or gowns, masks, shoe covers, and caps. Indeed, seeing their husbands garbed in hospital greens or blues often delighted and amused the birthing women. As one physician noted about one father, "He (as well as his wife) enjoys his medical appearance in surgical gown, cap, and mask."[35]

Very gradually hospitals began to change their policies and practices—or bent existing policies—to allow some men into delivery rooms. Hazel Corbin observed that "doctors, nurses, and administrators are learning to adjust to the husband's active part in helping his wife to relax in the labor room and the delivery room. Often this causes extreme difficulty because hospitals were not built or organized to accommodate the husbands during their wives' labor and delivery."[36] Even though delivery rooms were quite spacious, physicians feared the men might wander about and be in the way. Thus, men's presence was sometimes virtual rather than real. One woman described her delivery with this interesting depiction of her husband's presence: "Bob was standing at the peep hole so we yelled back and forth through the glass and grinned at each other."[37] At another hospital, there seemed to be no problem at all accommodating the husband, who was in the delivery room "with his cameras dangling all over him."[38]

Some hospitals experimented in the 1950s with allowing fathers greater latitude. One physician related how the practice worked at his hospital:

> In the delivery room the prospective father wears a complete gown with cap and mask, of course. He is given a stool to sit on just beside his wife where he can lend his support as needed. An easy exit from the delivery room is always provided, but to date this has never been used. As the baby's presenting part begins to crown, the husband is called to a vantage point where he can clearly see what is taking place. The obstetrician's description of the process is directed to both mother and father to be, and frequently the father is not only a passive observer but lends his vocal interpretation to each step. After the actual delivery the new father returns to his stool beside his wife and their enthusiasm seems to know no bounds.[39]

The physician's observation that the father is not "a passive observer" is important. Not only were some fathers allowed into the delivery rooms, but when there, they may have actively engaged and showed their emotions. A new father said, "Obviously I could not experience Natural Childbirth in the same way in which my wife could as she gave birth, but being with her through the delivery I could share her experience on a feeling level as well as on an intellectual plane. . . . Being present in the delivery room was the culmination of the long time we had shared vital life experiences." He continued,

> I was frankly very curious and wanted to know just what childbirth was actually like. Above all, I had a deep abiding desire to do whatever would make my wife happier and more relaxed. It is difficult to recapture in words the thrill, elation, awe, mystery, and sense of the miraculous I felt all in one wave of emotion when I saw my daughter actually born. I felt immensely close to my wife for having shared this experience with her. My baby was more real and closer to me than she could have been seen through a glass partition hours after

her birth. I felt myself immeasurably fortunate. I did not have to pace the floor for hours, waiting for news.[40]

The men who wanted to abandon the stork clubs for labor and delivery rooms in these years did not see their increased participation as a challenge to physicians' authority. The fathers-to-be at Wesley Memorial Hospital, for example, wrote with great admiration about the medical aids available to their suffering wives in the modern hospital and embraced these benefits. The only thing they wanted to change was to be with their wives to support them and help them through the difficult time. One man, not wanting to offend his wife's physician, blamed God rather than hospital policy for his predicament of not being permitted into the delivery room: "It is horrible not to share in this as we have in everything else but God didn't see fit to arrange it that way."[41]

A nurse delivered two of her own babies separated from her husband and wished things otherwise: "We are still hoping for one thing—that before we have had our last baby, it will be possible for fathers to actually be with their wives to assist and share in the joy of witnessing the birth of their children if they so desire."[42] Another woman separated from her husband obviously thought about him: "My obstetrician praised me for the very nice things I had said about my husband while under the anesthesia."[43] Couples, sharing other intimacies, were ready to experience childbirth together.

During the 1950s, despite a growing number of couples who were beginning to achieve their desire to be together during delivery, the majority of hospitals continued to keep the two apart. A woman who had three babies in 1952, 1954, and 1956 in different hospitals in southern California wrote that "fathers never were admitted to the delivery room and only sometimes into the labor room."[44] Corroborating this observation, attendees of a California conference on maternity practices in 1955 generally agreed that men should not be allowed in the delivery rooms, in line with state law at the time. "The objection to the husband's presence was not that he presented an infection hazard, but rather his presence created administrative problems and responsibilities for the physician and the hospital. The idea that the husband's presence might interfere with the physician's efficiency was also expressed." One conference member recalled an experience during which he had allowed the father into the delivery room—the man fainted, fractured his skull, and later sued the hospital for his injury. Another said, "That is no place for a father from a psychological standpoint. Remember, you have the sex life of this family which follows for many years after; that is a problem. I am also certain that it would not help the physician to have a nervous person standing in back of him."[45]

Physicians voiced quite a bit of worry about fathers' fainting in the delivery room and taking nurses away from their other duties to tend to them. One account in the *New York Times*, lightheartedly discussing such reactions to childbirth, concluded, "As a matter of fact, expectant fathers have fainted in almost every nook and cranny of the maternity pavilion. They have passed out in the waiting rooms, in the corridors, in their wife's room during labor, and in the delivery room in those rare instances when they were granted permission to enter."[46] While some fainting fathers have been reported, the vast majority of men stood up well for the event.

Stories of couples happily together in the delivery room practicing natural childbirth began to appear in popular magazines in the decade of the 1950s. The *Ladies' Home Journal* published one exuberant account written by Margaret Hickey in 1953. Hickey quoted new mother Edith Patten: "I held John's hand; above the surgical mask his eyes were the happiest eyes I have ever seen. Everyone seemed excited and happy—the whole world was a joyous place. . . . And of all the bright sweet moments in my life and John's, I felt that was the best." Hickey reported that one hospital in Seattle "consistently allows papa to be present at delivery" and that others do so "by special request when business is not too brisk. Faced with such requests, the trustees of one hospital held several meetings and decided to cut a window in the delivery-room door so the determined father could at least watch."[47] Specifically connecting the practice to natural childbirth, an article in *Cosmopolitan* publicized that "some doctors . . . even encourage fathers to be in the delivery room."[48]

Fathers' presence in the delivery room during the 1950s was often but not always associated with natural childbirth. Use of caudal anesthesia,

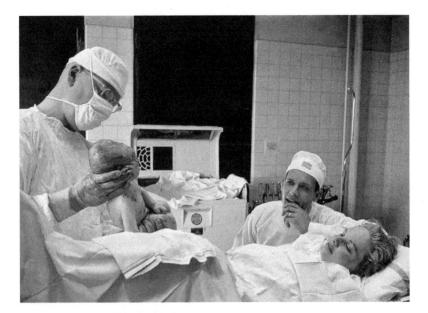

John Stouffer watches with his wife as their baby is born in a hospital delivery room. "A Father Sees His Child Born," *Life*, June 13, 1955, 136–37. Photograph by Burton Glinn. Burton Glinn/Magnum Photos.

which left women awake and relatively pain-free, prompted some hospitals to allow the men to join their wives for both labor and delivery. *Life* ran a photo spread on the birth experience of Mary and John Stouffer at the Virginia Mason Hospital in Seattle in 1955. John summed up the experience, "I feel like I had that baby myself." The caption to one photograph read, "DRESSING HIMSELF in a surgeon's smock, John prepares to enter delivery room. But first he braced himself with a gulp of coffee, a few puffs on a cigarette." For the big double-paged photograph, the caption stated: "JOHN'S MOUTH FALLS OPEN AS, WITH CAREFUL HANDS, THE OBSTETRICIAN LIFTS ONE-SECOND-OLD, 7-POUND 5-OUNCE JOHN ALAN STOUFFER INTO THE WORLD."[49]

Despite this kind of publicity about the joys of couples sharing birth, and even given her fame, actress Julie Harris could not convince her hospital or physician to allow her husband to be with her during her delivery in 1956. She and her husband had triumphed and shared labor together but, Harris told Betty Friedan:

Then suddenly they were lifting me onto a table with wheels; Manning's hand was gone. I begged, but they wouldn't let him go with me to the delivery room. The doctor was holding my hand. The feeling wasn't the same [as her husband's hand]. They were wheeling me into bright white light, lifting me on to another table, strapping my legs down in long white leggings, clamping my feet and hands in stirrups. For the first time in my whole labor I felt helpless and afraid. And then the doctor tried to clamp an ether mask on my face. I was terrified, then angry. They were going to make me miss the climax. I wanted to *be* there when my baby was born. I fought so that when they took the mask off I was still conscious.[50]

Harris's experience of not being permitted to be with her husband was typical for American women during the 1950s. Many hospitals followed the rules when they excluded the men. The Wisconsin Administrative Code, for example, stated very clearly in 1956: "Visitors . . . shall not be admitted to the delivery room or the nursery."[51] Genne's handbook for fathers published in the same year told the men why:

Most hospitals have regulations prohibiting husbands in the delivery room. The reasoning behind them is somewhat like this: . . . The doctors, nurses, and most of all, your wife are very busy. You are not needed and you are apt to be in the way. . . . No man can tell exactly how his autonomic nervous system will react. Many times husbands, big husky ones, too, will faint at the sight of blood. This is especially true when it is someone they love. Since the doctors and nurses already have their hands full, they have no time to be picking husbands up off the floor.[52]

Notwithstanding this advice to stay out of the way, Genne did inform fathers-to-be who read his handbook that the subject of men in the delivery room was contested and that many physicians believed that the men could be helpful to their wives during delivery. He told the men to consult with their wives' physicians, learn the local regulations, and then "co-operate wholeheartedly with the physician you have asked to assume responsibility for your wife and baby."[53]

Men contemplating accompanying their wives into delivery received encouragement in popular magazines. Peter Browne told his story about when he joined his wife in the delivery room. He wrote in *Readers' Digest*, "At that moment I felt fear. I was more scared than I had been when I flew as an air gunner with the Royal Air Force — and I was pretty scared then." He said his legs were shaking as he entered the room, but then, "I saw her wince as a contraction gripped her, and I forgot to be frightened any more. I sat on a stool by her side and took her hand." After the delivery, he continued, "Today I had the most wonderful experience of my life: I saw the birth of my son. . . . All day I have been . . . telling myself how lucky I was to be there. I have a new and deeper admiration for my wife, and I think that perhaps I am a better person for seeing what I saw. God knows I am a humbler one."[54] Browne, who felt all the emotions of "amazement, amusement, tenderness, pride," related that the day contained "the most powerful emotions I have ever known." He wanted to tell every father-to-be: "If you possibly can, do as I did. There is, I know now, nothing to be afraid of — the moment of birth is too wonderful a thing. At such a time your wife needs you as never before. From her suffering comes a miracle, and to witness it will be the greatest privilege you will ever have."[55] Such powerful stories led other men and women to want to share the same experiences.

Robert and Muriel Goldfarb similarly revealed in the popular *Ladies' Home Journal* how important to the birthing woman a husband's presence in delivery could be. Muriel had delivered her first child under the usual midcentury hospital procedures, suffering her long labor and delivery alone and lonely, while her husband waited outside. "I had awakened on the delivery table in an empty, white room. The baby was gone and I was tied to the table." Not wanting to repeat that alienating experience for the birth of their second child, the couple tried to arrange to be together in the delivery room. Informed by their hospital that the board of health "would never permit [Robert] staying in the delivery room," the couple researched the regulations and found there was no such restriction in their county. But the health board said "the hospital would object." People also told them that Robert would view her as "less attractive" after seeing her during delivery. "Would I ever think of her as romantic and pretty again? I wondered, too, though I don't believe I ever admitted it," Bob revealed later. When the time came, they were together. Bob donned a surgical suit, cap, and mask and rushed down the corridor to the delivery room. Muriel said, "Once he came into the delivery room, I felt nothing could happen to me. . . . I was safer or stronger or maybe just more secure with him beside me."[56] And Bob answered all his former doubts: "I know this now. Those few minutes in the delivery room made her more beautiful and made me love her more than ever before. . . . A family is supposed to share everything. . . . This time we were together—the three of us."[57]

Grantly Dick-Read encouraged the men to join their wives in delivery: "I have never seen anything lovelier, or more likely to establish the emotional security of married life than that look which is exchanged between husband and wife when each has just seen their baby born. A father may be nervous at first at the thought of seeing his wife's delivery and his baby's birth, but nearly every father will admit that he resents the role he is usually expected to play—that isolated figure in the hospital corridor."[58]

The Goldfarbs' 1958 story offered a concrete and successful example for those growing numbers of couples who wanted to be together in the delivery room. When women who had recently delivered babies were surveyed about their preferences in a study published the same year, 40 percent said that their experiences would have been more satisfying if hospitals allowed "their husbands in the delivery room where they could share the experience of childbirth together, and where the husband could add moral support." Fred Kartchner concluded his study with the prediction that with more women awake during their deliveries (either because of natural childbirth or because of caudal anesthesia) "there is going to be an increasing demand for the husband to be with the wife."[59] Gladys Denny Shultz, who in the same year wrote the "cruelty" exposé in the *Ladies' Home Journal*, agreed with the woman who said that birthing women should not be shuttled "off to delivery rooms among brusque strangers like sacks of potatoes for the A&P." Rather, Shultz concluded, "if the wife wants her husband in the delivery room—not all women do—he should be permitted to be there. . . . Many mothers who had their husbands with them tell us in lyrical terms of the help this was."[60] Many husbands, she

felt, "instead of a grim, gruesome spectacle," found "a deeply spiritual experience, increasing immeasurably the tenderness they felt for both wife
and new baby." But Shultz had to admit that "for every hospital which
permits a husband to be with his wife through labor and delivery there
are many, many others where he is just barely tolerated and kept strictly
confined to a fathers' room."[61] University Hospital in Minneapolis was
one such hospital where the fathers could not be with their wives in the
delivery room; they could observe the birth through glass from a "viewing
booth" nearby.[62]

With all the publicity, increasing numbers of couples wanted to be
together through labor and delivery. However, the usual scenario at the
end of the 1950s was that even if the man did finesse staying with his
wife throughout labor he was not permitted to follow her to the delivery
room.[63] "Stayed with Carolyn in labor room from 9:30 AM to 5:15 PM.
[She went] into delivery room. . . . [I am] waiting. . . . Nurse informs
me we have a fine baby boy."[64] Policies and practices of exclusion were
only beginning to change as men and birthing women — health care consumers — directly challenged them.

Medical and Nursing Perspectives, 1960s

As the men tried to find ways to enter the delivery room, physicians worried that the men's presence would inhibit their ability to perform well
and would also challenge their authority. One doctor wrote that he was
glad to practice in a military hospital where family members were not
present. He thought doctors who allowed patients' families to participate
in labor and delivery would suffer "a loss of will power and fortitude" at
the hands of these lay intruders.[65]

Physicians remained divided and conflicted about how to respond
when men wanted to enter delivery rooms. Nurse Bonnie Miller recalled:

> I remember that one physician, particular, oh, he just talked and
> talked about he just thought it was totally out of the question. But his
> one partner really thought it would be neat and it just so happened

that when it was going to be instituted the original physician I'm speaking of, was on [call] for the liberal one, for that weekend and the first one [the first patient] came in. All the arrangements had been made with her doctor that the husband was going to be present for the delivery and apparently . . . in the group they had agreed that they would deliver these for each other if they got stuck with one and so, he did do it. And it was beautifully done, beautifully handled. But before and afterwards the physician just carried on, just something terrible.[66]

Miller said that the "big concern was something terrible was going to happen." In one case she remembered, there was a problem during delivery, and the baby did not immediately respond. Miller said, "Of course, he [the father] was seated there by his wife's head and we were working like crazy on that baby. . . . [Finally the baby cried.] We were absolutely, you know, so drained. . . . And the husband had just sat there quietly with his wife the entire time and he looked at me and he said, 'Gee, it takes a long time to get along doesn't it.' And I thought, 'He thinks this is what always happens.' He wasn't aware that there was anything wrong."[67] The story illustrates that men would not necessarily be in the way even in cases of medical stress. But it also provided the kind of story physicians would use to explain why fathers should be excluded.

In Springfield, Massachusetts, doctors in the Wesson Maternity Hospital, feeling under significant pressure from lay groups and their patients to allow husbands at deliveries, adamantly refused to give in: "The practice can constitute a serious potential hazard to the wife's well-being by unstringing the obstetrician or his team."[68] Because of this worry that physicians might not perform well under lay observation, the hospital continued to ask the men to wait for word of the birth while sitting in waiting rooms. In Merrill, Wisconsin, Dr. Betts wanted to be able to allow fathers into the delivery room, but "the other physicians got together and told him he could not do this." Betts left the community because of the restriction on his practice.[69]

As the debates raged at local conferences and medical meetings and in medical journals as well as in popular magazines, parents-to-be showed increasing interest in promoting a place for men in the delivery room. In the New York area, a couple delivering at Cornell University's New York Lying-In Hospital were able to be together for two deliveries in the late 1950s and early 1960s. When they moved to Long Island, they wanted to deliver their third baby, in 1962, at Hempstead Hospital and again be together during delivery. The hospital refused permission and told them it was against the rules of the board of health. When queried, however, the public health physician, Jean E. Schultz, told the couple, "This policy is not a policy of the Health Department but an individual policy established by each hospital Board." Dr. Schultz believed that the only hospital in Nassau County then allowing the practice was North Shore Hospital in Manhasset. She provided the reasoning of the hospitals. First, they feared infection and established "rigid controls" including "exclusion of all persons from these services except those actually giving medical or nursing care." A second reason, she explained, "is the severe nursing shortage." Since the hospitals and their staffs were unfamiliar with the practice, Dr. Schultz did "not foresee an early solution to this problem."[70]

Indeed, physicians continued to worry about what the father's presence would mean for their own autonomy. Dr. Roger Hoag of Berkeley, California, was sensitive about physicians' medical authority and autonomy. Repeating an argument physicians had used earlier, he wrote: "It may be difficult psychologically for the physician to share with the husband the approbation and affection of the patient which has been directed toward the obstetrician at the height of, and following this emotional moment in her life."[71] Another physician, nervous at the thought of the presence of an independent male in the room, put it this way: "The management of complications requires primarily that the physicians not panic in the presence of the husband."[72] Gender thus played a role in these debates and physician concerns. Male physicians could feel intimidated by another man in the room who might be critical of his actions.

Alongside the physicians' concern about loss of authority and their general skepticism, during this transition period many nurses also supported husband exclusion. Accustomed to following routines and procedures without interruption and already feeling overburdened with duties, some nurses found it hard to accommodate the new ways. Bonnie Miller, who specialized in obstetrics beginning in 1958, related how the men would go into the waiting room when their wives went into delivery. "But, eventually, of course we had the fathers present [in delivery] and . . . we were terrified at first." She told one very evocative story:

> We had a couple who had several babies here and she would be taken back to delivery and all of a sudden the husband would be standing there in the delivery room. I happened to be there for both of the deliveries where this happened. I was absolutely horrified, didn't know what to do. Asked him to leave. Tried to be very calm about it. No way. And so, we even mentioned calling security. He just stood there. "My place is at my wife's side." That's the only words that he would speak and then he would say a few words to her. And if you said anything, "My place is at my wife's side." And rather than do anything more with that we'd just let him stay there and we were just stiff during the entire delivery. You know, it was just a terrible thing that this husband was back there witnessing this birth. Did that to us two times. The second time I had forgotten them until just when they got on the delivery table and turned around and there he was and I thought, "oh, no."[73]

Nurse Joan Knudson noted that in 1965 in her hospital, fathers in delivery rooms were much discussed. "They still wouldn't allow them in. . . . I was really surprised when they [ultimately] did that [admit them] because I figured the husbands are going to be fainting right and left . . . passing out or being sick." Actually, when it came to it, however, "husbands have held up very well." She became an advocate for the practice.[74]

An obstetrical nurse who practiced in Madison, Wisconsin, at the same time said that as the practice of husbands coming into delivery rooms increased, "some of the [nurses] thought it was just a terrible idea. . . . They were going to be in the way, and what were we going to do with them."[75] She noted that nurses had some additional work connected to the changes. "We had to have consents signed and . . . father could not go in [to the delivery room] if the physician wasn't there. They couldn't go in if it was going to be a difficult delivery. They had to have the understanding that if something went wrong they would have to leave the room and there were a whole lot of rules and regulations that came from the physician staff on letting fathers into the delivery room. . . . [The physicians] were reluctant in the beginning." Explaining all these regulations to the men fell to the nursing staff: "The one we had probably the most trouble with is if the doctor was not there and they were going to deliver before he could get there. And some of the fathers would get upset with that. . . . There was only one gentleman that really got angry with us about it and I mean he was really, really angry."[76]

Ann Gunderson, an obstetrical nurse at University Hospital in Madison, remembered that during the 1960s fathers were not permitted to be in the delivery room. "We always used to keep the fathers in the hall . . . outside the closed door. . . . We used to let them stand at the door. . . . I think there might have been one or two that we might have let in but only sneaking around. We just didn't allow it. . . . I think most people were afraid of something happening and happening to mama, something being wrong with the baby."[77] At Methodist Hospital in Madison, too, fathers were not permitted to be with their wives, even in cases in which the physician wanted it. As one woman explained about her 1966 delivery, "Dr. Brew explained apologetically that Methodist Hospital had a policy against letting family members into the delivery room (fear they would faint, or something), so this was the one of our births [her husband] missed."[78]

Whatever private worries they had about the possibility of their own authority being challenged by the birthing woman's husband, physicians continued to emphasize safety issues in most public discussions. Primary among them was the question of whether fathers' presence increased the risk of infection. Other issues included the men getting in the way or initiating law suits. Robert Bradley reported on his eight years of experience letting fathers into delivery rooms at Denver's Porter Hospital in 1962, patiently answering in turn all the objections his fellow obstetricians had voiced. Bradley thought the regulations about fathers grew at a time when women were anesthetized for most deliveries, and he believed that the newer trends of conscious natural deliveries should work to overturn those rules. He reported that he included husbands in more than 95 percent of deliveries he attended. To the objection that husbands might get in the way, Bradley answered, "In our experience this is not true. They remain seated at the head of the delivery table on the stool formerly occupied by an anesthetist. They have been instructed not to leave this honorary seat, and do not present an obstacle to the functioning of the attending nurses." To the worries that the men would get sick, faint, or contaminate the area, Bradley responded merely that those things had not happened. Addressing the critics who worried that malpractice suits would increase if husbands were in the room, Bradley wrote, "On the contrary, we feel there is less likelihood of criticism when the husband is included." Bradley argued: "Complications of any conceivable nature can be handled by the obstetrician far more efficiently with a calm cooperative patient." He concluded that the husband is "a proud useful companion, who by his presence elicits peaceful cooperation from his beloved wife in the ennobling act of bearing his child."[79] The layman had a real champion in this physician.

Alongside such medical supporters, fathers-to-be made considerable headway in these midcentury years. In Grand Rapids, Michigan, Dr. Charles Aldridge remembered that he did not allow fathers in the delivery room because he worried about the man "looking over his shoulder," but by 1970 he had completely changed his mind. His hospital experimented with allowing fathers who had been trained in prenatal classes to sit on a stool at the head of the delivery table to watch and talk with their wives. The program was a complete success and led to a more open hospital policy.[80]

Yet practices and physicians' opinions still varied significantly. During a panel discussion of family-centered maternity care in the 1960s, one physician supported the idea but not its immediate implementation. He opined, "The matter of actually having the husband in the delivery room is important, yet I don't think we can accomplish this immediately." But another doctor added, "I think it depends entirely upon why the husbands are in the delivery rooms. If it's somebody who's curious, who just wants to see how a baby is born and what kind of stitches we are going to take and how we are going to do this and do that, I would say he should not be permitted to be present. If he's there for the support of his wife and if she's trying to have the baby by natural childbirth, I can see that completely." The way to ensure that voyeurism was channeled into support was described: "A chair is placed at the head of the table and that's where they sit. That's their place, with their wife, at the head of the table."[81] Another analysis of the situation found that "most New York City hospitals do not permit expectant fathers to be present in the delivery room." As reported in the newspaper, hospitals refused the men because "it adds another person to distract the doctor and the mother-to-be. In large cities, many doctors see very little of the husband and they cannot predict his delivery room behavior."[82]

Stuart Price's experience at Bellin Methodist Hospital in Green Bay, Wisconsin, demonstrated that some individual men were able to sidestep exclusion policies. As an ordained Methodist minister, he had some connections that helped in his effort to be with his wife during delivery. He promised to sit at the head of the table. The physician finally agreed, "if I promised not to tell anyone I had been allowed to be there." The physician did not want too many repeat performances.[83]

Dr. Roger Hoag summed up the variety of medical opinions and physicians' role in the decision:

> For many laymen, and indeed some physicians, labor and delivery is regarded as a somewhat earthy and unaesthetic, if not disgusting experience . . . better left unseen by both the patient and husband, solely in the hands of an experienced obstetrician. . . . I feel strongly that this is a matter that should be left to the final opinion of the attending physician in every case. If I had to vote whether to allow all fathers in the delivery room as a matter of right or unrestrained privilege versus allowing no fathers in the delivery room, I would favor[,] without equivocation, their exclusion. However, I feel there is an area of practice in which physicians should be able to admit to the delivery room selected fathers of selected patients in selected obstetrical situations.[84]

Hoag's choice of language, referring to birth as "disgusting," indicates the emotional power of this subject and how strongly some physicians felt about excluding the father. His repetition of the word "selected" indicated, probably, a bias in favor of educated middle-class men.

Allan Barnes, editor of the *American Journal of Obstetrics and Gynecology*, wrote an article for *Harper's* detailing to a lay audience some of his worries about the safety of inviting fathers' participation. He objected to the way that possible dangers to the baby were being overlooked and felt that concerns about having fathers in delivery took attention away from such risks: "Particularly in the past decade, the gospel of pregnancy and labor as a time of sweetness and light has been so widely preached that the hazards to the embryo [sic] are seldom mentioned. The American woman is likely to be more concerned with whether or not her husband can be in the delivery room than with the fate of her baby."[85] These words, which more than implied that women were not good mothers if they wanted their husbands with them, were not couched in terms to gain support among parents. Physician John Miller reacted negatively to the article, too. He wrote that Barnes "must come to realize that a woman's interest in her husband and her interest in her unborn child are not mutually exclusive interests, but that they are one and the same thing. . . . When 78 percent of our patients are in favor of such a program, it behooves the medical profession and the hospital people to take steps to provide it."[86] Many agreed that parents should have a voice in determining hospital obstetric practices.[87]

Standards issued by the American College of Obstetricians and Gynecologists in 1965 gave voice to the dilemma many physicians felt between meeting consumers' wishes at the same time as adhering to medically generated safety standards. It stated, "The decision as to whether or not a husband may be permitted into the delivery room . . . should rest with the attending physician and be in accordance with the policy and set-up of the particular department and in accordance with local public health regulations. It should be borne in mind that a husband's presence in the delivery room can be hazardous, particularly if an unforeseen emergency arises."[88] Their own understanding of safety concerns determined some physicians' stances.

An incident in a New Jersey hospital that ended in a court of law illustrated how contested practices still were during the 1960s. A man named John O. Keim gained "unauthorized" admission to the delivery room and was subsequently fined $150 "on charges that he acted in a disorderly manner when he refused to leave his wife's side in the delivery room at Plainfield's Muhlenberg Hospital." Keim appealed the conviction, contending "that he had caused no trouble and that he did not know three men, summoned to the delivery room to ask him to leave, were policemen." A nurse gave Keim "surgical garb" while she asked permission for him to enter. When permission was denied and he entered the room anyway, the nurse called the police. Keim "told the court that an earlier pregnancy of his wife ended in miscarriage, that his wife had German measles during the recent pregnancy, and that she was two weeks late in delivering this child."[89] He wanted to be there in case something went wrong again.

Physicians and nurses continued to debate the question throughout the rest of the decade. At one meeting of the American College of Surgeons, an obstetrician from Evansville, Indiana, where a successful family-centered maternity program was in operation, admitted that there were still "two physicians on our staff who refuse to allow husbands in the delivery room under any conditions." The obstetrician thought, "The husband-father can be and is helpful and supportive when he is given the opportunity. Fear, loneliness and panic leave the labor and delivery rooms and are replaced by concern and cheerfulness. The result is less analgesia, and fewer narcotized babies."[90]

Wesson Maternity Hospital in Massachusetts refused to change its exclusionary policies even in the face of significant lay pressure when "some 250 citizens of this area . . . [were] exhorting the [hospital] to allow husbands in the delivery room." The hospital surveyed regional practices and found that 81 percent of hospitals in the area "do not allow husbands in the delivery room." The upshot was "a unanimous confirmation of our hospital rule prohibiting witnessing of delivery by the husband." Physicians in the hospital worried that laymen's presence could "introduce a potential source of infection; result in possible lawsuits from uncomprehended procedures; and cause unfavorable psychologic reactions in the husband."[91] Most women and men across the country in the 1960s still did not have the choice of being together for the delivery of their children.

Some physicians and hospitals permitted the fathers to enter delivery rooms and liked it so much that they even initiated the practice. At Georgetown Hospital in Washington, D.C., in 1968, Donald Sheaffer helped his wife through labor with no plan to enter the delivery room. But when it came time to move her into the delivery room: "They asked me if I wanted to go with her. I must confess, I was caught up in the whole thing. I said yes." He quickly had to sign a consent form saying he would leave immediately in the case of an emergency and if he fainted the hospital was not responsible for any injury. His wife, too, at the height of transition, had to sign a form giving her consent to his presence.[92]

Childbirth educators in the 1960s understood that the efforts to get husbands into delivery rooms echoed earlier home childbirth experiences, where familiar faces surrounded the birthing woman, and they worked consciously to return to some of those practices. The difference was that in the hospital setting, instead of all the women's female friends and relatives, only the father would be included in hospital deliveries, his new role taking the place of women's traditional roles.

Hospital Topics in 1966 published a series of four articles on the subject of fathers in the delivery room. Despite the reality that most hospitals did not yet allow men in delivery rooms, three articles favored the practice and one dissented. The articles provide insight into the depth and breadth of the discussions at that time. One favorable article came from Virginia Mason Hospital in Seattle, where almost 90 percent of fathers participated in delivery. Robert Rutherford, who started the practice at his hospital, championed the cause and proclaimed its successes.[93] John Miller insisted in the second article, "We must restore some of the joy that home, familiar surroundings, loved ones and compassionate neighbors used to provide." He felt that incorporating husbands into the childbirth experience was the key to making hospital practice more family-friendly. He continued,

> It takes a husband about a minute to change into a scrub suit when his wife is ready for the delivery room. He will gladly help move her onto the gurney and proudly push the gurney to the delivery room. As he puts on cap and mask he will inevitably ask his wife how he

looks and she will almost certainly make a joking reference to Ben
Casey and thus smiling, perhaps through their tears, they approach
together the moment of bliss for which the last nine months has
been a prelude. When we are oriented to the joy of childbirth it is
unthinkable that at this moment we will shut the door on this man.[94]

Miller, a physician, portrayed the situation from the layman's point of
view: "He too has lived through nine months of pregnancy. . . . At the end
of a long arduous labor he is often as weary and drawn and concerned as
is his wife. If he then is forbidden to share the moment which transfigures
her—which makes it possible for her to start talking about next time—
but rather is relegated to a waiting room and further searing anxiety, his
reaction is very likely to be 'never again.'" Miller also wrote from his own
medical perspective: "The decorum of husbands in the delivery room is
above reproach. They are of tremendous comfort and reassurance to their
wives and frankly are often helpful when the service is busy or when personnel is spread too thin. . . . I write with conviction gained from having
participated in or having observed thousands of husband-attended deliveries in California."[95]

The third article, which also favored husbands' participation, was
more guarded in its support and perhaps more typical of the majority of
physicians in the mid-1960s. Carl Goetsch thought that husbands could
be helpful but that the conditions under which they enter the delivery
room should be carefully circumscribed. First, he wrote, "the physical
set-up of the delivery suite should be appropriate. Delivery rooms should
be isolated one from another in such a way that the privacy of a patient
in one delivery room is not violated by the presence of a husband in another." Next, he felt that "it must be made very clear that the presence of
the husband in the delivery room is a privilege to be granted, and not a
right to be demanded." He did not approve of husbands wanting to satisfy
"idle curiosity" and thought physicians must "want the father's presence
and find it comfortable."[96]

The series included one article against admitting fathers written by
California physician John H. Morton. He voiced strong medical opposition to letting men anywhere near the delivery room:

Along with the vast majority of obstetricians, we are opposed to the admission of non-medical people, including fathers, to the delivery room—which is an operating room. The day we are born is the most dangerous one of our lives. Everyone in the delivery room must have a definite duty to perform and do it as well as he can. Anything or anybody who might divert attention from the mother and baby is intolerable. This room is no place for sentimentality, sightseeing, sex gratification, or salesmanship. We believe in a strictly professional approach without any nonsense, and have ever since we saw our first mother die on the table.[97]

Among Morton's objections to the practice were his worries about the father's emotive state: "It is an emotional time for the father, and he may be having problems adjusting to fatherhood because of increased responsibility, latent homosexuality, threatened dependency relationships or unresolved parental attitudes." Morton also believed that "intimacy between two human beings should have limits. . . . A girl simply is not at her romantic best in a delivery room. . . . Delivery is a messy business at best. . . . We must set limits to intimacy in the interests of those for whom we care." Morton concluded that "visitors to the delivery room [should] be barred by formal statement in the bylaws of the hospital and its staff."[98] Morton represented a number of physicians who remained adamantly against fathers entering delivery rooms under any circumstances.

Although barring fathers from delivery became a losing battle, there were many physicians who echoed Morton's concern that attending women in childbirth was not a proper "masculine" activity[99] and that the men only wanted to be there for voyeuristic reasons.[100] Dr. George Schaefer of Cornell University Medical College believed, "I don't think this should be a commonplace event. . . . On the whole, it is not a show to watch."[101] Dr. Robert Stewart felt even more strongly: "The male attitude to the female genitalia is one of unconscious hostility. To him the charm of a woman is her mystery. It is inconceivable that a normal male watching the delivery of his wife could experience anything but revulsion at the vision of these genitalia under the worst and filthiest conditions." He figured only "sadistic instincts" of the woman or masochistic ones in the

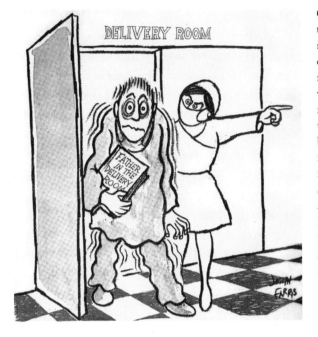

Cartoon showing that fathers may not be welcome in delivery rooms nor may they tolerate it well. Despite such messages showing their presence to be contested, many men were ready for the experience. *Science Digest*, August 1969, 24. Reprinted with permission of Joseph Farris and Science Digest.

man could lead them to want to be together at delivery. He continued, "As the charm of woman is in her mystery, it is inconceivable that a wife will maintain her sexual prestige after her husband witnessed the expulsion of a baby—a negligee will never hide this apparition."[102] In Madison, Wisconsin, a physician tried to dissuade Dan Wendland from going into the delivery room with his wife in 1967. "Dr. Baker was incredulous wondering why I would want to be part of this process, comparing it in these memorable terms: 'You wouldn't want to be in the same room while your wife was defecating, would you?'"[103] Many physicians, worrying that watching delivery would alienate the man from his wife's body and decrease his sexual interest in her, simply thought the men should stay out.

Men's Responses and Changing Policies

One reason that birthing women felt they needed their husbands to follow them from labor rooms to delivery rooms in the 1960s was that mothers themselves had to make the move from one room to the other at the "transition" point in labor—the most difficult part—when the cervix dilates from seven to ten centimeters and the urge to push becomes urgent and strong. The policy of moving the woman during these sensitive moments was built on ideas about the danger of infection and the possibility that surgical intervention (such as episiotomy, forceps, or cesarean section) might become necessary during delivery. While the woman could go through the whole of the first stage of labor—when the cervix was slowly effacing and dilating—in an unequipped labor room, physicians felt it was necessary for the birth of the baby to move her to a delivery room that was equipped for a surgical emergency. The medical rationale that made the transfer necessary was described in a book on hospital design: "The mother is moved from the labor room into delivery, sometimes via the prep room, on a stretcher or in the labor bed, which may be a special bed like a recovery room bed (a comfortable stretcher with side rails). When it is time for delivery, the procedure is much like that in surgery. The obstetrician and his aides scrub and don masks, gowns, and gloves, as does also the scrub nurse. Anesthetic may be given. Aseptic techniques are the same as for surgery."[104]

Those fathers-to-be who had been in the labor rooms understood the tension of the moments of transition, and many voiced their desire to stay with their wives through delivery. They were encouraged by the increasing number of articles in popular magazines in the 1960s that touted the benefits to the family. *Redbook*, for example, helped to increase interest in and demand for men to attend their wives in delivery with a story that championed family-centered childbirth; it quoted one father who wrote a letter to the hospital after accompanying his wife through labor and delivery: "I think of myself as a cold-blooded person. Maybe I am, but at that moment [in the delivery room], while the doctor was holding our baby, the cord still attached to my wife, I felt tears rolling down my face for the first time since we were married. I felt closer to my wife than ever before. The birth of this child has touched me as nothing before ever has and as nothing will again until we experience the birth of our next baby together. The whole delivery was beautiful beyond words. Not pretty, but beautiful in the sense of a God-given, natural beauty."[105] The *Redbook* authors sided with the young parents who wanted to be together.

Fathers in the 1960s who shared their stories publicly urged other men to experience birth themselves. Walden Crabtree, for example, admitted that the delivery room once had "a shroud of mystery cloaked about it. No more now; I've been there." He watched the birth of his fourth child: "I saw him pushing and poking to free himself from his maternal cocoon; I almost felt him struggling to thrust himself past the ties that had held him too long already; I saw him manifest, with pokes and shoves, then finally with an explosive, exuberant cry, his impatience at being immured too long and denied from beginning this job of living that would go on and on." Crabtree went on to say: "Perhaps the most cherished experience the father receives as he stands by the side of his wife is a greater understanding of her, a deeper knowledge of what pain she cheerfully, even joyfully undergoes to bring his children into the world. . . . Though immersed in pain, she stifles every complaint. Here lies a woman, bathed in pain, that some call excruciating, cheerfully laboring to give a part of her body that will be your son."[106]

With such compelling personal commentary, there was a lot of pressure on doctors and hospitals to expand the practice. The men who wanted to enter delivery rooms were supported by lay organizations such as the International Childbirth Education Association (ICEA) and increasingly by physicians who came to see the practice as beneficial to all. Many physicians, in fact, took the lead in inviting the men in. In Dodgeville, Wisconsin, in 1963, a physician invited a father-to-be into the delivery room. It was the couple's eighth child, but the man had never before been in the delivery room. Giving truth to the often fabled account of men's vulnerability, Dr. David R. Downs recalled, "The baby came with no trouble, and just as I was delivering the placenta, I looked up and asked him if this was his first time in the delivery room, and he didn't answer me, but let out a low moan and slid slowly off his stool at the head of the table and onto the floor." The physician said this was the only time a man had fainted in hundreds of husbands attending in delivery. Downs included the laymen because it "seemed the right thing to do, considering that they were there at the beginning of the pregnancy (hopefully), so logically they should be there at the end. It also seemed a good way for fathers to know exactly what their wives went through to bring new life into the world, and maybe would facilitate their commitment." The physician claimed that he never felt pressure from the fathers; rather, he "asked them if they would like to be with their wives, and about 99% did." The high percentage might have reflected that couples chose Downs to attend them in part because they knew he would welcome the men. The mothers were very appreciative to have the support of their husbands and told him so.[107]

The ICEA issued a major report on the subject of fathers in the delivery room in 1965.[108] The report reflected the organization's commitment to ·family-centered maternity care and to fostering both nuclear families and physicians' autonomy. While strongly committed to couples sharing the experience, the organization chose not to pose a direct challenge to medical and hospital authority. It explicitly agreed with statements by doctors that their own discretion should determine whether husbands could be present in the delivery room. The report included opinions and reflections from physicians, hospital administrators, and nurses, along with a list of hospitals that permitted husbands and some experiences gleaned from the practice. It provides a revealing snapshot of the situation at mid-decade, just as rules and regulations were changing.

The ICEA believed that "the husband has a most important place at the birth of his child when the physician is practicing family centered obstetrics and feels the husband is properly prepared."[109] It happily reported a big increase in the practice across the country. At the Alta Bates Community Hospital in Berkeley, California, husbands had been included for four and one-half months "without any problems—such as fainting, illness, or interference with obstetrical procedures."[110] Only 20 percent of physicians at that hospital refused to include the fathers. Other hospitals reported similarly positive experiences, including institutions as diverse as Yale's Grace–New Haven Hospital and the Children's Clinic of Black Mountain, North Carolina. The report quoted Robert Bradley, whose experience with fathers attending delivery then spanned eleven years, who said, "The value of such [policy] has been shown in the decrease in medication, the healthier babies, shortening of labor, and the emotional and psychological benefit of making birth a joyful spiritual experience."[111] Similarly, Michael Newton, chair of the OB-GYN department at the University of Mississippi School of Medicine, representing a part of the country where the smallest number of hospitals allowed the husbands entry, opined, "I feel that a husband should be allowed to stay with his wife during delivery if he has had some education for this event in the form of classes or adequate reading and if both he and his wife wish him to be there. Under these circumstances I have found husbands to be a real help to their wives and to myself as the obstetrician."[112] Prenatal education could teach the men what to expect, and nuclear families could be strengthened.

The 1965 ICEA report quoted many hospital administrators who made statements of cautious support for the practice of allowing the men into delivery rooms, always with the proviso that the decision was up to the physicians in each individual case. Sister M. Clarice, the maternity supervisor at St. Alexius Hospital in Bismarck, North Dakota, said that her hospital had allowed family-centered maternity plans since January 1962, under very stringent regulations, including that "permission from the physician must be written on the mother's chart. . . . Arrangements must be made between physician and patient before admission to the hospital. . . . The father must remain seated at the head of the table." The actual practice, she said, was rare. Her hospital had only about one request for this each month, or about one in every ninety-seven deliveries.[113] With similar regulations and reporting relatively new experiences, administrators from Denver; St. Louis; Dayton, Ohio; Cleveland; St. Paul; and Dallas made it clear that hospital practices were indeed changing, however slowly.

The 1965 report listed hospitals that allowed fathers in the delivery room under specified conditions, spanning eighteen states and the District of Columbia.[114] In California, physicians favoring the practice convinced the state's hospital advisory board and the state department of health to lift the state's prohibition of visitors in the delivery room to allow husbands in. A formal ruling on the issue came in February 1964, interpreting the term "visitor" to apply to any person who had no function to perform. The ruling was that the exclusion of visitors "does not preclude the presence in the delivery room of a trained participating husband provided that his presence is authorized by the attending physician, the prospective mother, and the hospital concerned."[115] Prenatal education moved the layman from the position of untrained visitor to someone with a role to play.

In 1967 the Illinois Hospital Licensing Act similarly allowed husbands to attend their wives in delivery rooms, with the consent of the birthing woman, her physician, and the hospital.[116] Such changes in the laws might have hastened fathers' entrance into the nation's delivery rooms, but progress was still slow and individual. In these years laws and court rulings established that a father's presence in the delivery room was a privilege to be allowed by physicians or by hospital policy, but definitely not to be considered the couples' right.[117]

An account by a physician who tried to insert fathers into the delivery rooms in his hospital revealed another dimension of the battle during the 1960s. John Miller "began routinely inviting husbands to accompany their wives to the delivery room" when he was in his last year of residency training at the University of California. When he entered private practice, he continued to do so. For nearly thirteen years, "this altogether pleasant policy continued and I was blissfully unaware that trouble was brewing." His life, he said, was "tranquil," although he was not successful in his candidacy for the San Francisco Gynecological Society. "Then February 6, 1963 arrived, a day I think I will remember as vividly as Pearl Harbor day. Before that day passed a set of regulations was propounded at the hospital to which I had given my entire effort and loyalty for many years, which among other things forbade the presence of fathers in the delivery room."[118]

Miller fought the regulation, with the help of the ICEA and other physicians, until the attorney general's 1964 ruling allowed the practice again. He argued, "We are servants. We serve people. People are different. Our job is not to judge them, to say you are OK because you see things my way and you are crazy because you don't." He felt it was "an act of unspeakable cruelty to tear [the couple] apart in a crisis like childbearing. It makes no more sense than dragging a husband in who really doesn't want to be there." Miller did not think it necessary to exclude the husband even if something went wrong. "If a husband sees what is going on, realizes why one must resort to forceps or whatever; if he sees clearly that the [baby] which is deformed came from his wife's womb and that it's not the doctor's fault; not only does he understand and save long difficult anguished explanations, but also he is in a position to comfort his wife." Miller concluded that not only is the man's presence better for his wife but "it is infinitely better for the husband. He is at this moment supremely the head of the household, caring for and comforting his wife in her finest hour, proud of her and proud of the care he has enlisted for her help. . . . Thus the husband is given a manly place in this happy hospital event."[119] Evoking the characteristics of masculine authority and strength emphasized the point.

At Cornell's New York Lying-In Hospital, couples could arrange to be together during both labor and delivery in 1963, when Jane Kavanau had her first baby. Her husband was with her throughout labor, and she was "extremely pleased" to have him with her during delivery. But when the couple had their next child, in 1966, he stayed with her through labor but chose not to go with her into the delivery room. "I was surprised that Joe didn't want to come with me but I felt all along that it had to be his decision and it was okay with me."[120] Having the choice was the crucial issue, but not all men would choose to be there.

Robert Bradley pointed out that popular support of husbands had already led to significant increases in the practice of allowing the men to join their wives in the delivery room. He told the story of a Portland, Oregon, bus driver who "refused to be confined to the 'immature nursery,' as he labeled the fathers' waiting room. He went to civil court to get permission to be with his wife at the birth of their child . . . [and] received applause and a standing ovation from the courtroom crowd after he had explained his reasoning." Bradley thought anesthetized women and cigarette-smoking fathers waiting in their own room "present an old-fashioned picture that is obsolete in our more advanced hospitals."[121]

Couples who were able to be together waxed eloquent in support of the practice. One woman told an interviewer, "The *presence* of my husband made me feel like a person, or a personality whereas if I had just been with the doctors I would've been just another body having a baby." Another woman said, "The whole thing, both of us have said, this was probably the most thrilling experience of our lives."[122] Men's responses in concurrence were even stronger. One man wrote, "The experience in the delivery room was for me . . . a full fifteen minutes + [plus] of intense peak-experience. Slowly I began to feel a kind of holiness about all of us there, performing an ageless human drama, a grand ritual of life. . . . [I experienced] intensities of joy and excitement that I cannot possibly adequately describe them . . . a sense of profound participation in a profound mystery."[123] Gerry F. wrote to Elisabeth Bing about the immediate aftermath of delivery: "They left us alone for a time. We looked at our son. He was so beautiful. I felt a sense of ecstasy. And a love and warmth for Sharon that was thick and palpable and alive. In my head I kept seeing the birth, the body of my son emerging from Sharon's body. I didn't want to lose that image ever. The colors. His crying. Sharon's sounds of joy. We kissed and kissed again and looked at our son. What a woman, what a woman she is, I thought. And she is my wife and she loves me."[124]

The practice of husbands entering delivery rooms became increasingly accepted by physicians and hospitals, yet it was far from universal in the 1960s. One study found that 61 percent of the 162 husbands whose wives were having their first babies "had no desire to be present, even in support of their wives," and 58 percent of the 286 husbands of wives who had previously had a child also "were not interested in being in the delivery room."[125] In Colorado, hospitals worried that labor coaches could create problems "not the least of which is their legal rights and privileges on the obstetrical service of the hospital. . . . [They can create] liability problems." Calling such people "trespassers in the delivery room," a nurse warned hospitals to be "sufficiently alert to the delivery room 'traffic' to be certain that the highest quality of service is maintained. . . . Hospitals would be well advised to put the legal damper on efforts [to let labor coaches into the room]."[126]

St. Mary's Hospital in Grand Rapids, Michigan, began a "trial program" in 1968 to include fathers in delivery if physician, patient, and husband wanted it.

The following routine has been established: . . . The father is not brought into the delivery room usually until after the mother has been prepared and draped; and often after a pericervical block has

been administered. He sits on the stool at the head of the table. . . .
He is given some simple instructions regarding watching in the mirror and how he might communicate with his wife by word or touch
without contaminating the field. It is important to explain to him
that he may excuse himself any time he wishes. Verbal support to
both father and mother is an important part of the delivery room
atmosphere. . . . Immediately after birth the baby is shown to both
parents. Then, before the episiotomy repair, the father is asked if he
would like to leave, — 'to make a phone call' or — 'to fill out the questionnaire.' At this point, the need for him to stay with his wife has
passed and he is usually perfectly willing to go.[127]

In the first year, 150 couples participated, a figure that accounted for
9 percent of the total deliveries in that hospital; in the second year, the
number of participating couples increased, accounting for 15 percent of
that year's deliveries.[128]

In Wisconsin, hospital codes banned all visitors, including husbands,
from delivery rooms until 1960 but thereafter allowed hospitals to set
their own visiting rules.[129] As the codes changed, increasing numbers of
physicians joined the debate on the fathers' side. In Madison, Wisconsin,
physicians in the main community hospital pressed to allow fathers into
the delivery room. The young Dr. James Lindblade, arriving in Madison
in 1969, motivated by his patients and also by his own experiences during his wife's delivery when he was excluded, worked with a committee
of physicians and nurses at his hospital to write policy that would allow
fathers into the rooms. Lindblade remembered that the policy change
went through channels rather easily by 1971.[130]

A nurse who worked at St. Mary's Hospital in Madison said that when
the men were admitted "it was not a real relaxed atmosphere. . . . It was
'Get the white scrubs on and wait down the hall and when the doctor says
you can come in, you can come in and if he says leave, you leave,' and you
had the smelling salts ready for anybody that was going to faint. . . . Everybody was so afraid that he was going to upchuck, or contaminate somebody, or something, or breathe on the wrong object."[131] Routines were
established whereby physicians maintained the authority they wanted or

needed and nurses had their own specified roles to play. Fathers in the delivery room during these years were kept in a carefully defined place.

Nonetheless, men found the experience exhilarating. Steven Barney recalled his experience at Madison General Hospital in 1969, when he accompanied his wife through labor and delivery. He described what happened when his wife was ready to go to the delivery room: "At this point the doctor makes the final decision about Father. Everything looked dandy for the Barneys and the doctor gave the OK. . . . Dressed from head to foot in green, I rushed to the hallway that enters the delivery room area. I was told to wait until Karen was properly prepared. In a moment the doctor called out, 'Father can come in now.' At the head of the delivery table was a chair. . . . From this position I could talk to Karen and look up into the same mirror through which she would watch the delivery."[132] He was so thrilled with the whole process that he wrote up the story for his newspaper, the *Wisconsin State Journal*.

Many happy new fathers corroborated the positive aspects of the experience. John Roberts stayed with his wife throughout labor and delivery at the Wilmington, Delaware, Medical Center in 1969. He publicized his reactions:

> The impact on me of that day was tremendous. For one thing, I came out of the delivery room knowing why the word labor is used to describe bearing a child. It is hard work. I don't think any man can come near appreciating just how hard, unless he watches his wife deliver their child. . . . The second main revelation for me was in the significance of this event in Julie's life. This, too, is something I don't think most men can fully appreciate unless they witness the miracle of childbirth. I can't imagine anything more marvelous than the whole sequence of growing and bearing a child.

Roberts concluded, "When the moment of birth came, it was Julie who did it. I was a bystander—no more. But that was enough. And never again will I laugh to myself condescendingly when two mothers start talking about their childbirth experiences. Instead, I'll just try to join the conversation."[133] Demonstrating that paying African American couples now had access to shared delivery, entertainer Oscar Brown Jr. witnessed the birth of his daughter in 1969 and told *Jet* magazine, "It was a gas. It was a great spectacle. . . . It was like a great big beautiful explosion. Imagine it. Here comes somebody, life, from nothing. And we did it. The whole thing was larger than life."[134]

Physicians and hospitals felt pressure from their women patients and from natural childbirth groups to be more flexible in their practices and to let married couples experience delivery together. They also felt it very pointedly from their patients' husbands. Fathers-to-be did not have their own organized movement, but they met one another in prenatal classes and also got strength from connecting to other men through published writings. Individually men worked in their own communities, with their wives and their wives' doctors, and through local hospitals and childbirth educators to bring about changes. They wanted to be with their wives to support them through the difficult time of delivery; they also came to experience childbirth as a rewarding time for themselves. The male voices ultimately became a chorus and, in unison with women and childbirth education groups, were effective in cracking open delivery room doors. These men did not defy physicians' authority; they were the same men who repeatedly praised the doctors and their medical acumen. The delivery room opened to laymen because of pressures that were grounded in support for the nuclear family and respect for medicine. Thus, the conflict was waged without challenging basic cultural values and institutions. By 1970, men's presence in hospital delivery rooms was not yet routine, but it was no longer remarkable.

7 * WE DID IT

Together in Delivery and Birthing Rooms

In 1973, Representative Martha Wright Griffiths (D-MI, 1955–74) introduced a bill in the U.S. Congress to allow biological fathers to attend the
birth of their children. Congressional attention to the subject indicated
that fathers attending the birth of their children had become an issue of
national importance but was not yet a common reality. By the middle of
the 1980s, the contentiousness of the topic finally resolved into a new
standard practice in American hospitals. The new practice evolved with
the help of various court cases, the women's movement, and childbirth
reformers — including significant continuing active participation by the
fathers. By the mid-1980s, most hospitals in the United States welcomed
fathers into delivery rooms, and many actually pressured the men to attend the momentous event.

As hospital practices evolved to allow fathers to participate more
closely in the births of their children, cultural depictions mirrored the
changing experience. The popular television show *All in the Family* addressed Americans' growing interest in natural childbirth and men's place
with their wives during labor and delivery. For five years during the 1970s,

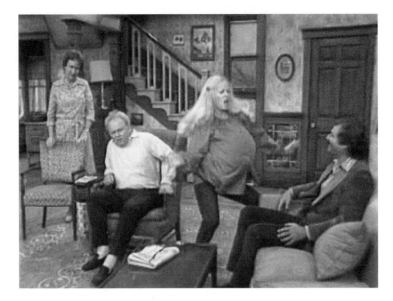

Archie Bunker has a conversation with his daughter, Gloria, and son-in-law, Mike,
telling them he thinks laymen do not belong in the delivery room. When Mike
seems to agree, Gloria protests. *All in the Family*, "Mike's Pains," October 6, 1975.
All in the Family, © 1971, 2008 ELP Communications, Sony Pictures Television.

the show was the top-ranked television series. It dealt with timely and
controversial issues including race, homosexuality, and women's liberation. In an episode titled "Mike's Pains," which aired on October 6, 1975,
liberal son-in-law Mike Stivic, usually pitted against conservative Archie
Bunker, this time faced his own traditional bent. His wife, Gloria (Archie's
daughter), was pregnant and planning a natural childbirth. Archie had a
conversation with the young couple:

ARCHIE: I understand that fathers are not supposed to be in the
   delivery room! Jesus, even doctors are not supposed to be in
   there. That's why they wear those masks.
GLORIA: Daddy, you're being very silly. Michael's looking forward
   to this, aren't you honey?
MIKE: Right.
ARCHIE: I'm warning you, you'll pass out in there. Did you ever
   see them snip an umbiblical [sic] cord?

GLORIA: Would you stop trying to scare him. Michael can't wait
   for the baby to be born can you?

MIKE: Right.

ARCHIE: Well you two are crazy. . . . The whole world is going
   to hell in a bucket.

MIKE: Ah, well, to be perfectly honest with you, I, uh, I never.
   I don't know how I'm going to react, I've never been in a
   delivery room before.

GLORIA: Neither have I!

MIKE: Yeah, but you'll be there for a reason, me I'll just be standin'
   around getting in everybody's way.

ARCHIE: Get in the way in there, and you're liable to lose an organ
   or something. . . .

MIKE: . . . To tell you the truth, I don't think I can be in the room
   when you deliver.

GLORIA: You didn't mind being in the room with me when you
   placed the order! Now you want to back out.[1]

As it did with other pressing social issues of the period, *All in the Family*
faced fathers' fears and ambivalences about an increasingly popular
middle-class American trend. The show's message was that men should
overcome their fears for their wives' sake.[2]

Practices Still in Flux

A 1970 survey of California hospitals by county revealed how varied practices were at the beginning of the decade. In twenty-two hospitals in two
counties, for example, five did not allow husbands at all; one allowed
husbands to watch the delivery through a window; and three had policies
that allowed husbands in only with special permission. Another five hospitals routinely allowed fathers into delivery, while five more said it was
becoming a more frequent occurrence. The remaining three allowed it
occasionally. Many hospitals apparently did not encourage the fathers to
attend but also did not fight them when they insisted; the Bay Area Chapter of the American Society for Psychoprophylaxis in Obstetrics noted in

1970: "Policies are changing with demand." French Hospital in San Francisco, trying to discourage couples from choosing home births in order to be together, had the most liberal policy: "Husbands are allowed to be with their wives from start to finish . . . are allowed to take photographs at will, and to tape record the delivery if they wish."[3]

Individual California hospitals were gradually changing their policies and admitting the men. Earl Withycombe, who had been made to sit in the lobby during his wife's first birth in 1969, in 1971 was welcomed into the delivery room in a small town in California. Withycombe wrote, "[The doctor] outfitted me with a hairnet, mask, and drape, and asked if I had observed a birth before. . . . He positioned me behind his right shoulder as he sat facing the birth canal, and gave me and Leslie a running dialogue as the baby was born. . . . I watched in awe at close range as our second daughter . . . was born. . . . The doctor . . . handed her to me with a big grin. . . . I walked to the side of her gurney and handed the baby to Leslie." Withycombe concluded that his "experience as a father was vastly enriched by this opportunity."[4]

Tom Clark wrote about his experiences at the Kaiser Foundation Hospital in Oakland. During the delivery of his first child, he helped push his wife's gurney down the hall as far as the swinging doors into the delivery room. "As she is wheeled through[,]the doors close behind her and tears well up in my eyes. I want so much to stay with her, to help her, to see my child born. For a moment I am dizzy with rage and despair; I feel like destroying the entire hospital in a fury of vengeance for denying my right to see my child born."[5] Things were different for him during his wife's second birth. He entered the delivery room, uninvited, and "a nurse spies me and demands shrilly, 'Who are you???'" He managed to stay, nonetheless, and wrote about it:

> Never having been in a delivery room before, I am somewhat disoriented by all the glitter of stainless steel, bright lights, and gleaming Buck Rogers equipment. Are we going to the moon or is my wife having a baby? . . . I feel ecstatic to be at Jo's side, but it's hard to believe that I am actually witnessing the birth of our child. The event is at once entirely natural and completely improbable. . . . I wipe her

brow . . . and marvel at the beauty of the whole experience. . . . As though in a dream I watch the head of my child emerging from the womb . . . beautiful because he is ours. . . . I feel very peaceful and satisfied—the whole experience has been good, and now there is a sense of completeness not present [during the first delivery].[6]

In Madison, Wisconsin, having made the leap to allowing husbands in the delivery room, hospital administrators were reluctant to go any further. Dr. Gloria Sarto remembered that she met with Lamaze instructors and thought the method was "logical," and so she delivered her patients who wanted to use the method and allowed the husband to be present: "I just did it." But in the early 1970s, caring for a pregnant woman whose husband was a truck driver and frequently out of town, Sarto agreed to allow the woman's female friend, who had also taken the prenatal classes, to coach the birthing woman through delivery. The day following the delivery Sarto received a letter from the chief of staff of the hospital revoking her hospital privileges for this breach of acceptable behavior. Only the birthing woman's husband was permitted to be there. In time, the issue was sorted out, and Sarto went on delivering babies in the hospital; the story provides insight into the power of the marriage bond inherent in policies that admitted laymen.[7]

Many men in 1971 still had to remain outside. In Waukesha, Wisconsin, Jean Truesdale delivered her second child without her husband despite their wishes to be together. The couple had trained in Lamaze, but their obstetrician "did not allow fathers in the delivery room because he'd once allowed a veterinarian friend in and the man fainted at a critical moment, gashing his head. We argued that my husband had had training that his friend hadn't had but of no avail. . . . My husband had to stay out."[8] Other physicians in the same hospital allowed men to attend. Practices were changing, slowly, one physician at a time.

The men who were included in their wives' deliveries in this period wrote poignantly about how much the experience meant to them. Alvin Berndt, for example, enjoyed the couple's first birth in 1970 at University Hospital in Madison, Wisconsin, and proudly took a photograph of his son when he was twenty seconds old. In 1973, at a different Madison hos-

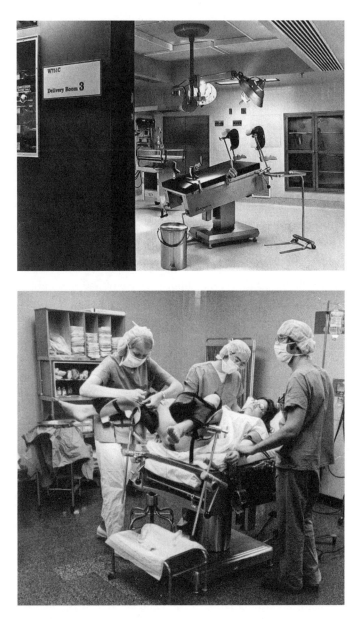

TOP A late twentieth-century delivery room, showing delivery table with stirrups in place, lights, and updated equipment, Medical College of Georgia Hospitals and Clinics, Augusta, Georgia. Reprinted with permission of Ross Planning Associated, *Perspectives in Perinatal and Pediatric Design* (Columbus, Ohio: Ross Products Division, Abbott Laboratories, © 1988). BOTTOM Woman being positioned for delivery with her legs in stirrups and her husband standing by to help. © Suzanne Arms.

pital, Berndt participated more directly. "Our daughter had to be rotated in the womb, and I applied muscle relaxant gas to Pam via a small tank and mouthpiece. This was incredibly intense for me, but again, the ability to actually do something useful helped keep my mind focused on that activity and not on any fear of birthing problems." Thirty-five years later, he remembered that, even with his Lamaze training, "I was in a daze during and after the birth[s]. Even today the exhilaration of that time in the delivery room and the humility I felt seeing what my wife went through remains with me and will, I expect, forever."[9]

Some hospitals made the decision to allow fathers in delivery rooms out of economic necessity. Madison General Hospital in Wisconsin, for example, opened the delivery room to fathers after St. Catherine's Hospital in Kenosha and St. Joseph's Hospital in Milwaukee already allowed it. One nurse believed this came about because of fear of competition.[10] Childbirth educator Sandra Eiseman, who began to teach Lamaze pre-natal classes in Madison in 1967, thought competition with Columbus Community Hospital, which was thirty miles away and had a flexible policy about laymen, encouraged Madison hospitals to permit the fathers to be in the delivery rooms. Although not many Madison women traveled to Columbus to deliver, Eiseman herself did in 1968.[11]

By 1975, fathers' presence in Madison delivery rooms had become commonplace but not yet universal. Alice Robbin described her delivery at Madison General Hospital: "Joel was part of everything that happened. What I remember most about the delivery room was how packed it was with people. Doctors, nurses, residents, nursing students. This is after all a university teaching hospital. Joel was there, looking over everyone's shoulders, and very excited." She still remembered "his running up and down the delivery room yelling excitedly, 'This is the greatest thing that has ever happened!'"[12] But another man in the same hospital, who was able to be with his wife in labor in 1969 and again in 1975, "was ushered out to the waiting room" when she entered the delivery room. He felt he had been treated badly: "It seemed to me that the doctor thought my involvement was completed 9 months before the births." His memory of both births was "of major trauma for my wife and for me."[13]

In 1975, the International Childbirth Education Association (ICEA) repeated its study of ten years earlier and surveyed fathers' participation in labor and delivery in hospitals around the country. Its findings revealed that some progress had been made but that significant regional variation still existed. Western states led the country in allowing fathers in delivery rooms: 81 percent of hospitals permitted laymen to be with their wives in the delivery room. The East followed with 78 percent and the Midwest with 68 percent. But the South still lagged far behind the rest of the country: only 28 percent of hospitals in that region allowed the men to attend their children's births. Access to sharing the childbirth experience depended very much on where you lived, in addition to race and class. Respondents to the survey identified the advantages to fathers' presence, emphasizing that the mothers were calmer and more cooperative and that the men's presence led to a more united family. They also cited some disadvantages: birth would be more time consuming and upsetting if complications arose, there was a potential third patient if the father fainted, and some fathers were not well prepared. All regions responded that physicians' objections were the primary reason for rejecting the practice.[14]

Fathers' reactions to being at their children's births in the 1970s were generally positive. Daniel P. B. Smith's experiences were typical. His wife delivered their first child at St. Mary's Hospital in Madison, Wisconsin, in 1974 and the second at Norwood Hospital in Massachusetts in 1976. The couple trained in Lamaze and found that St. Mary's was very familiar with natural childbirth and husbands' presence at delivery. Smith wrote, "I was delighted by the experience and by the *celebratory* atmosphere. Being a teaching hospital there were plenty of interns and residents and so forth, and the labor and birth experience almost felt like a party or athletic event with people cheering Jean on. . . . It was an overwhelming experience for me, it felt religious and frankly the only word I can use is 'miracle.' Everyone who knows me says I was walking on air for days afterwards." Two years later, his wife delivered in a hospital where most women had spinal anesthesia, but there, too, he was able to accompany her during her unmedicated delivery. "If I had not been present at these births I would have missed out on what simply were THE two greatest moments of my life."[15]

Medical Responses

Despite the increasing liberalization of practices, an important theme of the 1970s was continuing medical resistance to the presence of fathers-to-be in the delivery room. Tom Clark had been able to worm his way into the delivery room, but many other men who wanted to be with their wives instead waited in fathers' waiting rooms. It is worth looking closely at the medical opposition to fathers in delivery rooms during this period when some physicians and some hospitals still refused to allow the men in. In some respects the opinions of the physicians who opposed the practice, although a smaller group, hardened from what they had been during the 1960s and often applied specifically to less educated couples who frequented public hospitals. Dr. Narinder Sehgal, who practiced at the Sacramento Medical Center in California, felt strongly about the issue. He favored admitting men to labor rooms, where they could keep their wives company and offer some emotional support, but he said the delivery room was "something else again! There, his presence affects not only his wife, but several other people—the obstetrician, the anesthetist, other doctors, nurses, and even other patients in adjacent delivery rooms." In complicated situations especially, he thought, "the physician's performance could well be adversely affected by the watchful presence of the husband." [16]

There was more to Dr. Sehgal's worries. He said that while most deliveries were normal and uncomplicated, some develop into unpredictable emergencies. Because of the husband's emotional attachment, he "may become too excited—even faint—from the sight of blood, mother's pains, baby's color and appearance at birth, 'delay' in breathing, forceps delivery, etc." Although some of these situations could be anticipated and dealt with in a private practice with paying patients, in a teaching hospital often serving the poor, Sehgal felt the situation made it out of the question for laymen to attend delivery.

> With attending staff, interns, residents and medical students, it's difficult to get the same rapport between patient and doctor as it naturally develops in private practice. . . . Just imagine what it would be

like to have a husband in the delivery room—along with medical students, interns and residents! The husband couldn't possibly understand any teaching discussions among the house staff about the management of the patient—and you can almost read his mind: "These guys don't know what they're doing!" [or] "They're treating my wife like a guinea pig!" In other words, clinical training of house staff in the labor and/or delivery rooms would be just about impossible with a husband hanging around and "listening in."[17]

Sehgal was most concerned that what he called the "professional ability of the obstetrician" would be compromised. He concluded, "No physician should be forced to let a husband stay in the delivery room."[18]

Sehgal was not alone. Other physicians worried that their own ability to make decisions essential for a happy outcome—their medical autonomy and authority—would be compromised if the laymen were there to challenge what they might not fully understand. An obstetrical nurse remembered that a physician told her about an experience in his practice when the "husband was in the room and he would not let him put on forceps, wouldn't let him cut his wife and said he would kill him if the baby and the wife weren't okay."[19] Another nurse, working in Missoula, Montana, related that a physician told her, "The first time a father gets in my way" or "The first time a father faints" or "The first time a father tells me what to do, . . . I'll just kick him out." One physician approached her one morning and said, "Carolyn, one of your G[od] D[amn] fathers was at a delivery this morning and he wouldn't let me give Pitocin. He said that we could put the baby to breast [to get the same effect of encouraging uterine contractions]." The physician called the police and had the man removed.[20] This kind of pressure, real or anticipated, revealed some raw attitudes about the fathers and explained why some physicians in the 1970s continued to believe men might interfere with their medical practice and held out against letting them into the delivery room.

An obstetrics nurse who practiced in a large teaching hospital in the South wrote that the first time she "brought a father into the delivery room in 1972 [she] was met with alarm and active resistance on the part of the senior OB resident. The [resident] engaged the authority of the department's head nurse to exclude the father as a safety issue. This capable, soft-spoken young woman disarmed the situation by pleasantly assuring the resident that the father's presence with his wife was 'alright' with her. . . . The father, fully aware of what had transpired, remained quietly and helpfully at his wife's side throughout. I think he was afraid to look up, lest he draw more attention to himself."[21]

As increasing numbers of physicians came to accept laymen's presence in the delivery room, some of them realized a gendered bond with women's male partners. Physicians might consult men about certain procedures, enlist their help in gaining the woman's cooperation for such interventions, and even solicit their silence in not revealing to the birthing women what was happening. One example provided a sense of how things were for some as fathers became a more routine participant in birthing. Eric Luft, who had actively participated in his wife's delivery at Bryn Mawr Hospital in Pennsylvania but fainted right after it—from "sheer happiness" he thought—related that his wife's (male) physician "asked ME how tight I wanted [him to sew up the episiotomy]. . . . Neither of us consulted Jennifer about her OWN vagina." Luft was so happy that the meaning of the question was slow to emerge. "Later it dawned on me what I had done, so I apologized to her. Jennifer then said that she had indeed been upset about two guys discussing the future of her vagina without consulting her, but added that she was too happy to get mad at anything just then."[22] I did not find a lot of evidence of such specific consultation about sexual matters between fathers-to-be and male obstetricians, but examples like this one reveal an important dimension of delivery-room interactions. As more women joined the ranks of obstetricians by the 1980s, the dynamics of such exchanges probably changed to become more inclusive.[23]

Throughout the 1970s and early 1980s, as changes were occurring, physicians themselves retained the decision-making authority about whether the men would be allowed into delivery. Nurses helped to make judgments about particular couples. Some nurses apparently "thought it was okay if the father of the baby was with the mother if they were married, but if they weren't married they didn't belong back there in that delivery room." But usually the nurses kept their opinions to themselves and carried out physicians' wishes. With the help of hindsight, one obstetrical nurse recalled events:

> The doctor really still had power. . . . At the physician's discretion . . . [the father] would wait in the hallway until the physician said, "Okay. It's ok for him to come down here, now." And that used to bother me so much because I would think, "Here are these two people. They're working as a team together. Why are they separated now at this most crucial time of second stage labor when she probably needs him now more than ever and he's waiting out there in the hallway for her to be draped and pudendal block to be put in and for the physician to bring out his cotton balls and decide when the exact time for a husband or the father of the baby to come into the room." And there was one in particular . . . who almost made it a game. A power game. And it was so obvious and it was so irritating.[24]

Pressures for Change, Organizational and Legal

Men could get quite insistent with physicians about their place at their wives' sides. Margaret Gamper, a childbirth educator and strong advocate for men's attendance during delivery, told a story of one father "denied access to the delivery room unless he submitted to a battery of costly tests, including stool examination, throat culture, and X-rays." The man took the tests, and then he insisted that everyone else who was to be in the delivery room do the same and have the results sent to his lawyer. "Needless to say," Gamper said, "that father was allowed to witness the birth of his child without any further hindrance."[25] In fact, many instances of individual physicians giving in to individual men occurred, meaning that some men learned how to get their way; men who did not put up a fuss might still be excluded, an indication that education and class gave men an advantage.

One reason physicians worried about threats to their autonomy in the 1970s was that medical authority was in fact directly challenged by the language about women's rights that characterized the women's movement as second-wave feminists joined the battle to admit men into the delivery room. For example, Representative Martha Griffiths used such language in the bill she introduced to the Ninety-third U.S. Congress in January 1973, which tried to force hospitals and physicians to allow biological fathers into delivery rooms if the women wanted them there. The bill insisted, "It is the natural human right of a woman to determine the manner of her child's birth." Although it never came to a full House vote, the legislation would have mandated that hospitals and physicians "allow the biological father to be in attendance during all phases of childbirth if consent is first obtained from the woman involved."[26] Historians of the feminist movement Rosalyn Baxandall and Linda Gordon found the women's rights language of this bill significant because it took "for granted that the right to determine the manner of childbirth is so fundamental that it should be written into law."[27]

The same natural rights language that was in Griffith's bill was articulated at the First International Childbirth Conference in Stamford, Connecticut, in 1973. Educator Kathy Linck addressed the conference about legalizing a woman's right to choose who could attend her during labor and delivery, finding that "the cruelest practice of our maternity system is that of depriving laboring women of the loving support of their husbands or some other person of the woman's choice." Adding that last phrase "or some other person" went beyond the Griffith bill and beyond the married, heterosexual norm that was central to family-centered maternity care. Linck found, "This emotional isolation among indifferent strangers is devastating to a woman, compounding her pain and fear." She continued, "We are viewing the situation very wrongly when we say that a hospital 'allows' fathers in delivery. This is a woman's natural human right and *it is not enough that hospitals grant as a conditional privilege what is a natural human right*."[28] A birthing woman echoed the language: "I want to be free [to choose] to have my babies with dignity and joy with my husband's help."[29]

The women's movement of the 1970s helped to embolden laywomen and their partners to demand a greater voice in decision making regarding childbirth. The authors of one article wrote that the women's movement wanted "a redistribution of power between the gynecologic spe-

93D CONGRESS
1ST SESSION

H. R. 1504

IN THE HOUSE OF REPRESENTATIVES

JANUARY 9, 1973

Mrs. GRIFFITHS introduced the following bill; which was referred to the Committee on Interstate and Foreign Commerce

A BILL

To provide for hospitals to allow the biological father to attend the birth of his child if the woman consents.

1   *Be it enacted by the Senate and House of Representa-*

2   *tives of the United States of America in Congress assembled,*

3   That any hospital, clinic, or similar establishment set up for

4   the purpose of fostering, restoring or observing a person's

5   health and which receives Federal funds under a grant, con-

6   tract, or loan or which has loans guaranteed under any Fed-

7   eral program shall allow the biological father to be in

8   attendance during all phases of childbirth if consent is first

9   obtained from the woman involved.

I

Copy of U.S. House of Representatives bill 1504, 1973, 93rd Congress, 1st session, intended to allow the father to attend the birth. The bill never got out of committee. Courtesy of Milwaukee Public Library.

cialist and the patient." They observed, "Women have realized that the doctors on occasion abuse their power and exploit their patients' ignorance and helplessness."[30] An article in *McCall's* put it this way: "As a rule, hospitals and doctors don't ask women how they would like their babies delivered, but lately women have been telling them."[31] The feminist activity to encourage choice in childbirth received a boost from the many books and manuals that were published in the 1970s in support of women who wanted to use natural childbirth methods. One was the very popular *Immaculate Deception* by Suzanne Arms. Filled with emotionally potent photographs and evocative stories, the book helped to bring many couples into the fold.[32] Much of the childbirth reform movement was informed by feminism in the 1970s.

The argument about women's rights was powerful, but it was only one perspective used by childbirth reformers and birthing women in the decade. The majority of women who became interested in natural childbirth and having their husbands with them during delivery and the majority of men involved in childbirth reforms did not directly challenge medical authority or couch their argument in terms of rights. Generally a pronatalist group, they voiced a considerably less threatening message, emphasizing the joys of birthing and parenting and that women needed the company of their husbands throughout labor and delivery.

Many communities worked proactively to gain a place for fathers in hospital delivery rooms. In Broward County, California, for example, a group of concerned citizens, including parents, lawyers, and physicians, organized to make presentations and speeches to convince the Board of Commissioners of North Broward Hospital District to liberalize its policies for public hospitals and allow the men to participate in delivery. As a result of this pressure, the board did change its policy to allow the practice.[33] Similarly, childbirth change came to Boulder, Colorado, after Roberta Scaer and Diana Korte surveyed maternal birth preferences in order to give the Community Hospital of Boulder information about the services women wanted in its new maternity wing. The volunteer efforts of about forty people were aided by the Northern Colorado Chapter of the March of Dimes. Scaer and Korte polled 694 women, drawn from records of La Leche League (a group promoting breast-feeding), childbirth training classes, and a random sample of new mothers found from newspaper birth announcements. One of the strongest findings of the survey demonstrated that 98 to 100 percent of respondents wanted fathers-to-be in delivery rooms.[34]

There were a number of lawsuits claiming injury brought by men who witnessed what they believed to be a negligent childbirth, and they help us understand why some physicians continued to refuse to come under the laymen's close observation. Even though the men usually did not win such cases because they were judged to be voluntary witnesses to any accidents, legal concerns played an inhibitory role.[35] In one important case, *Justus v. Atchison*, two sets of parents brought suit against a hospital because of the "wrongful" death of their children and for the men's shock at having witnessed those deaths during delivery. In this case, the judge ruled, "We must assume that each husband was in the delivery room by his own choice. Surely, a layman who voluntarily observes a surgical operation must be prepared for the possibility of unpleasant or even harrowing experiences. This is no less true of the procedure of childbirth."[36]

Many of the issues of concern to physicians about having laymen in the delivery room were settled in the courts during the 1970s. The decade started with a direct challenge to a Chicago regulation banning fathers. Attorney Barry Gross and his wife, Merle, about to have their second child, decided to fight a 1933 Chicago Board of Health regulation that banned "lay visitors, including relatives," from the delivery room. They filed suit in the U.S. District Court for the Northern District of Illinois to be permitted to be together. Their physician, Dr. Allan Charles, joined the suit and supported the couple's wishes. The Grosses made sure their childbirth experience received wide publicity. Three reporters waited with other fathers in the waiting room while Barry was with his wife during labor and delivery. At one point the couple walked into the waiting room, and flashbulbs popped. "We were cheered on by other fathers who were excited for us and a bit envious," Barry noted. The event propitiously occurred just before Father's Day, and Barry made media headlines as he showed off his new son before the cameras. "It was delightful . . . awe-inspiring," he emoted to reporters. "I can't think of anything more appropriate or masculine or husbandly than seeking to protect and comfort one's wife during childbirth, as during the rest of life." The court overturned the Chicago Board of Health regulation, paving the way to future attendance by the fathers in Chicago.[37]

However, in response to the "rights" arguments, courts determined that "the presence of fathers in the delivery room is a privilege, rather than a right."[38] In one significant case in 1974, *Hulit v. St. Vincent's Hospital*, Michael and Michele Crowley, a couple in Billings, Montana, trained in Lamaze and wanting to be together during labor and delivery, used their "right of marital privacy" to challenge the prohibition against husbands in delivery. They were joined by their physician, Bob E. Hulit, and the Lamaze group in their town to argue also that the physician's right to practice medicine should not be constrained. The hospital had debated Hulit's request but, worried about malpractice suits arising from the men, had decided not to allow the practice. The question before the court was whether the law should intrude itself into the administration of the hospital on such decisions. Hulit wanted to "be allowed to bring husbands of his patients into the delivery room to participate in what is referred to as the Lamaze or psychoprophylactic method of childbirth."[39]

Reversing an initial decision of the trial court, the judge in the Montana Supreme Court ruled that the hospital had acted in good faith and on medical advice: "Licensed hospitals have the authority, acting on the advice of their medical staffs, to adopt rules of self-regulation governing the hospital's physicians. Licensed physicians must live according to the rules adopted by their colleagues." He further ruled that "the increased possibility of infections, concern about malpractice suits, inadequate physical facilities . . . increased costs . . . greater tension in the delivery room . . . lack of privacy to other women who are preparing to deliver, and the strict policy concerning visitors in surgical areas" all warranted the restriction against fathers.[40] Groups of physicians could make decisions that individual physicians then had to follow.

In the landmark 1975 case *Fitzgerald v. Porter Memorial Hospital*, the Seventh Circuit Court allowed to stand a hospital policy "prohibiting the presence of any person or persons in the Delivery Rooms located in the Obstetrics Ward other than members of the Medical Staff and Nursing Staff."[41] Evelyn and Bruce Fitzgerald, a married couple from Valparaiso,

Indiana, trained in the Lamaze method, brought the case and argued that the hospital policy violated their civil rights to "marital privacy" and also that it violated their physician's right to practice medicine as he determined best. But the court ruled, "We hold that the so-called right of marital privacy does not include the right of either spouse to have the husband present in the delivery room of a public hospital which, for medical reasons, has adopted a rule requiring his exclusion."[42] Giving full authority to the hospitals, the opinion continued, "This is the classic example of the kind of situation in which individual hospitals should be permitted to make individual choices, rather than having an inflexible rule imposed upon all hospitals in the nation by federal judicial decision."[43]

To address any legal issues that might arise and based on these decisions, those hospitals willing to allow the men into their delivery rooms adopted the policy of insisting that couples who wanted to be together during delivery sign consent forms agreeing to abide by hospital rules. Such permission forms became common practice in American hospitals. For example, Lakeland Hospital in Elkhorn, Wisconsin, required fathers to sign a release form like this one:

> My wife and I both desire that I be present in the Delivery Room
> during the birth of our baby. I have received the doctor's permission.
> I agree to maintain a position at the head of the delivery table so
> that I can support my wife. I also agree to leave the Delivery Room
> immediately if the doctor or nurse asks me to do so. I hereby certify
> that I release Lakeland Hospital and the attending physician . . . from
> all liability for any claim for damages which may arise because of my
> presence in the Delivery Room during the birth of our baby.[44]

Increasing numbers of couples shared their birth experiences with their physicians' approval even as the procedures to arrange for men's participation became quite bureaucratic. Yet some hospitals and some physicians in the 1970s continued to discourage such practices: men and women did not have the right to choose who would be in a hospital delivery room over medical objections. The court rulings or new laws made it clear that legally hospitals and physicians could still determine who could enter a delivery room.

Proper Roles for Fathers and Family Togetherness

In response to continued pressure to let the men into delivery rooms, hospitals and physicians developed principles about the man's proper role in his wife's birth experience. He was to be there primarily to provide emotional support but also because their togetherness would strengthen the marriage bond and help ease the pain of labor. One researcher who analyzed the experiences of ten middle-class, white, college-educated couples concluded that childbirth indeed could constitute a test of the marriage's success. Max Deutscher wrote, "The emotional presence, encouragement and admiration of the husband for his wife's labors—spontaneously expressed in his sense of pride in her and the expected child—clearly assisted in the reduction of pain and ease of delivery."[45] Similarly the authors of an obstetric textbook wrote that "most husbands can be very helpful in this psychologically trying situation."[46]

Physicians carefully delineated proper behavior for the father in light of their worries over medical autonomy, cultural norms, and their fear about the men contaminating a clean delivery room. George Schaefer wrote in the 1972 revised edition of his handbook for expectant fathers that some doctors did not allow fathers inside the delivery room because "each person in the delivery room is a member of a well-trained and highly coordinated team and must perform his job quickly and efficiently. In a misguided attempt to be helpful, you might get in the way at a crucial moment. If, for example, you were inadvertently to touch the clothing of a sterilely clad nurse or doctor, that person would have to take time out to change."[47] If you were allowed into the delivery room, Schaefer told the men, "your place is next to your wife at the head of the table so that she can talk to you and you can help her during the actual delivery. You should not wander around the delivery room or try to look over the doctor's shoulder unless you are specifically asked to do so."[48] Many hospital polices insisted that men stay at the head of the table.

Joan Beck wrote a series for the *Chicago Tribune* in May and June 1972 exploring fatherhood issues and advocating what she called a "contemporary style of masculinity."[49] She supported fathers watching the births of their children. Describing Chicago hospitals, Beck noted, "Fathers are no longer rarities in the delivery room."[50] She said that increasingly "the father is expected to be present during labor and delivery, not only as an emotional support and coach for his wife, but also so he can share the joy of a peak moment in their relationship."[51] An active role for fathers during delivery could lead to their more active domestic and child-rearing participation.

Men emoted about their joy at being part of the birth. One man, after missing the deliveries of his first three children, finally was permitted to be with his wife during the delivery of their fourth child and wrote, "It is an experience that no father should miss."[52] Another happy man wrote: "Joshua was born at 6:50 am. I watched him being born. Out-of-sight!!"[53] Another: "There is not a moment on Earth to compare with seeing your baby come into the world, to really live, to breathe!"[54] Yet another: "Just had the thrill of my life, I saw my first baby son born."[55]

Lee Epperson publicly wrote about his son's birth, when he donned a "medical monkeysuit" and joined his wife, Dale, in the delivery room. "It's difficult to describe the completeness you feel as a family . . . when you experience the birth of your child," he wrote. "Love unites. I don't think there was ever a stronger bond between Dale and me than at that moment. If the child is to be part of our life, how could we not both share this moment of birth? . . . I sat there and held my son tight. Dale says I had a tear in my eye. I did—a tear in my eye, a prayer in my heart, and a thousand thoughts in my head and a respectful wonder in my whole being."[56] Actor Donald Sutherland had an equally positive experience and wrote about it for *Ms.* magazine: "It was the most incredible, wonderful, terrifically joyful, sexual, sensual, loving time of our lives. It was so intensely personal. . . . It was extraordinary for us because we did it together."[57] The family-building rationale became the most powerful of the debate.

Although increasing numbers of fathers attended delivery in the 1970s, throughout this period, too, there were still men who did not want to be in the delivery room and some women who did not want their husbands with them. One woman wrote about her conflicted feelings. She wanted her husband there, but she knew he had his work deadlines in mind and would be looking at the clock. She was happy with just doctors and nurses helping: "There was the OB between my legs; [his] craggy, hook-

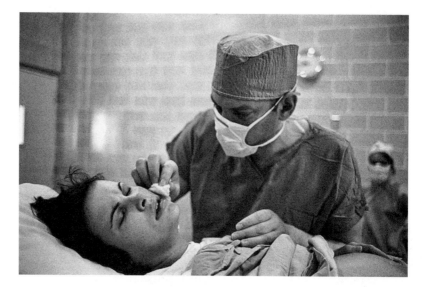

Donald Sutherland helps his wife through delivery, wiping her face and giving her
comfort. Donald Sutherland, "Childbirth Is Not for Mothers Only," *Ms.*, May 1974, 49.
Photograph by Mary Ellen Mark. Reprinted with permission.

nosed, heavy-bearded face was very beautiful. He was not the enemy.
Two strong-featured OB nurses were my friends, too, amazingly calm but
plain-spoken and firm about what I needed to do."[58] In a similar vein,
Barbara Grizzuti Harrison, the feminist journalist, wrote to *Esquire* about
how much her two deliveries hurt and admitting that she believed men
could not understand that pain and therefore could not be of very much
help to birthing women. "Birthing used to be the business of women,"
she noted, but now "the man who once paced the corridors is likely to be
inside the delivery room taking home movies. Men now want to be part
of the mysterious inner-sanctum action. They want to 'share the experience.' . . . They want to be able to say—and they do say—'We gave birth.'"
Harrison wanted none of it. "I think that bred in the bone and marrow
of a woman is a still, deep knowledge that giving birth is, like dying, an
experience that one does not ever truly 'share.' A man may be there—a
woman who loves a man may be happy to have him there—but his consciousness is a separate consciousness. . . . The arena for the act of birth

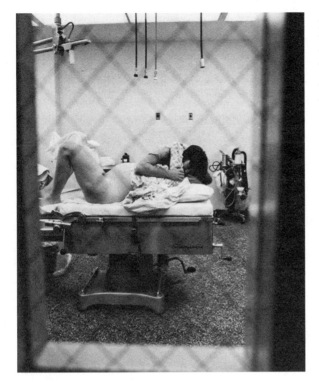

A man embraces his wife as she lies on the delivery table. Suzanne Arms, *Immaculate Deception* (Boston: Houghton Mifflin, 1975), 128. Photograph by Suzanne Arms. © Suzanne Arms.

is a woman's body, and no man can fully comprehend or share it."[59] As a feminist, Harrison supported a woman's choice about who should be with her, understanding that there would be varied feminist positions on the subject.

Far more women—feminist and not—publicized their desire to share birth with their husbands and stressed the importance of sharing. Katherine Wolff of Nampa, Idaho, shared her birth story: "Because my husband and I had each other, we could keep in control and accept what was happening," she wrote. "I thank God my husband was with me. He was my source of strength. . . . My husband's presence eased the emotional pain."[60] Another woman wrote that her husband raised her shoulders and "together we pushed—the head was born! It felt SO GOOD to push. . . . The baby's head was born! What a tremendous feeling of accomplishment and relief—WE DID IT! . . . We were awake and aware together.

We made it! . . . The joy and beauty we shared, my husband and I, the effort, the planning, classes and practicing—it all paid off in the most rewarding of births."[61] "We" was the important word.

Some men revealed that they attended the deliveries only because their wives wanted them to be there (supporting Harrison's point that men did not understand the event in the same way women did). "My wife wanted us to be together in this," one told an interviewer. Often the men who attended at their wives' insistence nonetheless proudly remarked afterward, as this one did: "She couldn't have done it without me," or "I would go through it again." Most of the men in one study admitted they "wanted to participate because they felt their wives needed them."[62] Another study of participant husbands concluded that more men than women wanted the man to be in the delivery room.[63] Interviewed men in a different study said the experience was "great and moving," "most amazing thing I've ever seen," and one remarked, "I'll never forget it."[64]

The *Las Vegas Review-Journal* published an article in its Sunday supplement in 1974 that revealed men's reactions to childbirth. It followed Jim Fox, "one of the new breed of fathers that think childbirth has a lot to do with them, too." He went into the delivery room "totally covered in blue paper clothing." He watched his baby's birth and wrote later, "I was paralyzed. I couldn't move. It's such an emotional experience seeing your child come into the world." His wife said, "He was the most important person there." Jim concluded, "It's beautiful teamwork."[65]

Ozell Bonds, who wrote his story alongside his wife's in the pages of *Essence*, started out reluctant to attend the birth but changed his mind. He visited the delivery room on a hospital tour with his pregnant wife and thought to himself, "It looks like a torture chamber. . . . The setting was a cold, huge room with brick walls and a hard, tile floor. In the middle was a glinting, stainless steel table with brackets on each side for the metal stirrups. . . . Suddenly, I wasn't sure that I wanted to 'watch the whole thing.' I wasn't even sure that I wanted to be there when it happened." He hoped he could "ease out" of the delivery. But when the time came, he "began to realize that I really wanted to be there. It was no longer a case of catering to my wife's whim nor of me heroically striving to rescue her from the jaws of lonely suffering. Our child was about to be born and I wanted to be a part of it." Once beside his wife and holding her hand and seeing her smile at him, "I wanted to see it all. Lifting, lowering, talking—my eyes were riveted on the mirror." When the doctor handed the new baby to his wife, a new family configuration was born. Ozell wrote, "Abruptly, the talking ceased and the three of us were in a world all by ourselves. In a quiet place, a peaceful place, an almost-sacred place—we met."[66] The new family configuration started in the delivery room.

Another father demonstrated how difficult the experience could be. After witnessing his baby's birth, he said, "Despite all the films I saw, the sight of the baby's head completely shook me up. . . . It took all my strength to keep down my ten cups of coffee."[67] Another man wrote that two things bothered him during delivery: "First, the forceps. Even though I was a medic in the army, I never saw such a large surgical instrument. And second, cutting the umbilical cord. It seemed so final an act, and I said so." His wife's reaction was "Oh no, nine months is enough. The baby's not going back in."[68]

A study of fathers' engrossment with their newborn children, comparing fathers who had been in the delivery room with those who had not, found that those who had attended delivery had an enhanced bond with the child and "felt more comfortable holding their baby." The men had very positive reactions to attending the birth. "Mr. C," for example, stated, "I took a look at it and I took a look at the face and I left the ground—just left the ground! I thought, 'Oh! Jesus Christ! This is marvelous!'" Many new fathers articulated a closer attachment to the child. One man commented on his child's birth: "The kid was born—and I was there—and I really had a strong feeling towards her."[69] Many observers concurred that the more men participated in birth, the higher was their participation in infant caretaking activities.[70]

As more and more hospitals around the country opened the delivery-room doors to fathers, academic studies of the effects of the practices proliferated. One study out of Harvard University looked specifically at middle-income couples and found that the very large majority of men reported positively on the experience, using language like "It was the greatest thing I've ever done," or "It meant a lot to each of us to start our lives as parents together." One man told his interviewer, "It was very powerful.

There we were — my wife pushing and I pushing with her — then the baby slipped out. . . . I held her, my bright-eyed little child, and she looked right at me and quieted in my arms."[71] But a different study found some men who described feeling that they had been "abandoned" or "deserted" during their wives' labor and were "shocked" at the newborn's appearance, finding it "ugly," "like a newborn rat," and "ghastly." That study found such remarks exceptions to the more common positive responses.[72]

As fathers became more routine and accepted within the walls of delivery rooms, their roles became more clearly defined. Most commentators felt the men were primarily there to support their wives: "The father's role in the delivery room is very specific. He is there as coach, supporter and reporter to his wife. . . . He is there to remind her to use all of the mechanisms of pushing that she was taught and they practiced together. He is there to tell her she is doing a good job. He is there to share the joy, the excitement and the sense of accomplishment when their baby is born."[73] He was there, thus, in service to his wife and his family.

Holy Family Hospital in Manitowoc, Wisconsin, began letting fathers attend deliveries in 1973, and its experiences underscored the importance of planning ahead to determine fathers' place. In a "no frills delivery room," and very atypically, the men at Holy Family were positioned to watch the delivery, not to support their wives. One nurse recalled some of the issues that emerged: "Many of the husbands had a difficult time in this position. The room was cold & sterile appearing. They were perched on a stool where all they could see of their wife was her bottom stretching out to deliver. Normally episiotomies were performed. . . . I remember many deliveries with my scrub nurse . . . positioning her leg to catch the father as he suddenly lost it and fainted." Later, Shirley Oswald remembered, the situation was corrected, and the men sat at the head of the table next to their wives to offer comfort and share "the birth miracle."[74]

Research in the 1970s revealed that fathers' presence during labor and delivery could significantly reduce women's reports of pain and their need for pain medication.[75] Identifying this very practical positive effect of men's participation gave boost to the childbirth reformers. Interestingly, as birthing women felt more relaxed, the men were the ones to show more emotion. An obstetrical nurse who witnessed these changes noted that women used to cry in the delivery room but that once fathers were present that behavior was less frequent. "It's very rare that women cry in the delivery room anymore and they do not ask about fingers and toes. . . . Fathers cry quite a bit in the delivery room, a lot of tears, quiet ones. . . . I think her partner has taken over some of that responsibility to worry about [fingers and toes] and women now are much more serene after delivery. You know, they watch and they look, but they aren't as anxious."[76]

Providing support and comfort for the birthing women during labor and delivery helped build family ties and bind the man more closely to his wife and children. As one nurse wrote, "Early contact between father and child is important for fatherliness to develop. Not allowing the man to have physical contact with his baby may stultify and inhibit such feelings from developing."[77] Steven Strassberg reported that "fathers who were present during the delivery engaged in more activities with their infants, spent more time with them."[78] One man who witnessed his son's birth put it this way: "Between me and that tiny but tough, sweet but stubborn, guileless but clever little one year old, there exists a special kind of bond."[79]

Robert Price wrote of his experiences in the pages of *Essence* in 1975, reaching a black middle-class audience and similarly revealing how important delivery could be in strengthening the family bond. Price believed that "fathers have a greater responsibility in the birth process than we are presently accepting," and he urged others to assume that responsibility. Physicians might treat "fathers like meddlesome children who have to be tolerated," but it was worth the pursuit to find the right situation. He found the delivery very satisfying: "This event allowed me to confirm firsthand the beauty of birth and has instilled in me a new respect for the entire process. . . . I am closely linked to this star child for I have been with him from the start. I did not have to sit in a hospital lounge and wait for him like a doll from a department store. I shared the responsibility for his first breath and this sharing has deepened my sense of fatherhood."[80]

If another story in *Essence* the following year is any indication, practices in integrated hospitals had changed for both black and white couples.

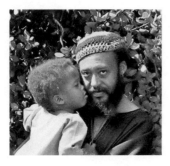

Robert Price with his child, whose birth
he wrote about. Robert Price, "A Father's
Labor Pains," *Essence*, December 1975, 52.
© Barbara DuMetz.

Patricia Patterson delivered her baby in Oakland, California, and the hospital required only that the couple enroll in prenatal classes. After dressing in a sterile gown, her husband, Jimmy, entered the delivery room.
"With each contraction, he held my shoulders up a little and I pushed
down a lot. . . . A boy . . . Jimmy leaned over me and said, 'We did it!' We
both smiled and laughed. They wrapped up our joy and let Jimmy hold
him." At the end of her article about her "total" experience, Patterson
wrote, "It did something for us as individuals and as a couple. I gained
knowledge of myself and what can be done through effort and will power.
. . . Hopefully more and more of my sisters and brothers will share this
experience."[81] By the mid-1970s, natural childbirth and husbands' participation in delivery had reached middle-class couples regardless of race.

Newspapers and popular magazines frequently reported happy
couples' experiences in the 1970s, and such stories encouraged others to
be together for the birth event. For example, the *Eau Claire (Wis.) Leader-
Telegram* ran a story about Tim and Connie Relyea. When they had a child
in 1972, Tim was with his wife in the labor room but not allowed into delivery. But during their 1975 delivery, they were together the entire time.
Connie commented to the newspaper, "Just knowing that he was there
helped me, and he knew it was a girl as soon as I did. That seems to be
something that the parents should share rather than the nurse going out
to tell the father what they had." Her husband added, "I could see everything that happened. It's really exciting. I think most men who haven't
gone through it just can't imagine what it's like. It was fascinating and I
really enjoyed it." The Relyeas said that the hospital helped make the birth
a family event.[82] Many men likewise wrote favorably about their experi-

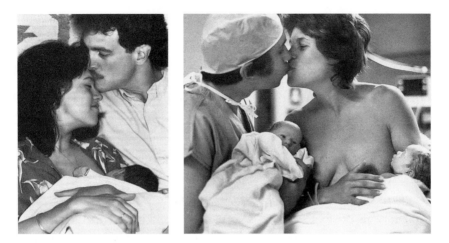

LEFT The new family unit: mother, father, and baby. Suzanne Arms, *Immaculate Deception II* (Boston: Houghton Mifflin, 1994), 148. © Suzanne Arms. RIGHT The family doubles in size: mother and father with new twins. © Suzanne Arms.

ences in the delivery room in terms of supporting their wives and bonding with the family. One wrote, "We experienced the most supreme moment a couple could experience. Watching our son pop out of her womb was an experience, a moment of joy I will treasure the rest of my life."[83]

There were already some critics in the 1970s, presaging what would become a larger movement in the 1990s, who wanted more than just the men's presence in the delivery room. They wanted the father's own needs to govern his participation, instead of only his wife's wishes or family-centered needs. One wrote that men sometimes occupied "only a peripheral position during the child-bearing experience." This was not always comfortable. Mark Bernheim, whose wife delivered their first child in 1974 in New Brunswick, New Jersey, wrote that while he considered it a "great privilege, a miracle really," to be able to help his wife through labor and delivery, "I felt in some sense I didn't 'belong' there as I had no medical training and might end up in the way. . . . There was not much for me to do. . . . While I would not have left for anything, I was not sure really what being there 'meant.'"[84]

Thus, even as fathers were establishing themselves in birth rooms around the country, some observed that they wanted more. One observer noted that the man should be "seen as an integral part of the whole drama, free to choose from a gamut of roles — from nonparticipant to exclusive coach. In our eagerness to include the father in the labor and delivery experience, I think we also have to respect his wishes if he chooses non-participation."[85] Getting the man into delivery was only one step in child-birth reform concerns. As one nurse put it, "The focus of family-centered maternity care must be broadened in order to more directly reflect the needs of the father."[86] And another observer commented, "It seems increasingly likely that many men across the country, now initiated into fatherhood in the delivery room instead of in the waiting room, are looking for support to develop roles as nurturant and involved fathers."[87] A handbook for expectant fathers did not pass over the more ambivalent and even negative remarks that men made. For example, one man who accompanied his wife throughout wrote, "At times when I couldn't do anything I felt like an 'innocent bystander.' At times I felt helpless. In spite of this, it was comforting to me to know I was helping her by being there and doing little things, and she would let me know I was helping her." Another man felt, "I was invading a sacrosanct area. . . . I was part of the program because I wanted to be, but still I had to push myself to do it."[88] The door, once opened, created varied responses from the fathers-to-be, especially as the experience led them to examine their own transition to fatherhood.

A study published in 1976 directly addressed the subject of fathers' mixed responses. Identifying a "crisis of expectant fatherhood," Jacqueline Rose Hott recognized that when expectant couples planned their childbirth, they had to ask whether the father-to-be should be in the delivery room. "Suppose his wife wants him to, and he doesn't?" she asked. "One may speculate that some of the emotional crises faced by the expectant father are associated with his fears about being pushed, literally and figuratively, into the delivery room where he is afraid he cannot cope." Hott concluded, "It is the evangelical zeal of some of the 'natural' or 'prepared' childbirth educators which may be a factor in exacerbating additional crises in the expectant father whose ambivalence about participating has not been carefully examined and who has to be swayed to participate when not emotionally ready to do so."[89]

A study in 1978 tried to determine what differentiated the men who chose to be in the delivery room from those who did not. Eileen DeGarmo concluded, "In terms of age, race, marital status, birth order, experience with children, and experience as a hospital patient, the fathers who went into the delivery room paralleled those fathers who did not witness birth." She found, however, that the two groups of fathers differed with regard to education levels. Those who attended during delivery had at least a college degree; those who did not had, on average, a high school diploma.[90] As education is a good predictor of class, which DeGarmo did not specifically identify, it is clear that during the 1970s shared birth experiences were still mainly the prerogative of middle- or upper-class couples.

One role that became very common for men attending their wives' deliveries was that of photographer. Men brought camera equipment and tape recorders with them into the birthing room, causing hospitals additional worries about keeping the room clean. One man wrote that he was aware that many hospitals do not permit "the father to introduce a camera into the process." He was grateful that he could bring his camera to New York Hospital's Lying-In division: "I'm aware for the first time of how fantastic it is that I can be present at the birth of my own child, assisting my wife and recording it all on film."[91] "Terri F." delivered her second baby accompanied by her second husband, for whom it was a first birth, and understood that the camera helped her husband to be more comfortable with his participation. "At first he was reticent about [coming into the delivery room]. He said, 'I don't want to do that' but then . . . he fell in love with the whole concept. Pictures, still pictures at the time . . . And we had the album, from the pregnancy test, the positive pregnancy test, to all the labor and delivery pictures through her first year." Years later Terri recalled, "I can remember just going into the delivery room. I can remember my husband with a camera. Sort of ignoring me at this point because he was taking pictures of the baby emerging and to him it was just unbelievable. . . . He went home after the birth . . . and put 2001 A Space Odyssey on. You know that music and just listened to it, and reenacted the birth for my mother."[92]

During the late 1970s, a growing interest in mother-infant bonding, which could be fostered by immediate physical contact following deliv-

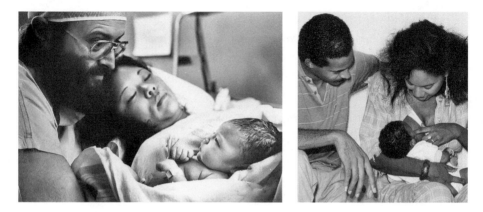

LEFT Following delivery, a man makes eye contact with his newborn as his wife rests. © Suzanne Arms. RIGHT A father watches as his wife breast-feeds their new baby. © Suzanne Arms.

ery, supported and led to increased numbers of fathers attending birth so that they, too, could immediately bond with their children.[93] By most accounts, fathers' attendance at labor and delivery by 1978 became, as Lamaze activist Elly Rakowitz put it, "the expected norm, rather than an unusual oddity."[94] Indeed, in 1978, family-centered maternity care, which included the father's participation, was promoted by the American Association of Psychiatry, the American College of Obstetricians and Gynecologists (ACOG), the American Nursing Association, the American College of Nurse Midwives, and the Nurses Association of ACOG and endorsed by the American Hospital Association.[95] A survey of 1,354 residents of Baltimore in 1978 found that 73 percent of new mothers had been accompanied through delivery by the father of the baby.[96] This result suggests that the practice had spread widely.

Despite the Baltimore numbers, other studies made it clear that attendance at prenatal classes, which was often a prerequisite to attending delivery, was still class- and race-dependent even in the early 1980s. Working-class people for reasons ranging from the price of carfare to working two jobs and larger families did not have the flexibility in their schedules to attend prenatal classes. One researcher claimed, "Families from lower socioeconomic levels are far less likely than middle or upper-class families to attend childbirth preparation classes and this fact tends to preclude their participation in the birth experience." Helen Gabel set out to study black family men with a high school education and blue-collar jobs to see whether they were included in the family-togetherness activity of birth and what they thought of it. The men had attended their children's deliveries without preparation and with some "negative expectations." Gabel provided some voices of men who had previously remained hidden. One man told her, "I was nervous. I didn't know, how could I help her? How could I do anything? I'd just be lost and scared. Not know what to do. Maybe even panic or something. Do the wrong thing." After the birth, however, the new fathers said they had found the experience "meaningful and positive." Ninety percent of the men interviewed spontaneously indicated they felt pride and self-esteem. One said, "Yeah. I was brave. I was pretty brave. When she told me to cut that cord I wasn't shaking. Well, she gave me the scissors and I cut it. The cord! I liked it! I felt like I was a doctor or something. Wearing those green clothes. Felt pretty good." Another man believed being at the delivery deepened his relationship with his wife: "When they were sewing her up, you know, it just brought me much closer to her. . . . It made me grow in having much much more respect for her throughout our life."[97]

Most of the men in the study found the experience a rare and important marker in their own lives. One said, "I would tell any man that it would be one of the most exciting experiences he would ever face." Another, "I feel honored and blessed to know that this is something that I was actually part of and perhaps it's the paramount experience of my life." One put it in religious terms, like so many men who had written in the fathers' books in the 1950s and 1960s: "It was a great experience to see life coming into this world seeing what my wife and I and God produced together." One man gave advice: "Go ahead in! The lady needs you! . . . If his woman's there, well, he should be there too, with her." Gabel's study provided evidence that by the end of the 1970s the delivery-room door had opened to working-class black men who had not previously been present.

Fathers' attachment to their newborns became an increasingly important issue for childbirth reformers. Elisabeth Bing had noted at the beginning of the 1970s, "Without sounding sentimental, I am convinced that such a shared experience makes a marriage into a very real and deeply felt partnership. The husband is not left out to see his baby only after birth, through a glass window. He has actually helped in the birth of his child. . . . He can immediately relate to his child and he shares with his wife the wonderful feeling of a great achievement."[98] By the end of the decade, studies corroborated this observation and revealed that men who participated in birth were more likely to continue that participation in family activities during the child's infancy. One study of forty-six middle-income couples tested the hypothesis of greater father involvement and concluded, "The father's participation in the birth and his attitude toward it were found to constitute the most significant variable in predicting father attachment." The authors of the study said their results suggested that hospitals could enhance fathers' bonding with their children by helping the men overcome any inhibitions they might have about being involved in the birth process.[99]

A 1980 research study explored father-infant attachment in the hours following delivery, comparing men who had attended the delivery with those who had not. The researchers found that "fathers who were present at delivery demonstrated more social attachment behavior than fathers who were not present."[100] Repeatedly, research demonstrated that men who attended their children's births had more interactions with their infants and spent more time taking care of them.[101]

The emphasis on fathers' nurturing roles by the 1980s seemed to fit the changing times. Fathers were no longer just providers for their families, especially since women had entered the workforce in increasing numbers (50 percent of married women were working outside the home in 1980), and they sought greater family involvement.[102] Close bonding with their children, which many believed began by attending delivery, became increasingly common among the new fathers. Carmen Sorvillo, a high school teacher in Howard Beach, Queens, New York, admitted that attending his children's deliveries had been his wife's idea and that initially he had been disgusted by the thought. But after attending the births of his three children, he said, "It was very beautiful, very exciting, no less

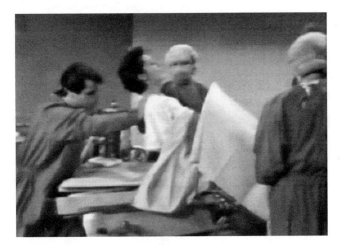

Fonzie, having entered the delivery room reluctantly, supports Lori Beth as
she pushes during delivery and is entranced by the newborn and happy to be a
part of the event. *Happy Days*, "Little Baby Cunningham," November 3, 1981.
Happy Days, courtesy of CBS Paramount Network Television.

exciting the third time around." He felt closer to his children as a result
and participated more in their care.[103]

To understand how deeply into American culture the practice of including men in delivery had reached by the beginning of the 1980s, we
can return to the television version of events. Just as *Happy Days* included
an episode in which Fonzie accompanied Lori Beth, his friend's wife, to
prenatal classes, the sitcom's camera also followed Fonzie to Lori Beth's
delivery. The nurse tried to get Fonzie into a hospital gown, but he resisted until Lori Beth screamed out, "Fonzie, where are you? Fonzie, I
need you!" In the delivery room Fonzie stood behind Lori Beth, supporting her back and telling her to take breaths, relax, and push.

> FONZIE: Lori Beth, Lori Beth, you listen to me now. This is your
> coach talking. There's a little baby in there, and it wants to see
> Milwaukee. If I can wear a gown, you can push.
> . . . [She does and the baby is born.]
> DOCTOR: It's, it's a boy.
> FONZIE: Oh Lori Beth. You did it. It's a boy, Lori Beth, you made
> a beautiful little boy.

DOCTOR: A beautiful healthy baby boy.

FONZIE: You made a baby. A baby boy, it's a baby boy. [Doctor hands baby to Fonzie.] What's that?

DOCTOR: The kid who wanted to see Milwaukee.

Being present at the delivery turned Fonzie into a convert advocate of laymen's attendance at birth. He was touched by the delivery and overwhelmed with the emotion of it. The *Happy Days* episode left the clear message that men had significant roles they could play for their partners but also that they themselves could benefit from childbirth. It was, the Fonz said, "one of the highlights of my LIFE."[104]

Cesarean Sections, the Last Frontier

The last hurdle for fathers-to-be to overcome during the 1970s involved their participation during cesarean sections. At midcentury, rates of such operations rose dramatically, and accusations were made that nonmedical reasons sometimes determined who would be operated upon. Differences in the rates by race and class indicated that social and educational considerations entered into the decisions doctors made about when to operate.[105] In the 1950s, fathers-to-be had little say about such operative procedures from their position in the waiting room. "Have been here all day Sat & Sun afternoon," wrote one weary father from the waiting room. "Doctor Benaron informed me that a cesarean section will be performed in a half hour."[106] One father sat through his wife's long labor only to learn from his wife's doctor "that a Caesarean Section must be performed."[107]

There were, however, instances in the early fathers' books that made it clear that sometimes consultation with the fathers occurred. One man wrote, "The doc came in and told me that he thought it best to perform a cesarean—the word alone made me shiver. I didn't quite know what to say but finally we agreed to it."[108] Surgery was definitely a collaborative decision in this entry: "Due to an extreme disproportion, Dr. Bayly has suggested scheduling a Cesarean Section. After much concentration we decided against waiting any longer."[109] Communication or not, men whose wives had C-sections seemed relieved, as this man put it: "No real sweat this time — cesarean deliveries are calm cool and collected. . . . We are thankful that all went well."[110] Examples from the 1970s illustrate that sometimes physicians consulted with the couple and even may have colluded with the birthing woman's husband in order to gain his help in dealing with his wife. Ozell Bonds talked with his wife's doctor "outside of the room," where he learned the physician was considering a cesarean section because of an irregular heartbeat detected in the fetus. Bonds kept the information from his wife. Ultimately his wife delivered vaginally.[111] In almost all instances before the mid-1970s, men waited outside the delivery room when physicians performed cesarean sections.

In 1976, some hospitals allowed the men to be in the room during the surgical procedures. One physician noted that "actually the outcome of a Caesarean section is more predictable than with vaginal delivery. And so it's somewhat paradoxical to permit husbands to be present during the vaginal delivery and not for Caesarean." Because of this, he gave his approval to the O'Connors, delivering at Terrace Heights Hospital in Hollis, Queens, New York, to be together for the operation. Mr. O'Connor stood at the head of the operating table, reassuring his wife throughout. "I was able to comfort her. I told her they were doing everything they could. . . . I was hoping that I wouldn't faint, and it turned out that I didn't. She said I should keep talking to her. Every once in a while I'd peek over and see what was going on." The birthing woman recounted, "The most important thing was that my husband was there. One thing is for certain. I would move to another state if I couldn't find a doctor to allow my husband to be with me."[112]

Yet most hospitals did not move quickly to permit the men to attend during the operation. One woman sadly reported that she had had an emergency cesarean section: "I just wish that my husband had not been suddenly rushed out of my labor room which upset both of us not knowing what was happening. My husband should have been allowed to see the birth of our child — Cesarean or not."[113] A parents' committee in Westchester, New York, in 1977 worked to allow the fathers to attend cesarean section deliveries. One woman explained, "My husband and I were prepared for natural childbirth. We suddenly went from a birth situation to a surgical one. My husband was isolated from me. My child was placed

in an isolette away from me. And I was sent [alone] to a recovery room."
Dr. Douglas Robertson of Mount Kisco, New York, said, "Having a father
in the operating room is like having your mother-in-law in the kitchen."[114]
Indeed, some physician responses to the idea of laymen attending cesarean sections in the 1970s resembled some of their objections to the
men attending vaginal deliveries.

In 1977, Dr. George H. Nolan spoke at a meeting of the Michigan Society of Obstetricians and Gynecologists and discussed his study of forty-
eight women who delivered by cesarean section. He had wanted to know
whether the presence of the husband affected the experience and concluded, "The presence of the father in the delivery room during cesarean
section poses no threat to safety." He reported that the women who did
not have their husbands present felt "loneliness, inadequacy, and helplessness, and [were] more anxious about their own and their infants' health."
During the discussion of the paper, a physician in the audience asked
whether obstetrics had "prostituted itself" in trying to meet consumers'
demands. Nolan objected to the terms of the question and offered this
curt reply: "Consumer satisfaction is what medicine should be about."[115]

Connecticut hospitals piloted a program in early 1978 allowing fathers
to attend cesarean births.[116] The same year, the U.S. Supreme Court, in re-
fusing to hear an Illinois case, settled the legal issue of men's participation
in their wives' cesarean section deliveries. The court left intact a previous
decision that parents had no "fundamental right" to have the men present
for a cesarean delivery, but it said that practices could vary according to
individual hospitals or physicians' wishes.[117] In 1979, for example, in a
small town in Iowa, a couple had hoped to have a natural childbirth, but
labor did not progress. The woman remembered, "My husband's hand
was swollen and bruised due to my squeezing of it all day." The physician
suggested a cesarean section; the woman was given a spinal anesthesia
and rushed to the delivery room: "My husband was to wait outside the
room—the fathers were not allowed in for C-sections. . . . I was pretty
frantic about the idea of him not being there, and they relented and said
he could stand inside the room, but at the doorway—not close to the
'action.'" In subsequent deliveries, he was permitted to sit at her side for
the operation.[118]

During a cesarean delivery in Methodist Hospital in Madison, Wisconsin, the doctor allowed the father to enter the operating room, but, as the birthing woman recounted, "he had to stay seated at my head, basically behind the drape. My husband, never really being one to follow the rules, half crouched so he could actually witness the miracle of his son's birth."[119] In 1980 a National Institutes of Health advisory panel recommended that hospitals allow fathers in the room during cesarean sections.[120] But in that year, a study noted that "a majority of our hospitals continue to dictate: 'Fathers cannot enter the delivery room while a cesarean delivery is in progress.' Shockingly, in spite of parental wishes it takes only one disapproving obstetrical staff member to prohibit a husband's participation."[121]

By the end of the 1970s, when fathers' presence at delivery was well secured in most American hospitals, the issue of their attendance during cesarean sections continued to demonstrate that some of the same concerns faced earlier about risk of infection and the men's (in)ability to understand what they were seeing had not yet been resolved. A physician and his hospital brought suit in the Seventh Circuit Court against state and city health officers to allow men to attend cesarean births, basing their case on the *Fitzgerald* decision. The court held, as it had in that previous case, that the right of marital privacy did not include having the husband in the operating room. The court considered whatever rules hospitals wrote for medical reasons to be reasonable.[122]

Men and women continued to crusade to allow men into their wives' cesarean section operations. In 1981, the *New York Times* reported that some hospitals encouraged the practice, providing classes for the men to learn about what they would be witnessing. Dr. David Shobin of Nassau Hospital, where all fathers were so encouraged, said, "Most fathers enjoy and appreciate being with their wives." However, Dr. Joseph Rovinsky of Long Island Jewish Hospital disagreed, arguing (while inadvertently revealing what might characterize some surgical procedures), "The operation is a tense process. Doctors should be free to throw instruments, curse or ask the resident to help, and not be inhibited by the presence of the father."[123] Apparently, covering up such behavior was more important than changing it. The example reveals another concern physicians may have had about letting fathers observe cesarean (and perhaps also vaginal) deliveries: hiding flaring tempers or medical errors. Extremely reluctant to discuss this aspect openly, physicians may have wanted to hide such incidents from the family.[124]

In Beaver Dam, Wisconsin, one couple's efforts changed local hospital practices by 1981. Their first baby had been born in 1978 by emergency cesarean section, and William Sandberg was left alone and outside. His wife related, "I was alive, my daughter was alive, but my husband was a wreck. No one informed him what was happening, whether I was alive or not or anything about the baby. He asked and asked, but nothing." When she was again preparing to deliver in 1981, Beaver Dam Hospital allowed them to be together after they took childbirth classes. "Bill was seated where he could see everything. I was given a spinal and of course I had a drape so I could not see. But Bill was there. He was ready. He saw Hans born and he was delighted. . . . He got to hold Hans right there, in the operating room. Hans was alive, I was alive and Bill was happy."[125] Gradually, the practice became more common.

As rates of cesarean section soared in the 1980s—from 6 percent in 1970 to 25 percent of all births in 1988—demand for men's attendance at the operation also rose.[126] In 1982 a new edition of an advice book for fathers supported men's attendance at cesarean sections, arguing the fathers had as much right to be there as they did to attend vaginal births.[127] At University of Utah Medical Center in Salt Lake City in 1983, however, Marc Williams was allowed to be with his wife during her cesarean section only because he was a pediatric resident in the hospital. He was permitted to stand at his wife's head "next to the anesthesiologist."[128] In 1985, New York hospitals reported significant variation in practices, but the trend to include the men was clear. New York City's Presbyterian Hospital, affiliated with Columbia University, increasingly allowed fathers to attend cesareans, reporting that of about 900 women having C-sections in that hospital over the last year, 200 "chose to have the fathers present." "We've had good results with the fathers present," a physician in the hospital noted, adding ironically, "And we haven't lost one [father] yet."[129] Increasingly, hospitals seemed inclined to allow the practice under regulated conditions, and physicians, most of whom no

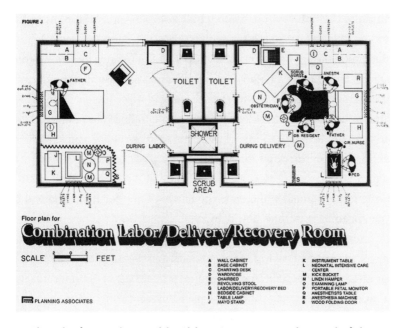

Floor plan for a combination labor/delivery/recovery room, showing the father
as an integral part of the architectural design. Reprinted with permission of
Ross Planning Associated, *Perspectives in Perinatal and Pediatric Design*
(Columbus, Ohio: Ross Products Division, Abbott Laboratories, © 1988).

longer viewed fathers as threats, allowed them full access to labor and
delivery rooms, even to witness cesarean operations.[130]

Birthing Rooms

During the decade of the 1970s, many hospitals created combination labor
and delivery rooms, called birthing rooms or alternative birthing suites,
which dramatically changed the physical spaces to better accommodate
birthing couples. Birthing rooms helped to make family-centered care a
more widespread reality. The ability of hospitals to incorporate the new
physical facilities varied greatly around the country, with public hospitals
slower than private institutions to meet the new space challenges.

The new spaces made it easier for hospitals to compete with the growing number of out-of-hospital alternative birthing practices.[131] Inside the
hospital, obstetrical nurses' duties expanded to include quite a bit of at-

tention to the father-to-be, helping him in his coaching duties as he encouraged his wife through the whole process.[132] Nursing journals provided guidelines to help nurses help the father, enhance his self-esteem, improve the couple's relationship, and heighten parent-infant bonding.[133] Many articles urged nurses to understand and meet the changing needs of the father: "The father's potential role in childbirth has evolved from one of an unnecessary source of infection to an essential source of affection for both mother and newborn." The authors encouraged nurses to support the man's role in labor and delivery and to be sure to allow time for the father to hold and cuddle the newborn and for the parents to be alone together with their new baby.[134]

Combining labor and delivery spaces decreased the traffic in the hallways of the maternity wing and accommodated the new delivery practices that included laymen.[135] This arrangement made it more comfortable for the women because they did not have to move during the moments of transition. It also made it easier for the men to participate, since they could stay in the room the entire time, instead of having to leave to don surgical attire and wait at the delivery-room door for readmittance. These combined rooms harked back to the home-birth era; they were designed to be more homelike than delivery rooms, and they usually hid any emergency equipment behind cabinet doors or curtains. The rooms contained the same technology as delivery rooms, with the possible exception of general anesthesia, but they were painted in warm colors, the windows were covered with drapes, and there were pictures on the walls. There would be a comfortable chair (maybe one that could be made into a bed) for the father and a rocking chair for the birthing woman. The bed could transform into a delivery table with stirrups if necessary. As one man noted, "Everything was much more relaxed in the birthing room. The whole time I felt I was right where I should have been. I think the last time . . . I was just standing around watching the [fetal monitor] machine. This time I felt like I was involved really because I could participate in what was going on. . . . We weren't separated even for a minute."[136] Hospitals like Manchester Memorial Hospital in Manchester, Connecticut, and Booth Memorial in Cleveland, Ohio, made the transition to birthing rooms quickly during the 1970s.

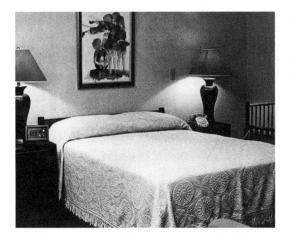

A birthing room at Booth Memorial Hospital in Cleveland, Ohio, set up like a home bedroom where the couple can relax together. Reprinted with permission of Ross Planning Associated, *Perspectives in Perinatal and Pediatric Design* (Columbus, Ohio: Ross Products Division, Abbott Laboratories, © 1988).

Michael and Joan Bahn participated in labor and delivery together in such a birthing room, the first time in 1975 at Family Hospital in Milwaukee and the second in 1979 at Sacred Heart Medical Center in Spokane, Washington. Milwaukee's Family Hospital initiated the family-centered combined labor-delivery room — and sometimes also offered the services of a nurse-midwife — when its declining admission rates forced the hospital to try more innovative practices.[137] Michael Bahn felt himself to be "a true partner" in the whole effort. During his wife's first and long labor, "We walked around, we talked, we read, we discussed what to name the baby, and we did the breathing when the contractions hit. I effleuraged [gently massaged], and effleuraged, and effleuraged her proud abdomen for hours it seemed. At one point I fell asleep with my head on the edge of the bed and my arm across her stomach." When Joan was ready for delivery, "the birthing team of the Bahns and the hospital staff was formed, and went into action. I was positioned by the attending nurse for effective assistance to Joan. . . . I saw the head appear and the baby slide out. I was overjoyed and amazed. Joan was relieved and exhausted. . . . Tears, a crying newborn, overwhelming joy, relief, excitement, exhaustion, the feeling of pride of our accomplishment, the quick camaraderie we had with the nurses and doctor, created an emotional vortex." The second delivery demonstrated family-centered childbirth even more strongly. The couple convinced the Spokane hospital to allow their four-year-old to witness the delivery, which it had never before done. With another friend as a chaperone for Elizabeth, the child, and lots of curious staff members stopping by, "a new era was started at Sacred Heart." Bahn wrote, "As before I watched with awe the birthing and cut the umbilical cord. . . . As much as I was observing and relating to Joan, I was watching Elizabeth's reaction to this whole process. Joan, even while under the stress of the contractions and the final push effort, was aware and relating to Elizabeth. . . . The whole event was amazing."[138] Admitting children to the delivery rooms was rare at the time, but birthing rooms paved the way for it to become a more common practice.

Some physicians thought birthing rooms constituted a step backward, a return to the time when babies were delivered at home; others found them the perfect solution to bringing home comforts into the hospital.[139] Most birthing women and their husbands were extremely positive about the new rooms. One woman who delivered the older way said that the next time she planned to "deliver in a hospital that has labor-delivery beds, so that my husband will feel more at ease (he was very uncomfortable in the 'sterile' delivery room setting)."[140] Another woman noted that her "labor experience went smoothly until the 'rush' to the delivery room, transfer (awkward, uncomfortable, distracting to me) to delivery table, and draping, etc. During this time, my husband was not allowed to be with me. I worried about him 'missing the delivery' and I missed his coaching-support during the time all this was taking place."[141] She would have preferred the birthing-room option had it been available to her.

The woman's observation that her husband was not comfortable in the sterile, well-equipped delivery room is especially interesting. Instead of laymen being isolated from the event as they waited in stork clubs, they found a place in the labor room, where they could help their wives through the ordeal and communicate with doctors and nurses about procedures. When they moved into delivery rooms, they increased their voice even further. They often demanded their way in, and once in, they interacted with and affected procedures. But some men remained ill at ease in what was clearly the physician's domain. Thus the switch to hospital birthing rooms, which were designed to be more comfortable for the birthing woman and her family, gave the husbands their highest comfort level and allowed them the most freedom of movement and involvement in decisions. Adding drapes and domestic comforts to hospital rooms might seem to "feminize" them and might appear to be a trivial change, but such alterations made the men feel more at home and more in control. At the Stanford University Hospital's new family birth room in 1980, "many families indicated their desire to have as much control and as little distraction as possible, in order to be less intimidated about coming to a hospital to have their babies."[142]

Hospital birthing rooms emboldened the birthing woman and her husband to take more control over events, even though they still utilized hospital nursing and medical care. One study of mothers' responses to birthing rooms reported that the women

> described the importance of their husbands' presence with them during the birthing process. They said: "We were never separated," "He was there all the time," "He supported me constantly without interruption." . . . Particularly [the women] noted the physical "closeness" of their husbands: "My husband was able to participate fully in the birth—helping to hold my legs—just more close to the whole situation." "He was not just standing there at my head but actually supporting me physically." Mothers used the word "intimate" repeatedly in their writings and frequently spoke in plural terms to indicate that they and their husbands experience birth as a pair.

The mothers also credited the nurses who staffed the birthing rooms for helping "the expectant parents maintain control of their birthing experience." One woman said, "My husband and I felt that the labor was 'our thing.'"[143]

One obstetrician built his practice on not just welcoming fathers into the delivery or birthing room but in encouraging them to deliver their own babies. His argument was that "letting dads 'catch' their own babies is simply a logical extension of the family-oriented approach that helps this practice flourish." Dr. Robert Block admitted that some fathers did not want such responsibility but the majority did. Laymen delivering babies constituted as much as 70 percent of Block's practice. Instead of pacing in the waiting room, the father was the first to see and touch his baby.

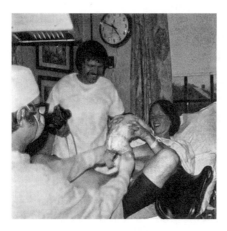

This couple is active in their child's birthing-room birth, as the mother lifts the baby and the father looks on happily, with a camera in hand. Philip E. Sumner and Celeste R. Phillips, *Birthing Room: Concept and Reality* (St. Louis, Mo.: Mosby, 1981), 16. Photograph by Susan Moore. © Elsevier.

Block believed, "The good effects carry over after the birth. Time after time, when a mother comes back for her six-week checkup, she'll say, 'I never imagined Charlie could be this good a father. He's so different with this baby than with the others.'"[144] *Parents* wrote an article about Block's practice, which he shared with two other physicians, Myron Levine and Robert Dilks, at Washington Memorial Hospital in Turnersville, New Jersey. The author of the article, Leah Yarrow, wrote about one couple's experiences: "The baby's head crowns, emerges and Dr. Dilks shows Jim where to place his hands. Jim keeps steady pressure on the head of the dark-brown hair and the shoulder slips out. Within seconds the entire baby is out, suctioned, and bellowing his indignation at being born. Jim's tears flow into his beard as he holds his firstborn, then places at his wife's breast his child he has delivered." The physicians believed the experience formed the "cement of the family unit."[145]

Birthing rooms became the ultimate step in men's move through hospital spaces. They were the culmination of the movement of childbirth reform that worked to free fathers from the confines of the waiting rooms and admit them to labor rooms and then to delivery rooms, and they provided the newest options within hospital walls for parents who wanted to share the childbirth experience.[146]

The 1975 circuit court decision in *Fitzgerald*, which left the decision about whether fathers could attend deliveries in the hands of hospitals and the individual attending physicians, did not actually inhibit the prac-

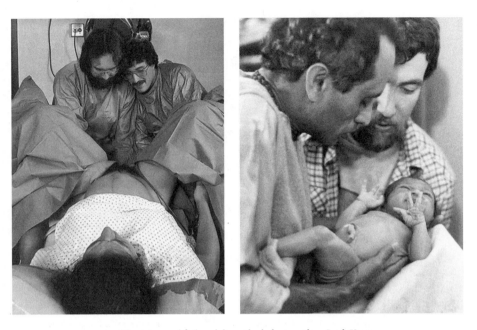

LEFT Physician and father deliver the baby together. Leah Yarrow,
"Fathers Who Deliver," *Parents*, June 1981, 62. Photograph by J. T. Miller.
© J. T. Miller. RIGHT Physician hands the baby over to the father
following delivery. © Suzanne Arms.

tice. Physicians increasingly realized that the men's presence did not adversely affect procedures and sometimes added a positive element, and
they let the fathers don scrub suits and sit and watch, if not actively participate.[147] By the mid-1980s, the overwhelming majority of physicians
and hospitals allowed, and even encouraged, husbands to stay with their
wives throughout labor and delivery. Worries about infection, fathers'
confusion or missteps, malpractice liability, lack of privacy for other
patients, or even challenges to authority or possible diversion of attention away from the work at hand, all of which had been earlier concerns,
became worries of the past. Men accompanying their wives throughout
labor and delivery became routine.[148] In a 1983 survey of eighty-seven
teaching anesthesiology departments in forty states, respondents said
that fathers were allowed in delivery rooms during vaginal deliveries in
97 percent and for cesarean sections in 86 percent of hospitals. One anesthesiologist wrote, "My staff doesn't like this, but have mellowed with

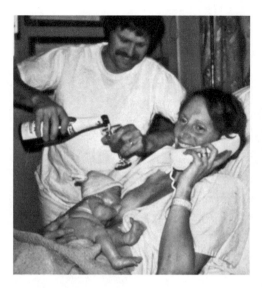

Birthing-room togetherness allows for immediate celebration and the calling of friends and relatives to give the good news. Cover of Philip E. Sumner and Celeste R. Phillips, *Birthing Room: Concept and Reality* (St. Louis, Mo.: Mosby, 1981). Photograph by Philip Sumner. © Elsevier.

time." Indicating that significant variability by socioeconomic class still existed, however, another noted that in his town the fathers were allowed into delivery rooms in the private hospital but not at the city hospital.[149] The manual of standards issued by the American College of Obstetricians and Gynecologists in 1985 fully supported fathers "and support persons" in the delivery room, as long as they were appropriately attired and educated, but its recommendation about such a person being present during a cesarean birth still "depend[ed] on the judgment of the obstetric staff, the individual obstetrician, the anesthesiologist, and the policies of the hospital."[150]

Not until the 1980s did new concepts emerge about what constituted "family" and who could accompany a birthing woman through delivery if her husband or a designated "relative" could not attend. In 1983 a Michigan court ruling in *Whitman v. Mercy-Memorial Hospital* cleared one very important hurdle in this regard. An unmarried heterosexual couple, in which the man was the acknowledged father of the expected child, attended prenatal classes together and wanted to be together for the entire labor and delivery. The hospital in which they were to deliver the baby, Mercy-Memorial Hospital in Monroe, Michigan, had a policy prohibiting an acknowledged father not married to the mother from being present in the delivery room (although it allowed a man married to the woman to be there). The hospital policy allowed one nonmedical person to support the woman but stipulated that that person had to be "a member of the mother's immediate family." The couple in question resided together, and the man supported the woman and her son from a previous marriage. They considered themselves to be "a family unit." While the case was debated, the woman delivered at a different hospital, with her partner present. The court went ahead with its deliberations because of the general importance of the question of whether the hospital policy about immediate family was "impermissibly discriminatory." It concluded that it was discriminatory because "a married woman has one relative that no unmarried woman has: a husband."[151] The ruling opened the way not just to unmarried fathers but also to lesbian couples. In 1985, hospital regulations about laypeople attending cesarean sections noted that women delivering at Columbia's Presbyterian Medical Center in New York City could have their husband with them " — or if the mother chooses, a relative or close friend—to be present."[152] The major textbook *Williams Obstetrics* in its 1989 edition stated unequivocally that "great benefits can be obtained by women and their spouses — or 'significant others' —who attend childbirth education classes [and share delivery]."[153]

Times had indeed changed. Sometimes gradually and sometimes with great rapidity, fathers moved from the waiting rooms to the labor rooms and ultimately to the delivery rooms and birthing rooms, where they were joined by "significant others." Pushed and pressured by their birthing women patients, by a family-oriented natural childbirth education community, by the women's movement, and equally strongly by many fathers-to-be, physicians had learned to live and practice within a more diversely populated delivery room.

EXPECTANT FATHERS' EXPECTATIONS

With the presence of fathers in delivery and birthing rooms across the country well established by the mid-1980s, except in some crowded public hospitals that continued to be pockets of inequality of access, laymen had conquered all the important spaces of hospital obstetrics. They had moved out of the constraining waiting rooms into the rooms where their wives labored, and they had also managed—with a lot of help from their wives, childbirth educators, the women's movement, supportive doctors and nurses, and community activity—to find a place for themselves amid the equipment-filled delivery rooms to be there for the event of birth itself. They had helped the transition from separate labor and delivery rooms to homelike birthing rooms. They had also helped to open the doors to nonhusbands, those others, including male lovers, lesbian partners, adoptive parents, and other friends, family members, and siblings, whom the woman had identified as necessary to her well-being.[1]

Hospital delivery rooms in the early twenty-first century often contain large numbers of people, as many women want to share the experience widely. As one author put it, "The door to the delivery room has swung wide open. Even the most traditional hospitals now allow multiple guests." Opening new facilities in 2005, Prentice Women's Hospital in Chicago included a "Family Zone" — extra space — in the delivery room near the head of the mother's bed in order to have room for all the people the birthing woman might want to have with her.[2] Indeed, a professor of family medicine at the University of Wisconsin teaches her medical students and residents how to "manage a crowd" around the delivery bed. Dr. Cynthia Haq said, "It is not now uncommon to have half a dozen people or even more with the mother in the room at the time of birth."[3] Multiple visitors and observers have become so common that some birthing couples feel pressure from their friends to attend. In a syndicated newspaper column, "Letter to Prudie," a "Private Parent" wrote that she and her husband wanted to limit attendance in the delivery room but worried that "friends and family have been talking about the day as if they plan to be in the delivery room with us." Prudie was "stunned" and opined that "giving birth is neither a party nor a social occasion. . . . Just tell anyone and everyone that you will not be entertaining on the day the baby is born."[4]

Television again helps us to understand some of the trends that are common at the turn of the twenty-first century. The popular NBC show *Friends*, for example, demonstrated the new use of hospital spaces. When the character Rachel gave birth on the May 16, 2002, episode, Ross, the father of the baby and not married to Rachel, remained with her throughout labor and delivery. And the fathers' waiting room was transformed from the space where the man paced alone and anxious into a place where lots of friends and relatives could gather. It became a staging area from which they all could visit the laboring woman and into which the father could retreat from the emotional activity to get revitalized by the support of his friends.[5]

Most of the men who fought their way in to their wives' delivery rooms and those who walked in on the coattails of others who preceded them were glad to be there. They wanted to support their partners, they wanted to be witnesses to the births of their children, and they found that both motivations helped them to bond with their families in new and mutually beneficial ways. Men have helped one another through the event, and

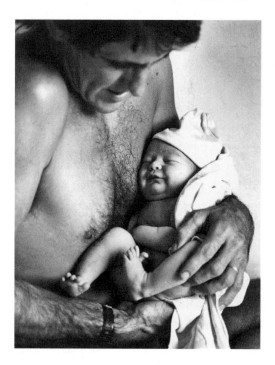

New father happily, if somewhat awkwardly, holds his baby skin to skin following his wife's cesarean section delivery. © Suzanne Arms.

many have formed support groups on the Internet and in local hospitals around the country to teach others meaningful ways to participate in childbirth.[6]

How has making "room for daddy" mattered in childbirth history? We can never know, of course, how things might have changed without the active participation of the men. But we do know that the men—often spurred on by their wives and by changing cultural perceptions of proper male behavior—made a difference. They created unprecedented new roles for themselves to participate in a traditionally women's event; they helped to make hospitals more flexible in how they handled birth; they accompanied birthing women through difficult hours, enhancing their experience; they attended prenatal childbirth classes alone or with their partners; they increased their own role not just in childbirth but in what it led to, increasing male participation in family domestic activities; they broke down some of the mystique of modern medicine and further opened the world of obstetrics to lay participation and interpretation; they opened doors and broke down partitions that had previously kept them out. We cannot possibly understand the full story of twentieth-century childbirth without the feelings, perceptions, and actions of these actors.

The history of childbirth is a study in changing medical practices, but it is also a study of changes in family and social history. Recognizing the role that fathers played in this particular human drama adds a new dimension to its rich and complex history and demonstrates that this female activity can be more fully comprehended by including the men in the analysis. After the Second World War, the move of middle-class families to the suburbs and men's search for masculine ways to participate in family activity came together to encourage men to play a bigger role in their wives' labor and delivery. The women's movement played an important role in furthering this increased participation, especially by demanding that women have a choice about who supported them through childbirth.

Despite the argument of women's rights, however, the childbirth reform that led to increased participation of laymen actually helped to reinforce the nuclear family and men's domestic authority. The reforms that succeeded were those that promoted women's roles as mothers, fathers' roles as breadwinners, and physicians' roles as childbirth experts. Hospitals reflected in their practices not just changing medical knowledge and ability but also cultural practices, evolving health care consumer interests, and men's and women's changing desires. We see in the history of childbirth in the mid-twentieth century the inequalities of the larger medical system, particularly with regard to class and race, and understand how incorporating men into hospital labor and delivery came first for white middle-class patrons, then for all middle-class couples, and only slowly began to integrate all people with more equal access and opportunity.[7] The themes of place, privilege, and power characterized childbirth's changes in the middle of the twentieth century. The seemingly radical change of including men in hospital labor and delivery did not create an egalitarian environment in the hospital. Rather, childbirth reform reinforced physicians' authority and family gender hierarchies.

Childbirth practices continue to evolve in the twenty-first century. Men have organized to act collectively through social movements, many of which are Web-based, as laymen's roles in hospital childbirth remain in flux. While most men happily have found their places at the center of labor and delivery practices in American hospitals, many do not yet feel that the birth experience meets their expectations and needs.

Even in the mid-twentieth century as men found a great deal of satisfaction in being included in birth and having a voice in how it would be achieved, some people recognized new problems and issues emerging. Counterarguments and worries surfaced as early as the 1970s that made it clear that not all men wanted to be in the delivery room, not all men wanted to be included in the processes of their wives' births, not all men liked the experience. Philip Taubman, for example, wrote about his "doubts" in a *New York Times* article. Admitting he would not want to go back to the waiting room, he wrote, "I think I can do without some of the *cinema verite* sights and sounds, not to mention some of the volatile emotions that went with the natural births of our sons." He wished someone had taught him some breathing to relieve his own fears. When it came to the delivery itself, he wrote: "Witnessing the birth itself was like no other experience I have had. Even in a hospital delivery room, with all the bright lights, shining surfaces and sterile equipment, the first sight of the living being seemed like a primeval vision." In his analysis, witnessing birth forced him "to live suspended somewhere among the roles of husband, lover, partner, protector, and father, not knowing which way to turn."[8] Childbirth educator Elisabeth Bing protested Taubman's conclusions: "But surely, this is what happens to all of us when we choose to share our lives with another person—we function at many levels, whatever is demanded at a given time." Bing objected to Taubman's characterization of men's birth experiences because "it means a great deal to a woman if she knows that her partner will be there to help and support."[9]

Most of the responses to articles questioning men's attendance at birth followed Bing's model in the 1970s and 1980s. Significant numbers of fathers felt as did Stephen Harrigan, whose birth account was published in *Reader's Digest*. Harrigan participated in prenatal classes, practiced Lamaze breathing at home with his wife, and stayed with her through labor and delivery. Before the birth, he worried that his role was peripheral to the real activity of his wife. "Most of us," he wrote about his Lamaze classmates, "realized that our wives were going somewhere

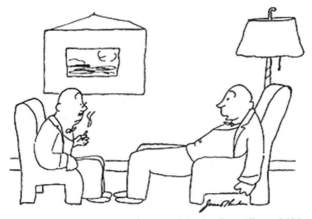

"I never really rallied after the birth of my first child."

Some men found that childbirth was not an entirely positive experience, a
point of view James Thurber captured in this 1935 cartoon. © 1935 by James Thurber.
Renewed 1963 by Rosemary A. Thurber. Reprinted by arrangement with
Rosemary A. Thurber and The Barbara Hogenson Agency, Inc.

without us. Childbirth was a crucible we could not follow them into." She
was an athlete who would finish the race; he would "be there cheering,
holding out the Gatorade." But when the time came, he said, his presence
"did not seem specious anymore." He was very glad he was there to experience birth, and he found it to be an emotional, meaningful transition
to fatherhood: "I was a man now, a father."[10]

Yet at the turn of the twenty-first century significant numbers of
fathers have voiced feeling at sea, abandoned, and out of control when
they entered into their wives' labor and delivery rooms. Many simply
did not want to be there. Others found a more complex picture as they
struggled to understand what a comfortable position for them might be.
Anthropologist Richard Reed, who interviewed fifty men after their participation in labor and delivery at the century's end, provided a comprehensive view of such ambivalent feelings. He wrote that the men found
the birth experience powerful and profound but that "a closer analysis of birth shows that few activities are defined by fathers themselves.
Mothers, nurses, obstetricians, as well as families and the general public, offer very specific sets of guidelines for fathers' actions in the hospi-

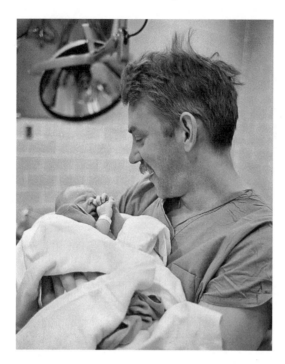

Donald Sutherland holds his new baby, looking very pleased after the hard work of his wife's labor and delivery. Donald Sutherland, "Childbirth Is Not for Mothers Only," *Ms.*, May 1974, 51. Photograph by Mary Ellen Mark. Reprinted with permission.

tal birthing room." Because of this Reed concluded that many men felt "peripheral to the birth of their babies."[11] He added that having fathers in delivery rooms "fails to provide for his needs. There are no notes in the chart about *his* progress; no nurses bringing him lunch; no physician's consultations about *his* blood pressure. There is no social support or even recognition of the fact that he was undergoing one of the most powerful events in a father's life."[12]

Reed criticized birth practices as they affected fathers: "It is not surprising that many fathers experience a deep ambivalence in the roles that they are offered in the rituals of labor and delivery. Trained to help mothers in labor, fathers are asked to ignore their own experience."[13] Rather than getting attention they might need, "fathers are at the bottom of the list of important people in the birthing room." New fathers feel an intense bond with their newborn at birth, but some of them also feel, in the end, unsatisfied with the experience of birth. "They walk away from the birthing room with a sense of distance from the event and their partners."[14]

In much the same way as men sitting in waiting rooms earlier, men at the turn of the twenty-first century have banded together to share experiences and strategize about how to effect change. One of the main messages of the new men's movement in this area is to reject the expectation that men need to be coaches at their wives' deliveries, and instead they are working to let men be women's companions without prescribed tasks. Many feel that gender barriers should fall so that a man can share and empathize with the woman's birth experiences and at the same time have space and time during the process to face his own new perceptions and relationships as he is becoming a father. "Mr. Dad," one Web site for expectant fathers, noted in 2005 that many health professionals, including physicians, nurses, and ultrasound technicians, "tend to treat [fathers-to-be] as though they're little more than intruders or spectators and the wife is the only one worth dealing with. . . . The fact that the dad-to-be might have some specific and important needs, concerns, questions, worries, or anything else of his own rarely seems to occur to anyone."[15]

Men feel they should not be in a position in which they need to control events or worry about what is happening to their partners but rather should be provided their own space in which to witness events and to begin their new fatherhood on their own terms. Birth transforms all who are a part of it, Reed believes: "working to birth their child becomes a passage rite into fatherhood" for the men.[16] A scholar of family history also emphasizes the fatherhood roles inherent in men's birth attendance: "The time to hook men on parenthood . . . was during pregnancy, at the birth, and in the crucial early months afterwards." Those who did not attend their wives in the delivery room, Jessica Weiss found, "had missed the boat of shared parenting."[17]

Midwife Rosemary Mander and others believe that the pendulum has swung too far and that men's childbirth role needs modification to accommodate men's particular concerns. Mander worries that in the late twentieth century many men felt pressured to attend their wives throughout the birth when they did not want to be there. She thinks that their role as a coach creates enormous pressure and worry and does not give a man the "opportunity to contemplate his own emotional needs."[18] Men's difficulties of, for example, watching their wives in pain and feeling unable to help, and their worries about feeling a decrease in sexual interest in their wives following watching them deliver, clash with a "conspiracy which enforces men's continuing presence."[19]

A dispute in the pages of the *New York Times* in 2005 corroborated the particular worry about sexual attraction—and perhaps exacerbated it. Psychiatrist Keith Ablow wrote about some of his male patients who suffered something similar to a post-traumatic stress disorder after watching their wives deliver, which "made it difficult for them to be attracted to their wives, at least in the short run." Some of them, he observed, never recovered their sexual interest in their wives.[20]

A week following the article's appearance, the newspaper printed a number of letters to the editor (mostly from women) commenting on this point. One wrote, "Maybe the [column] should have been called 'Man's inability to cope with reality and the inherent pain involved.' The fact that my body produced, delivered and eventually recovered from the making of two glorious human beings should be life-affirming—even for the fragile male ego that needs a tidy package with a pretty bow to stay attracted." Another woman wrote, "Cry me a river. It's too bad some men suffer from learning that their partners' genitalia has a function other than sexual." Some writers were more sympathetic to men's quandaries, but the published letters mostly supported the idea that the men should be there if the women wanted them.[21]

The debate continued. One woman wrote that she enjoyed reading all the letters, concluding: "Men aren't turned on by watching childbirth? I'm not turned on by nose-picking, flatulence, belching, etc., but most married men don't seem to think that those activities need to be censored. Relationships are a trade-off."[22] *Slate* ran an article that started, "A man who doesn't want to watch his wife give birth is a jerk."[23] Blogs took up the debate, too.[24] The subject remains sharp and relevant for many in the early twenty-first century.

Some observers have noted that women remain favorable about the men's presence, but they worry that men's influence might not all be positive. Mander thought that men's presence might lead to escalating pain and panic for the women because the men might be so upset that their feelings transfer to the birthing woman. Michel Odent, an influential physician and childbirth authority, similarly believed that a father's anxiety could be "contagious" and actually impede labor. He also questioned whether the participation of the father at birth could influence (adversely) the "sexual life of the couple afterward." He worried about whether men could "cope with the strong emotional reactions they may have while participating in the birth."[25] Indeed, Odent believed that men could not know what birthing women were experiencing as well as another woman could and that the men might be responsible for making the birth more difficult or longer and might even be implicated in the increasing rates of epidurals and cesarean sections.[26] While it is not necessary (or possible) to trace such interventions directly to the men who accompany their partners in labor and delivery rooms, it is important to remember that historically men did play a role in supporting the medicalization of childbirth, and this factor has to be considered as men's roles continue to evolve.

As an example of how concerns about the particulars of men's participation in childbirth filtered to the general public, psychologist Phillip Calvin McGraw, known to television audiences as "Dr. Phil," addressed fathers' delivery-room presence and gave advice to his large audience in January 2004. He talked about what men should do if they do not want to be there. "Perhaps he's the type of guy who gets squeamish when it comes to hospitals and medical procedures. Or maybe he's afraid he'll fall apart, making things harder on his partner. Or maybe he just doesn't want to see his wife in pain." He thought that as many as half of all expectant fathers had some ambivalence about participating in delivery. Dr Phil's advice was very clear. He said men should educate themselves, discuss their feelings with their partners, get a doula (a trained and knowledgeable laywoman labor and delivery assistant) to help, talk with other men; in the end, however, "if at all possible, tough it out. No matter how eloquently you explain your reason, missing the birth is probably going to hurt your partner. So if you're not absolutely at the panic stage, consider being there for the birth for no other reason that it'll probably make your partner happy."[27] Significant numbers of doulas now accompany birthing couples through labor and delivery, a trend that directly responds to and provides relief for some of men's concerns.[28] Training camps for expec-

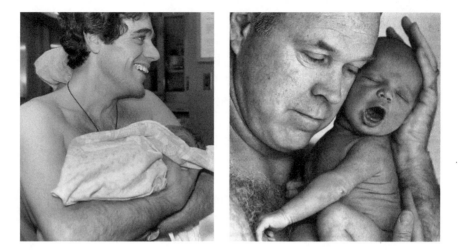

LEFT Looking extremely happy after his wife's cesarean-section delivery,
the new father holds his baby. © Suzanne Arms. RIGHT New father
holds his baby skin to skin. Suzanne Arms, *Immaculate Deception II*
(Boston: Houghton Mifflin, 1994), 172. © Suzanne Arms.

tant fathers have emerged to prepare men for fatherhood, including the
labor and delivery experience.[29]

It is not clear how many men in the twenty-first century find birth
problematic in the ways Reed, Mander, Odent, and others have identified; certainly many continue to wax eloquent on the miracle of birth. The
New York Times photo column "Lens" caught James Joyce, an executive at
an interactive television company, at his wife's delivery in 2005. Joyce had
taken prenatal classes with his wife and had studied books on the subject.
He said of this entrance into fatherhood: "The moment I saw the baby's
head appear I was in awe. When I held him I felt overwhelming love rush
all over me. I could feel the warmth on my chest—his skin on my skin.
There's everything before. And everything after."[30] Some men—probably
the majority of those who participate in labor and delivery—enjoy the
moment and find it meaningful.

A complex web of factors influenced and changed hospital childbirth
during the mid- to late twentieth century. Many different constituencies
tried to put their stamp on the hospital, including hospital administrators, who worried about liability, efficiency, and cost; insurance compa-

nies wanting hospital practices to maximize savings; physicians and specialists wanting to put into practice their own training experience and new procedures as they became available; birthing women who wanted to recapture some of the shared experiences of traditional home birth; feminist organizations that emphasized women's right to determine the manner of their children's births; nurses who found themselves caught between the worlds of men's medicine and its hierarchies and women's gendered bonds; lay groups such as the American Society for Prophylaxis in Obstetrics, the International Childbirth Education Association, and many local organizations that worked tirelessly to make hospital childbirth more flexible; and finally, but not least, the male partners of birthing women who wormed their way from outsider status in the waiting rooms into the inner sanctums of delivery and birthing rooms, where they became — if not always comfortable — insiders involved in the process of birth. All these groups and individuals had influence in changing practices and in bringing laymen into childbirth. The great variation in practices around the country, in specifics and in timing, existed because of the myriad influences at work in bringing about the changes.[31]

Men's roles in childbirth — their place in the hospital, their active participation in determining practices, and their own transitions to fatherhood — while often personally satisfying, continue to evolve. As I write in 2008, childbirth practices remain contested and in flux. Increasing numbers of women and men have opted for home deliveries or deliveries in alternative out-of-hospital birthing centers in the face of what seems to them intractable problems within hospitals. Men who accompany birthing women to the hospital still feel conflicted, and they are still trying to shape events to their particular liking. The cultural pressures that push them to be there for their partners are strong, yet some — perhaps many — resist. The reasons for men's attendance in labor and delivery, and their roles, are undergoing reexamination. Are men to be there to support their partners, in which case they must submerge any of their own issues that conflict with those of their partners, or, now that they have gained a place, can they define the event to meet their own needs even if they conflict with what the birthing woman might want or need? These questions exist today, and answers to them lie ahead. The historical experiences examined in this book can help deepen the analysis and improve the outcomes for all involved in the birth process.

Having earlier in this book told my mother's anecdote about Seymour, I conclude with another birth story that my mother used to tell, which well illustrates how much we need to pay attention to perspective. Apropos of some men's current concerns, the man in the story focused on his own experience: a father-to-be paced a hospital waiting room as he awaited the birth of his first child. A nurse occasionally entered the room, but never with news for him. The man sat, he paced, he smoked, and he worried. After many torturous hours, the nurse finally came to him and announced, "It's a girl!" "Thank God!" he exclaimed. "She'll never have to go through what I have just been through today!!" As demonstrated in this book, although the expectant fathers seemed to be just sweating it out in the waiting rooms and as they moved into labor, delivery, and birthing rooms, they were really hard at work contributing to changes in American childbirth practices; they continue that effort today.

A NOTE ON SOURCES

This project began when I visited the archives of Chicago's Northwestern Memorial Hospital to start research on a new project, a history of childbirth in the twentieth century. The archivist, Susan Sacharski, showed me a huge set of "Fathers' Books," once empty, thick journals that the hospital had kept in its mid-twentieth-century "Stork Club," or fathers' waiting room. In this stack of books that spanned the 1940s through the 1960s, men had written their thoughts and feelings as their wives labored and delivered elsewhere in the hospital and responded to other men who had earlier occupied the room. These books turned out to be a research windfall. From them I learned about men's powerful emotions as they waited, and I saw that men started to get more involved in the birth process from this perch outside hospital labor and delivery rooms. They were not just smoking and pacing; they were already part of the action of birth.

From that beginning, I narrowed my project's goal from childbirth during the whole century to a focus on the laymen in the midcentury period when their present-day roles were formulated. The fathers' books had revealed quite a bit about hospital policies and activities, but I needed a fuller context for the laymen's actions. The perspectives of the mostly middle-class men who had written in the books needed to be augmented to include a broader cross section of the population. I needed to be able to check the men's observations against as many other sources as possible in order to understand how fathers-to-be may have affected birth practices in twentieth-century hospitals. I looked first at hospital publications and policies and realized immediately that the men's jottings added significant dimension and detail to official hospital sources. Reading the literature by historians of medicine, the family, and social history in general confirmed my thinking that I was onto a subject that not only would be interesting but could also reveal some of the inequality of twentieth-century medicine and supplement what we know about hospitals, families, and childbirth.

Then I had to expand my searches considerably to try to get as full a story as possible. As the endnotes reveal, I searched medical and obstetrics texts and journals, nursing texts and journals, popular health and family magazines, handbooks, social science literature, newspapers, films, and television shows. Most important, I looked for men's own voices in all my research venues. I worked in collections and archives at the American College of Obstetricians and Gynecologists, the National Library of Medicine, the Wellcome Library for the History and Understanding of Medicine, and the Library of Congress. I used the wonderful collections in the University of Wisconsin Library System, including the Ebling Health Sciences Library and the Wisconsin Historical Society. I utilized extant oral histories and conducted a few interviews of my own. I sent out an author's query to my university's alumni magazine and various newspapers. I made use of a previous query I had placed with the *New York Times* Sunday Book Review section, when I was looking for women's birth stories, to see what the women had said about the men's roles. I searched for other hospital waiting-room fathers' books by writing to hospitals around the country. Many responded that they remembered having such books, but most could not locate them, although I was able to use one other set. In order to uncover men's experiences and emotions, I was comprehensive in my research and looked for birth descriptions from every vantage point, ultimately yielding multiple and sometimes complicated perspectives on men's historical childbirth experiences.

NOTES

Abbreviations

AQ, *NYT* Response to author's query in *New York Times* Sunday Book Review, July 24, 1983

AQ, *OW* Response to author's query in *On Wisconsin* 106, no. 2 (Summer 2005): 6

ASPON *American Society for Psychoprophylactic Obstetrics Newsletter*, Bay Area Chapter

BP The Birthing Project: Archive of Women's Birth Stories, interviews by Helen M. Sterk, Marquette University, Milwaukee, Wisconsin; transcripts quoted with permission

"Dear Diary" "Dear Diary . . . Thoughts from St. Mary's 'Father's Waiting Room,' 1969–1978," St. Mary's Medical Center, Madison, Wisconsin

ICEA International Childbirth Education Association

MNOHP Maternity Nursing Oral History Project, 1986, interviews by Sara Monkres (now Williams), typescript in Wisconsin Historical Society Archives, Madison, Wisconsin; quoted with permission

WHSA   Wisconsin Historical Society Archives, Madison, Wisconsin

WMH, FB   Wesley Memorial Hospital, Fathers' Books, Northwestern
Memorial Hospital Archives, Chicago, Illinois

Preface

1. For traditional accounts that make no mention of fathers, see, for example, Roy P. Finney, *The Story of Motherhood* (New York: Liveright, 1937), and Alan Frank Guttmacher, *Into This Universe: The Story of Human Birth* (New York: Blue Ribbon Books, 1937). For some recent examples of men getting some attention, see Richard W. Wertz and Dorothy C. Wertz, *Lying-In: A History of Childbirth in America* (New York: Free Press, 1977), and for a more popular account, see Jessica Mitford, *The American Way of Birth* (New York: Dutton, 1992). See also Jacqueline H. Wolf, *Don't Kill Your Baby: Public Health and the Decline of Breast Feeding in the Nineteenth and Twentieth Centuries* (Columbus: Ohio State University Press, 2001), and Laura Ettinger, "The Forgotten Man: New York City's Maternity Center Association Educates Expectant Fathers" (paper delivered at the History of Science Society annual meeting, Milwaukee, 2002). My thanks to Professor Ettinger for sending me an unpublished copy of this paper.

2. See Judith Walzer Leavitt, *Brought to Bed: Childbearing in America, 1750–1950* (New York: Oxford University Press, 1986), which emphasizes women's experiences.

3. My colleague Ronald L. Numbers has been pointing out this missing piece to me for years. I thank him for his prodding and encouragement. One early exception to this generalization is J. Jill Suitor, "Husbands' Participation in Childbirth: A Nineteenth Century Phenomenon," *Journal of Family History* 6, no. 3 (Fall 1981): 278–93. For more recent attention to this subject, see Richard K. Reed, *Birthing Fathers: The Transformation of Men in American Rites of Birth* (New Brunswick, N.J.: Rutgers University Press, 2005), and Rosemary Mander, *Men and Maternity* (London: Routledge, 2004).

4. Lisa Belkin, "The Selling of Fathers Day: A New Image Is Emphasized," *New York Times*, June 14, 1986, 33–34, quotation on 34. The editor believed that by 1985, 80 percent of American fathers were present in the delivery room. See also Rob Palkovitz, "Fathers' Motives for Birth Attendance," *Maternal–Child Nursing Journal* 16 (Summer 1987): 123–29. The Cosby book is *Fatherhood* (New York: Doubleday, 1986).

Introduction

1. Arnaz is quoted in Bart Andrews, *The I Love Lucy Book* (New York: Doubleday, 1985), 92. See also his *Lucy & Ricky & Fred & Ethel* (New York: Dutton, 1976), which contains synopses of all shows by airdate.

2. The details of the decision can be found in Andrews, *I Love Lucy Book*, 92–117, quotation on 94. For a broad look at television in this period, see James L. Baughman, *Same*

Time, Same Station: Creating American Television, 1948–1961 (Baltimore: Johns Hopkins University Press, 2007).

3. *I Love Lucy*, episode 50, "Lucy Is Enceinte," aired December 12, 1952, Desilu Productions. For more on this episode, see Andrews, *I Love Lucy Book*, and Michael McClay, *I Love Lucy: The Complete Picture History of the Most Popular TV Show Ever* (New York: Time Warner, 1995), 70–75.

4. The word "pregnant" appeared in the title of the second episode, "Pregnant Women Are Unpredictable," but not on the lips of any character during the shows themselves.

5. See, for example, Judy Kutulas, "'Do I Look Like a Chick?' Men, Women, and Babies on Sitcom Maternity Stories," *American Studies* 39, no. 2 (Summer 1998): 13–32. For a full discussion of popular culture and notions of motherhood in this period, see Elaine Tyler May, *Homeward Bound: American Families in the Cold War Era* (New York: Basic Books, 1988).

6. Jude Davies and Carol R. Smith, "Race, Gender, and the American Mother: Political Speech and the Maternity Episodes of *I Love Lucy* and *Murphy Brown*," *American Studies* 39, no. 2 (Summer 1998): 33–63, quotation on 49. See also Elizabeth Edwards, *I Love Lucy: Celebrating Fifty Years of Love and Laughter, the Official 50th Anniversary Tribute* (Philadelphia: Running Press, 2001), 84–90.

7. Davies and Smith wrote that this scene helped to "confer upon [Ricky] a fully mainstreamed white identity." They posited that its effect was to present Ricky, who could remove the costume, "as a fit American father." Quoted from "Race, Gender, and the American Mother," 49. On the use of comedy as a way of dealing with social concerns, see Stuart M. Kaminsky, *American Film Genres*, 2nd ed. (Chicago: Nelson-Hall, 1984), 135–65. Although I am not considering television audiences here, there has been much work done on this topic. For example, cultural studies literature in the 1980s revealed that situation comedies were favored by young black viewers even if all the actors were white. See, for instance, a review of this literature by Carolyn Stroman, "The Socialization Influence of Television on Black Children," *Journal of Black Studies* 15, no. 1 (September 1984): 79–100.

8. John Fiske, *Media Matters* (Minneapolis: University of Minnesota Press, 1996), 24. See also Gerald J. Baldasty, untitled book review of Bonnie J. Dow, *Prime-Time Feminism: Television, Media Culture and the Women's Movement since 1970* (Philadelphia: University of Pennsylvania Press, 1996), in *Signs* 24 (Winter 1999): 553–56; Todd Gitlin, "Prime Time Ideology: The Hegemonic Process in Television Entertainment," *Social Problems* 26 (February 1979): 251–66; and Muriel G. Cantor, "Prime-Time Fathers: A Study in Continuity and Change," *Critical Studies in Mass Communication* 7 (1990): 275–85.

9. Robert Price, "A Father's Labor Pains," *Essence*, December 1975, 52–53, 77, 79, quotation on 53.

10. For more on television, especially situation comedies, as a reflection of popular

social values, see David Marc, *Comic Visions: Television Comedy and American Television* (Winchester, Mass.: Unwin Hyman, 1989).

11. Both quotations from Andrews, *I Love Lucy Book*, 105, 106. The show *I Love Lucy* garnered Emmy Awards for best comedienne, best supporting actress, and best situation comedy in 1953. For an interesting analysis of Lucy, see Patricia Mellencamp, "Situation Comedy, Feminism, and Freud: Discourses of Gracie and Lucy," in *Feminist Television Criticism: A Reader*, ed. Charlotte Brunsdon, Julie D'Acci, and Lynn Spigel (Oxford: Clarendon Press, 1997), 60–73. The Winchell quotation appears also in Davies and Smith, "Race, Gender, and the American Mother," 40, where more is made of the juxtaposition.

12. Male doctors, of course, also are extremely important to the story, and I will consider them here as well. See also Judith Walzer Leavitt, *Brought to Bed: Childbearing in America, 1750–1950* (New York: Oxford University Press, 1986), which also discusses physicians' roles.

13. For a concise example of the richness and drama of this subject, see Judith Walzer Leavitt, "What Do Men Have to Do with It? Fathers and Mid-Twentieth Century Childbirth," *Bulletin of the History of Medicine* 77 (2003): 235–62, parts of which are reproduced in this section and in Chapters 2, 3, 5, and 6 and are used here with permission of the Johns Hopkins University Press. This book can be considered a meso-history of men's participation in childbirth at a particular moment in time. Meso-history is a bridge between the grand vision of macrohistory and the case study of microhistory. It is informed by aspects of both.

14. U.S. Public Health Service, *Maternity Care Utilization and Financing*, publication no. 947-4 (Washington, D.C.: U.S. Government Printing Office, 1964), and American Hospital Association, *American Hospital Association Hospital Statistics* (Chicago: American Hospital Association, 1987), table 1, pp. 2–7. See also Edith H. Anderson and Arthur J. Lesser, "Maternity Care in the United States: Gains and Gaps," *American Journal of Nursing* 66, no. 7 (July 1966): 1539–44.

15. To understand the history of the American hospital, see Morris J. Vogel, *The Invention of the Modern Hospital: Boston, 1870–1930* (Chicago: University of Chicago Press, 1980); David Rosner, *A Once Charitable Enterprise: Hospitals and Health Care in Brooklyn and New York, 1885–1915* (Cambridge: Cambridge University Press, 1982); Charles Rosenberg, *The Care of Strangers: The Rise of America's Hospital System* (New York: Basic Books, 1987); and Rosemary Stevens, *In Sickness and in Wealth: American Hospitals in the Twentieth Century* (New York: Basic Books, 1989).

16. David Barton Smith, "Addressing Racial Inequities in Health Care: Civil Rights Monitoring and Report Cards," *Journal of Health Politics, Policy, and Law* 23 (1998): 75–105, quotation on 79. See also his book *Health Care Divided: Race and Healing a Nation* (Ann Arbor: University of Michigan Press, 1999). Moses Cone Hospital is in Greensboro, North Carolina.

17. Jill Quadagno and Steve McDonald, "Racial Segregation in Southern Hospitals: How Medicare 'Broke the Back of Segregated Health Services,'" in *The New Deal and Beyond: Social Welfare in the South since 1930*, ed. Elna C. Green (Athens: University of Georgia Press, 2003), 119–37, quotation on 129.

18. Elizabeth S. LaPerle, "Study of Maternity Facilities in Cook County," Welfare Council of Metropolitan Chicago, May 1954. Typescript available from the University of Illinois Libraries, Urbana-Champaign.

19. For an excellent examination of patient demands changing medical practice in relation to breast cancer, see Barron H. Lerner, *The Breast Cancer Wars: Hope, Fear, and the Pursuit of a Cure in Twentieth-Century America* (New York: Oxford University Press, 2001).

20. Margaret Marsh, *Suburban Lives* (New Brunswick, N.J.: Rutgers University Press, 1990), xiv. For a description of the transition to men taking more of their leisure time with their wives instead of their male friends, see Kathy Peiss, *Cheap Amusements: Working Women and Leisure in Turn-of-the-Century New York* (Philadelphia: University of Pennsylvania Press, 1986). For more on men as well as women adopting family-oriented roles in the 1950s, see Stephanie Coontz, *The Way We Never Were: American Families and the Nostalgia Trap* (New York: Basic Books, 1992), and Jessica Weiss, *To Have and to Hold: Marriage, the Baby Boom and Social Change* (Chicago: University of Chicago Press, 2000).

21. Weiss, *To Have and to Hold*, 87.

22. Benjamin Spock, *Commonsense Book of Baby and Child Care* (New York: Duell, Sloan and Pearce, 1946). Pocket Books brought out a paperback version in 1951. By 1973, the book had sold more than 23 million copies. See also Benita Eisler, *Private Lives: Men and Women of the Fifties* (New York: Franklin Watts, 1986); Steven Mintz and Susan Kellogg, *Domestic Revolutions: A Social History of American Family Life* (New York: Free Press, 1988); and May, *Homeward Bound*. On Benjamin Spock, see Thomas Maier, *Dr. Spock: An American Life* (New York: Harcourt Brace, 1998); Nancy Pottishman Weiss, "Mother, the Invention of Necessity: Dr. Benjamin Spock's *Baby and Child Care*," *American Quarterly* 29, no. 5 (Winter 1977): 519–46; and William Graebner, "The Unstable World of Benjamin Spock: Social Engineering in a Democratic Culture, 1917–1950," *Journal of American History* 67, no. 3 (December 1980): 612–29.

23. Bernarr Macfadden, *Manhood and Marriage* (New York: Macfadden Publications, 1916), as discussed in Marsh, *Suburban Lives*, 81. Marsh located a 1916 edition of this book, but the first one I saw was published in 1923. See also his *Womanhood and Marriage* (New York: Macfadden Publications, 1929). Macfadden wrote many books on physical culture, right living, and marriage, many of which have been reprinted throughout the twentieth century. See Johnnie Lee Macfadden, *Barefoot in Eden: The Macfadden Plan for Health, Charm, and Long-Lasting Youth* (Boston: Prentice Hall, 1962). See also William R. Hunt, *Body Love: The Amazing Career of Bernarr Macfadden* (Bowling Green, Ohio: Bowling Green State University Press, 1989).

24. Stephanie Coontz, *The Way We Really Are: Coming to Terms with America's Changing Families* (New York: Basic Books, 1997), 37.

25. It should be remembered that postwar government funds for housing and education expanded the middle class and made it realistic for working families to aspire to and achieve owning their own homes outside the urban metropolis.

26. Sloan Wilson, *The Man in the Gray Flannel Suit* (New York: Simon and Schuster, 1955); film version produced by Darryl Zanuck and distributed by 20th Century Fox, 1956.

27. Betty Friedan, *The Feminine Mystique* (New York: Norton, 1963). The divorce rate fell slightly during the 1950s but rose rapidly in the next two decades. See Joanne Meyerowitz, *Not June Cleaver: Women and Gender in Postwar America* (Philadelphia: Temple University Press, 1994), for an examination of popular magazine articles that discussed nondomestic roles for women in the 1950s, and Wini Breines, *Young, White, and Miserable: Growing Up Female in the Fifties* (Boston: Beacon Press, 1992). Forty percent of women worked full-time during their pregnancies in the early 1960s. See U.S. Census Bureau, *Maternity Leave and Employment Patterns of First-Time Mothers: 1961–2003* (Washington, D.C.: U.S. Government Printing Office, 2008), table 1, p. 4.

28. Weiss, *To Have and to Hold*, 54.

29. For the plural use of the term in this context, see Athena D. Mutua, "Theorizing Progressive Black Masculinities," in *Progressive Black Masculinities*, ed. Athena D. Mutua (New York: Routledge, 2006), 3–42.

30. Mark Anthony Neal, *New Black Man* (New York: Routledge, 2006), 27.

31. For the *The Cosby Show*'s opposition to standard notions of black masculinity and its portrayal of nonsexist men, see Nathan Grant, "Mirror's Fade to Black: Masculinity, Misogyny, and Class Ideation in *The Cosby Show* and *Martin*," in Mutua, *Progressive Black Masculinities*, 177–89.

32. Neal dates the "new black man" later than I do here and sees it emerging more in response to and repudiation of the 1995 Million Man March, which celebrated traditional masculine and patriarchal values. But the black men who accompanied their wives in labor and delivery voiced similar ideas at least from the 1970s, as this book demonstrates. For more on black masculinity, see all the essays in Mutua, *Progressive Black Masculinities*. For a discussion of earlier twentieth-century ideas about black masculinity, see Martin Summers, *Manliness and Its Discontents: The Black Middle Class and the Transformation of Masculinity, 1900–1930* (Chapel Hill: University of North Carolina Press, 2004). For a related theoretical discussion, see Patricia Hill Collins, "A Telling Difference: Dominance, Strength, and Black Masculinities," in Mutua, *Progressive Black Masculinities*, 73–97, and Patricia Hill Collins, *Black Feminist Thought: Knowledge, Consciousness, and the Politics of Empowerment* (New York: Routledge, 2000).

33. See, for example, Katherine Beckett, "Choosing Cesarean: Feminism and the Politics of Childbirth in the United States," *Feminist Theory* 6, no. 3 (2005): 251–75.

34. Feminism was certainly not monolithic: individuals who identified as feminists differed in their positions, but many would have believed that the childbirth reformers yielded too much to medical authority. On differences among feminists, see, for example, Linda Gordon, "On Difference," *Genders* 10 (Spring 1991): 91–111; Sandra Harding, *Feminism and Methodology: Social Science Issues* (Bloomington: University of Indiana Press, 1987); and Elaine Marks and Isabelle De Courtivron, *New French Feminisms* (New York: Schocken Books, 1981).

35. Sandra Eiseman emphasized the conservative nature of La Leche League, a group that focused on breast-feeding, an important component in changing childbirth practices in the 1970s; Eiseman, interview with author, July 8, 2005, Madison, Wisconsin. On La Leche League, as an example, see Jule DeJager Ward, *La Leche League: At the Crossroads of Medicine, Feminism, and Religion* (Chapel Hill: University of North Carolina Press, 2000).

36. Jane E. Levey, "Imagining the Family in Postwar Popular Culture," *Journal of Women's History* 13, no. 3 (Autumn 2001): 125–50, quotation on 125. See also the rest of the "Dialogue" on "Reimagining the Family" edited by Nancy E. Cott and Jill Lepore in ibid., 151–68, and its introduction, 122–23. Middle-class manhood had been in "crisis" earlier in the twentieth century, too. For that, see, for example, Mark C. Carnes, "Fictions and Fantasies of Early-Twentieth Century Manhood," *Reviews in American History* 24, no. 3 (1996): 448–53, and Gail Bederman, *Manliness and Civilization: A Cultural History of Gender and Race in the United States, 1880–1917* (Chicago: University of Chicago Press, 1995). For a general and well-illustrated history of women in the middle years of the twentieth century, see Elaine Tyler May, *Pushing the Limits: American Women, 1940–1961* (New York: Oxford University Press, 1994).

37. See, for example Bederman, *Manliness and Civilization*.

Chapter One

1. Much of this chapter is based on my book *Brought to Bed: Childbearing in America, 1750–1950* (New York: Oxford University Press, 1986) and on my article "The Medicalization of Childbirth in the Twentieth Century," *Transactions and Studies of the College of Physicians of Philadelphia*, ser. 5, 11, no. 4 (1989): 299–319, which are used here with permission. For current birth statistics, see Joyce A. Martin et al., *National Vital Statistics Report* 55, no. 1, "Births: Final Data for 2004" (Washington, D.C.: U.S. Department of Health and Human Services, Centers for Disease Control, 2006). Midwives and nurse-midwives now attend about 8 percent of deliveries, most of which occur in the hospital.

2. Louis B. Wright and Marion Tinling, eds., *The Secret Diary of William Byrd of Westover, 1709–1792* (Richmond, Va.: Dietz Press, 1941), 79.

3. Francis G. Walett, ed., *The Diary of Ebenezer Parkman, 1703–1782* (Worcester, Mass.: American Antiquarian Society, 1974), 150, entry for February 16, 1747.

4. Mary Louise Fowler to Nettie Fowler McCormick, October 25, 1863, McCormick Family Papers, Incoming Correspondence, 1860–64, WHSA. See also, for the next generation, Nettie Fowler McCormick to Anita McCormick Blaine, August 1890, ser. 1E, box 459, and Anita McCormick Blaine to Nettie Fowler McCormick, August 14, 1890, ser. 2B, box 46, both in Nancy Fowler McCormick Papers, WHSA.

5. Malinda Jenkins, *Gambler's Wife: The Life of Malinda Jenkins, As Told in Conversations to Jessie Lilienthal* (Boston: Houghton Mifflin, 1933), 48.

6. Elizabeth Elton Smith, *The Three Eras of a Woman's Life* (New York: Harper Bros., 1836), 85.

7. See, for example, Nettie Fowler McCormick to Anita McCormick Blaine, August 1890.

8. Grace Lumpkin, *To Make My Bread* (New York: Macaulay, 1932), 12. My thanks to Mari Jo Buhle for calling this reference to my attention.

9. Mrs. W. H. Maxwell, M.D., *A Female Physician to the Ladies of the United States, Being a Familiar and Practical Treatise on Matters of Utmost Importance Peculiar to Women; Adapted for Every Woman's Own Private Use* (New York: published by Mrs. W. H. Maxwell, 1860), 3.

10. See, for example, Catherine Scholten, "'On the Importance of the Obstetrick Art': Changing Customs of Childbirth in America, 1760–1825," in *Women and Health in America: Historical Readings*, ed. Judith Walzer Leavitt (Madison: University of Wisconsin Press, 1984), 142–54.

11. See Leavitt, *Brought to Bed*.

12. William Allen Pusey, *A Doctor of the 1870s and 1880s* (Springfield, Ill.: Charles C. Thomas, 1932), 106.

13. Mabel Hobson Draper, *Through the Long Trail* (New York: Rinehart and Co., 1946), 278–79.

14. Diary of Daniel Cameron, May 25, 1853, 53, WHSA (emphasis in original).

15. For a fuller discussion of how fear of death and debility affected women's decisions about childbirth attendants, consult Leavitt, *Brought to Bed*, especially chap. 1.

16. William P. Dewees, *A Compendious System of Midwifery, Chiefly Designed to Facilitate the Inquiries of Those Who May Be Pursuing This Branch of Study* (Philadelphia: Cary and Lea, 1830), 359.

17. Historians who study this period believe that midwives, who could have learned to use forceps, did not use them because they believed that, as instruments, hands of "flesh" were superior to hands of "iron," as forceps were called. See, for example, Judy Barrett Litoff, *American Midwives, 1860 to the Present* (Westport, Conn.: Greenwood Press, 1978); Janet Bogdan, "Care or Cure? Childbirth Practices in Nineteenth-Century America," *Feminist Studies* 4, no. 2 (1978): 92–99; Janet Carlisle Bogdan, "Aggressive Intervention and Mortality," in *The American Way of Birth*, ed. Pamela S. Eakins (Philadelphia: Temple University Press, 1986), 87–92; and Jane B. Donegan, *Women and Men*

Midwives: Medicine, Morality, and Misogyny in Early America (Westport, Conn.: Greenwood Press, 1978).

18. Morris Fishbein, *An Autobiography* (Garden City, N.Y.: Doubleday, 1969), 25.

19. Helen MacKnight Doyle, *A Child Went Forth: The Autobiography of Dr. Helen MacKnight Doyle* (New York: Gotham House, 1934), 322.

20. S. H. Landrum, letter to the editor, *Journal of the American Medical Association* 58 (February 24, 1912): 576. I would like to thank Carolyn Hackler for calling this reference to my attention.

21. J. H. Guinn to editor, *Journal of the American Medical Association* 58 (March 23, 1912): 880.

22. J. H. MacKay to editor, *Journal of the American Medical Association* 58 (March 9, 1912): 720.

23. Samuel X. Radbill, M.D., to author, June 24, 1985, AQ, *NYT*.

24. By 1900 white married women, showing the ability to cut their fertility in half over the century, averaged 3.54 children, but there was significant variation through the population. White farm women living in the South continued to bear an average of almost 6 children at the end of the nineteenth century. African American women bore an average of more than 5 children. German and Irish women living in Philadelphia averaged more than 7. For more on fertility rates and mortality rates, see Leavitt, *Brought to Bed*, chap. 1.

25. Clara Clough Lenroot, "Journals and Diaries," pt. 1, 1891–1929, edited by her daughter Katharine F. Lenroot, typescript (May 1969) in family hands. My thanks to Katherine Vila, who shared copies of this diary with my class "Women and Health in America," University of Wisconsin, Spring Semester 1983, and who gave permission for me to use this quotation. Many more examples of women's worries about mortality can be found in Leavitt, *Brought to Bed*.

26. Lillie M. Jackson, *Fanning the Embers* (Boston: Christopher Publishing House, 1966), 90–91.

27. Hallie F. Nelson, *South of the Cottonwood Trees* (Broken Bow, Neb.: Purcellow, 1977), 214.

28. Quoted in "I Had a Baby Too: A Symposium," *Atlantic* 163 (1939): 764.

29. George I. McKelway, "Delivery through the Abdominal Walls vs. Craniotomy in Otherwise Impossible Births," *Journal of the American Medical Association* 19 (July 2, 1892): 8. For an expanded analysis of this issue, see Judith Walzer Leavitt, "The Growth of Medical Authority: Technology and Morals in Turn-of-the-Century Obstetrics," *Medical Anthropology Quarterly* 1 (1987): 230–55.

30. Unnamed woman quoted in M. F. Ashley Montagu, "Babies Should Be Born at Home!" *Ladies' Home Journal*, August 1958, 52–53.

31. Quoted in Gladys Denny Shultz, "Journal Mothers Report on Cruelty in Maternity Wards," *Ladies' Home Journal*, May 1958, 44–45, 152–55, quotation on 44.

32. S. Josephine Baker, "Why Do Our Mothers and Babies Die?" *Ladies' Home Journal*, April 1922, 32. See also, in the October 1923 issue of the *Journal*, her "The High Cost of Babies," 212–13.

33. See, for example, Margaret Charles Smith and Linda Janet Holmes, *Listen to Me Good: The Life Story of an Alabama Midwife* (Columbus: Ohio State University Press, 1996).

34. Marvin D. Muhlhausen to author, June 28, 2005, AQ, OW.

35. Ethel C. Dunham, Marshall Shaffer, and Neil F. MacDonald, "Standard Plans for Nurseries for Newborns in Hospitals of 50 to 200 Beds," *Hospitals* 17 (April 1943): 16–21, figures on 16. Figures for other groups are not available.

36. Quoted in Shultz, "Journal Mothers Report," 44.

37. Betty MacDonald, *The Egg and I* (Philadelphia: Lippincott, 1945), 163.

38. All quotations from J. P. McEvoy, "Our Streamlined Baby," *Reader's Digest*, May 1938, 15–18.

39. Philip A. Kalisch and Beatrice J. Kalisch, *The Advance of American Nursing* (Boston: Little, Brown, 1978), 343.

40. Leavitt, "Growth of Medical Authority," 230–55. See also, for example, Roy P. Finney, *The Story of Motherhood* (New York: Liverright, 1937), and Alan Frank Guttmacher, *Into This Universe: The Story of Human Birth* (New York: Blue Ribbon Books, 1937). For an overview of childbirth's move into the hospital, see Leavitt, *Brought to Bed*. The proportion of births that took place in women's homes declined from more than 50 percent in 1930 to only 12 percent by 1950. See Neal Devitt, "The Transition from Home to Hospital Birth in the United States, 1930–1960," *Birth and the Family Journal* 4 (1977): 47–58.

41. Finney, *Story of Motherhood*, 6–7. See also Guttmacher, *Into this Universe*, 192–267.

42. Eleanor Waddell interview, July 1, 1986, MNOHP, quotations on 8, 10. See also Sara Jane Williams, "Caught in the Middle: Maternity Nurses and the Natural Childbirth Movement" (M.S. thesis, University of Wisconsin School of Nursing, 1987).

43. Margarete Sandelowski, *Pain, Pleasure, and American Childbirth: From the Twilight Sleep to the Read Method, 1914–1960* (Westport, Conn.: Greenwood Press, 1984), 28.

44. See Larry C. Gilstrap, F. Gary Cunningham, and J. Peter Vandorsten, *Operative Obstetrics* (New York: McGraw-Hill, 2002), 89.

45. New York Academy of Medicine Committee on Public Health Relations, *Maternal Mortality in New York City: A Study of All Puerperal Deaths, 1930–1932* (New York: Commonwealth Fund, 1933), 213–15, 115–27, 113–17, 126–27. For a broader discussion of these issues, see Leavitt, *Brought to Bed*, 179–89.

46. Joseph B. DeLee, "The Maternity Ward of the General Hospital," *Modern Hospital Yearbook* 6 (1926): 67–72, and Joseph B. DeLee and Heinz Sidentropf, "The Maternity Ward of the General Hospital," *Journal of the American Medical Association* 100 (January 7, 1933): 6–14.

47. The quotations are from personal communications to the author in response to my author's query in the *New York Times* Sunday Book Review, July 24, 1983. I received about two hundred responses. Quotations here are from Katherine S. Egan, August 25, 1983; Marilyn Clohessy, September 9, 1983; Elsa Rosenberg, July 30, 1983; and women who wished to remain anonymous. My thanks to all of them.

48. The women are quoted in Shultz, "Journal Mothers Report," 44–45.

49. Robbie Davis-Floyd, *Birth as an American Rite of Passage* (Berkeley: University of California Press, 1992), 3–4.

50. Barbara Bridgman Perkins, *The Medical Delivery Business: Health Reform, Childbirth, and the Economic Order* (New Brunswick, N.J.: Rutgers University Press, 2004), 141–43. There are, as with any medication, some risks involved in using Pitocin.

51. B. C. Farrand, "After Office Hours: Elective Induction of Labor," *Obstetrics and Gynecology* 7, no. 6 (June 1956): 716–18, quotation on 716.

52. Barbara Ulfsparre to author, September 14, 1983, AQ, *NYT*.

53. Deb B. interview, June 26, 1996, BP, about her 1940s deliveries.

54. Carolyn Splett interview, April 24, 1986, MNOHP, 7–8.

55. Harvey Gabert and Morton A. Stenchever, "Electronic Fetal Monitoring as a Routine Practice in an Obstetric Service: A Progress Report," *American Journal of Obstetrics and Gynecology* 118, no. 4 (1974): 534–37.

56. Margarete Sandelowski, *Devices and Desires: Gender, Technology, and American Nursing* (Chapel Hill: University of North Carolina Press, 2000), 144, 135–75.

57. On women's resistance to fetal monitors and a thoughtful discussion of how such technology changes perceptions of birth, see Emily Martin, *The Woman in the Body: A Cultural Analysis of Reproduction* (Boston: Beacon Press, 1987), esp. 139–48.

58. Sandelowski, *Devices and Desires*, chap. 6.

59. Richard K. Reed, *Birthing Fathers: The Transformation of Men in American Rites of Birth* (New Brunswick, N.J.: Rutgers University Press, 2005), 182.

60. See, for example, Margot Edwards and Mary Waldorf, *Reclaiming Birth: History and Heroines of American Childbirth Reform* (Trumansburg, N.Y.: Crossing Press, 1984), 117–21.

61. Dr. Ralph Pomeroy tried to make episiotomy routine in 1918 ("Shall We Cut and Reconstruct the Perinium for Every Primipara?" *American Journal of Obstetrics and Diseases of Women and Children* 78 [1918]: 211–19), and Joseph B. DeLee emphasized its prophylactic benefits ("The Prophylactic Forceps Operation," *American Journal of Obstetrics and Gynecology* 1 [1920]: 34–44). For a fuller discussion of DeLee, see Judith Walzer Leavitt, "Joseph B. DeLee and the Practice of Preventive Obstetrics," *American Journal of Public Health* 78, no. 10 (October 1988): 1353–59.

62. Perkins, *Medical Delivery Business*, 41.

63. See, for example, Edwards and Waldorf, *Reclaiming Birth*, 142–45.

64. Jayne F. interview, July 12, 1990, BP.

65. Emanuel Friedman, "The Graphic Analysis of Labor," *American Journal of Obstetrics and Gynecology* 68, no. 6 (1954): 1568–75. See also his "Primigravid Labor: A Graphicostatistical Analysis," *Obstetrics and Gynecology* 6, no. 6 (1955): 567–89, and his "Synthetic Oxytocin: Critical Evaluation in Labor and Post Partum," *American Journal of Obstetrics and Gynecology* 74, no. 5 (1957): 1118–24.

66. Davis-Floyd, *Birth as an American Rite of Passage*, 51–59, 282.

67. As cited in Perkins, *Medical Delivery Business*, 37.

68. Roslyn Lindheim, "Birthing Centers and Hospices: Reclaiming Birth and Death," *Annual Reviews of Public Health* 2 (1981): 1–29, quotations on 5–6.

69. Quotations in this paragraph and the next from Shultz, "Journal Mothers Report," and Gladys Denny Shultz, "Journal Mothers Testify to Cruelty in Maternity Wards," *Ladies' Home Journal*, December 1958, 58–59, 135–38. For a fuller discussion of conflicts between birthing women and obstetrical nurses and some analysis of their meaning, see Judith Walzer Leavitt, "'Strange Young Women on Errands': Obstetric Nursing between Two Worlds," *Nursing History Review* 6 (1998): 3–24; reprinted in *Enduring Issues in American Nursing*, ed. Ellen D. Baer, Patricia D'Antonio, Sylvia Rinker, and Joan E. Lynaugh (New York: Springer, 2001), 180–200.

70. "Jean" quoted in Alissa Berman, Erin McCarthy, and Micaela Sullivan, "Childbirth in Chicago: Information and Expectations, a Generational Study" (paper written for History 483, Loyola University, Chicago, Dr. Kerr's class, April 8, 1984), 19. My thanks to Micaela Sullivan-Fowler for providing access to this paper and to some of her notes from the oral history interviews that she and her colleagues conducted.

71. Katherine Egan to author, August 25, 1983, AQ, *NYT*.

72. Ruth E. Owen and Lucille G. Denman, "Experiences in Childbirth," *Child-Family Digest* 4, no. 4 (April 1951): 27–32, quotation on 28.

73. Lotte Weininger to author, August 8, 1983, in AQ, *NYT*.

74. Shultz, "Journal Mothers Report," 155.

75. Gail Villotta, letter to the editor, *American Journal of Nursing* 72 (September 1972): 1576. My thanks to Naomi Rogers for this reference.

76. See, for example, E. Anthony Rotundo, *American Manhood: Transformations in Masculinity from the Revolution to the Modern Era* (New York: Basic Books, 1994); Robert L. Griswold, *Fatherhood in America: A History* (New York: Basic Books, 1993); Elaine Tyler May, *Homeward Bound: American Families in the Cold War Era* (New York: Basic Books, 1988); and Martin Summers, *Manliness and Its Discontents: The Black Middle Class and the Transformation of Masculinity, 1900–1930* (Chapel Hill: University of North Carolina Press, 2004). For an earlier period, see Gail Bederman, *Manliness and Civilization: A Cultural History of Gender and Race in the United States, 1880–1917* (Chicago: University of Chicago Press, 1995).

Chapter Two

1. For example, see Jessica Mitford, *The American Way of Birth* (New York: Dutton, 1992).

2. Dale Clark, "A Man's Crusade for Easy Childbirth: A Husband's Place Is Not in the Waiting Room, but Close to His Wife's Side," *Esquire*, October 1949, 51, 151–52, quotation on 151–52 (emphasis in original).

3. Edward F. Stevens, *The American Hospital of the Twentieth Century* (New York: F. W. Dodge, 1928); the maternity departments are discussed on 170–208, floor plan for St. Luke's on 179, floor plan for Chicago Lying-In on 180.

4. Norman Rockwell, "Maternity Waiting Room," *Saturday Evening Post*, July 13, 1946, 12.

5. For an excellent study of such practices and the history of historically black hospitals, see Vanessa Northington Gamble, *Making a Place for Ourselves: The Black Hospital Movement, 1920–1945* (New York: Oxford University Press, 1995).

6. William R. Rosengren and Spencer DeVault, "The Sociology of Time and Space in an Obstetrical Hospital," in *The Hospital in Modern Society*, ed. Eliot Freidson (Glencoe, Ill.: Free Press, 1963), 266–92, quotation on 278.

7. See, for example, E. Todd Wheeler, *Hospital Design and Function* (New York: McGraw-Hill, 1964), 135–39. "Near the entrance to the [maternity] suite provide a waiting room for fathers and other relatives" (138). See also, for example, an article about a new maternity suite at Memorial Hospital in Long Beach, California, which included a special fathers' room, in *Long Beach Independent*, June 9, 1960, 7.

8. U.S. Department of Labor, Children's Bureau, "Standards and Recommendations for Hospital Care of Maternity Patients," 13. Copy located in "Emergency Maternity and Infant Care Program," 1942, box 1, folder 7, ser. 2253, WHSA.

9. David Gruener to author, July 7, 2005, AQ, *OW*.

10. Greer Williams, "I Was a Father Once Myself . . . ," *Modern Hospital* 84 (January 1955): 68–72.

11. Stuart Price to author, August 11, 2005, AQ, *OW*.

12. WMH, FB, September 5, 1949. I am extremely grateful to archivist Susan Sacharski for showing me the books and her generous help with my research. The names of the fathers have not been used in the interests of patient confidentiality.

13. WMH, FB, August 27, 1959. The comedian Bob Newhart also used the phrase "torture chamber" in a monologue recorded live at San Fernando Valley State College, Northridge, California, December 17, 1963. It is available on his CD, *The Bob Newhart Anthology*, disc 2, track 5, "The Expectant Father." I thank Michele Lyons and Sarah Leavitt for calling this to my attention.

14. WMH, FB, March 13, 1949.

15. Ibid., January 5, 1950.

16. Louis Pollock, *Stork Bites Man: What the Expectant Father May Expect* (Cleveland: World Publishing Co., 1945), 122. This is a book for fathers written with humor. The story about the switchboard attendant continued, "And he turned and would have shuffled off if I hadn't called him. 'Wait a minute!' I stuttered. 'Is that the Pollock baby? . . . Well, I want to go up and see her,' I told him. 'I want to see her right away. . . .' The old man shook his head, 'Now there's no sense to that,' he said. 'She's sleeping now and all tuckered out. You'll see her in the morning.' 'How about the baby? Can I see the baby?' I queried. His head stopped shaking. 'What do you want to see the baby for?' he asked. 'He's all right and sleeping too. Why don't you go home and have some sleep. Everything's fine.' And he went back to his switchboard" (122–23).

17. Joseph B. DeLee, *Obstetrics for Nurses* (Philadelphia: W. B. Saunders, 1924), 196. For a later rendition of the same, see Edward Davis and Mabel Carmon, *Obstetrics for Nurses*, 16th ed. (Philadelphia: W. B. Saunders, 1957), 231: "The expectant father may be apprehensive when waiting in the husbands' room. He is concerned about his wife's safety and can imagine all types of complications. He feels threatened with the possible loss of his wife. The nurse can ease this anxiety by keeping him informed of his wife's progress."

18. Carolyn Conant Van Blarcom and Erna Ziegel, *Obstetrical Nursing*, 4th ed. (New York: Macmillan, 1957), 297.

19. Unidentified man quoted in Robert Allen Fein, "Men's Experiences before and after the Birth of a First Child: Dependence, Marital Sharing, and Anxiety" (Ph.D. diss., Harvard University, 1974), 189–90. Another man quoted in this study said, "They forgot to tell me what was happening. I waited and waited and waited for a word. The nursing staff forgot about me. It was really hard" (289).

20. William L. Hoffmann, "Papa Is All," *Herald*, March 1942, 8–9. Hoffman wrote the humorous account for the monthly magazine of the Junior Woman's Club of Orange, New Jersey. "Papa is all" is a Pennsylvania Dutch expression meaning he is finished, through, wiped out.

21. John Gould, "Pre-Natal Care for Fathers," *Esquire*, July 1947, 54–55, 130, quotations on 55, 130.

22. Mike Bitney interview, August 25, 1986, MNOHP, 3–4.

23. Sister Mary Stella, supervisor of obstetrics at St. Mary's Hospital in Evansville, Indiana, wrote this in "A New Approach," *ASPON*, February–March 1968.

24. Marie Baldwin to author, August 13, 1984, AQ, *NYT*.

25. Williams, "I Was a Father Once Myself," 70.

26. Helen Glixon to author, September 22, 1983, AQ, *NYT* (her ellipses). See also Gwen Gilmore to author, August 3, 1983, AQ, *NYT*, about her 1942 labor.

27. Jessica Gerard to author, no date, AQ, *NYT*. Girard sent a different woman's account of her delivery at the Maternity Pavilion at Milwaukee Lutheran Hospital.

28. J. C. Brierre, "History of Medicine in Shreveport: The Black Experience," *Journal of the North Louisiana Historical Association* 17, nos. 2–3 (Spring–Summer 1986): 91–96, quotation on 95.

29. See, for example, Edward F. Stevens, *The American Hospital of the Twentieth Century* (New York: F. W. Dodge, 1928), 172–73.

30. WMH, FB, May 15, 1951.

31. Ibid., July 14, 1954.

32. See Allan Brandt, *The Cigarette Century* (Cambridge, Mass.: Harvard University Press, 2007), 309.

33. Russell Baker, "Fathering," *New York Times* Sunday Magazine Section, June 20, 1982, 14.

34. Television critics of the situation comedy in the 1950s and 1960s have noted that more than two-thirds of domestic situation comedy series portrayed middle-class families and that those about working-class families often devalued the man, showing him as "an inept bumbler and even a buffoon," while his wife was more intelligent and sensible, a tradition that continued through the 1990s. It is tempting to try to read men's waiting-room behavior through this class-related lens: What does it mean that around birthing all men succumbed to the same behavior? See Richard Butsch, "A Half Century of Class and Gender in American TV Domestic Sitcoms," *Cercles* 8 (2003): 16–34, quotation on 20.

35. I am grateful to Steve Allen Productions for sending me a research copy of the skit, which I first watched in the Library of Congress film collection. It aired on NBC on June 1, 1958.

36. Quoted in Stuart M. Kaminsky, *American Film Genres*, 2nd ed. (Chicago: Nelson-Hall, 1984), 160.

37. *Rock-a-Bye Baby*, 1958, Universal Pictures, based on the screenplay *Miracle of Morgan's Creek* by Preston Sturges; Frank Tashlin, director; Jerry Lewis, producer; viewed from the video reproduction.

38. Some hospitals in these years allowed one person, usually the husband, briefly to visit a woman in labor. See, for example, Malcom T. MacEachern, *Manual on Obstetric Practice in Hospitals* (Chicago: American Hospital Association, 1940), 77. Men joining their wives in the labor room will be discussed in the next chapter.

39. Katherine Egan to author, August 25, 1983, AQ, *NYT*.

40. Deb B. interview, June 26, 1996, BP.

41. Muriel Goldfarb and Robert W. Goldfarb, "We Shared Our Baby's Birth . . . ," *Ladies' Home Journal*, December 1958, 140.

42. Shirley Ricketts to author, July 24, 1983, AQ, *NYT*.

43. August Stuart Clay, "Guidance in Maternal and Infant Care Two Months before and after the Birth of the First-Born," *Pediatrics* 2 (August 1948): 200–206, quotation on 202.

44. The Wesley Memorial Hospital Fathers' Books are available to scholars at the Northwestern Memorial Hospital Archives, Chicago.

45. Robert M. Yoder, "Let's Be Sick in Comfort," *Saturday Evening Post*, July 10, 1943, 22–23, 56, 59, quotation on 59. The article describes the new Wesley Hospital that opened in 1941. On the history of the hospital, see Vernon K. Brown, *The Story of Wesley Memorial Hospital, 1888–1972* (Chicago: Northwestern Memorial Hospital, 1981).

46. On Chicago neighborhoods, see Harold M. Mayer and Richard C. Wade, *Chicago: Growth of a Metropolis* (Chicago: University of Chicago Press, 1969); Dominic A. Pacyga, "Chicago's Ethnic Neighborhoods: The Myth of Stability and the Reality of Change," in *Ethnic Chicago: A Multicultural Portrait*, 4th ed., ed. Melvin G. Holli and Peter d'A. Jones (Grand Rapids, Mich.: William B. Eerdmans, 1995); Chicago Department of Development and Planning, *Historic City: The Settlement of Chicago* (Chicago: Department of Development and Planning, 1976); Dominic A. Pacyga and Ellen Skerrett, *Chicago, City of Neighborhoods: Histories and Tours* (Chicago: Loyola University Press, 1986); Louis Wirth and Eleanor H. Bernert, eds., *Local Community Fact Book of Chicago* (Chicago: University of Chicago Press, 1949); and David K. Fremon, *Chicago Politics Ward by Ward* (Bloomington: Indiana University Press, 1988). When the hospital opened in 1941, it contained five floors of private and two-bed semiprivate rooms and three floors of wards. The semiprivate rooms cost an average of eight dollars a day, single rooms as much as twenty-five dollars. Yoder, "Let's Be Sick in Comfort," 59.

47. *Wesley Memorial Hospital Yearbooks and Annual Reports*, 1942, 1943, 1945, 1946, 1947, located in the Northwestern Memorial Hospital Archives, Chicago.

48. Elizabeth S. LaPerle for the Welfare Council of Metropolitan Chicago, "Study of Maternity Facilities in Cook County," typescript dated May 1954, copy at the University of Illinois Libraries, Urbana-Champaign; see esp. 50–54. See also "Negro Births in Chicago, 1954–1955," *Journal of the National Medical Association* 49, no. 2 (March 1957): 124–25.

49. WMH, FB, September 5, 1949.

50. Ibid., February 9, 1950.

51. Ibid., April 4, 1954.

52. As quoted by Leonard Q. Ross, "Bards of the O.B. Floor," *New Yorker*, July 8, 1939, 66–70, quotation on 66.

53. Ibid., 68.

54. WMH, FB, January 28, 1950.

55. Ibid., November 11, 1951.

56. Ibid., November 13, 1951.

57. Bob Newhart, *I Shouldn't Even Be Doing This! And Other Things That Strike Me as Funny* (New York: Hyperion, 2006), 123. My thanks to Sarah Leavitt and Michelle Lyon for calling Bob Newhart's description to my attention.

58. "Tom" is quoted in Joan Beck, "Doodles by Daddies: A Waiting Room Diary," *Chi-*

cago Tribune, June 17, 1972, sec. 1, p. 11. For an understanding of "performing" gender roles, see Judith Butler, *Gender Trouble: Feminism and the Subversion of Identity* (New York: Routledge, 1990), and "Gender as Performance: An Interview with Judith Butler," interview by Peter Osborne and Lynne Segal, London, 1993, in *Radical Philosophy* 67 (Summer 1994): 32–39. Behavior is sometimes characterized as stereotypically masculine if it is active and feminine if it is passive. These categories fell away in the waiting rooms and also later in labor and delivery rooms. The men waiting in the Stork Club were not passive: they wrote in the fathers' books and together planned how to move out of the constraining rooms. Conversely, in the labor and delivery rooms, sometimes men did nothing but be there, sitting happily without activity.

59. WMH, FB, March 10, 1950.

60. Ibid., December 4, 1950.

61. On the domestic experiences of Americans during the Cold War, see particularly Elaine Tyler May, *Homeward Bound: American Families in the Cold War Era* (New York: Basic Books, 1988).

62. Ian Richie was quoted during Heidi Goldfein's National Public Radio report on the Fathers' Books, June 20, 1999.

63. In my efforts to find more fathers' books, I wrote letters of inquiry to many university-associated hospitals as well as to every hospital in two states (Georgia and Massachusetts). In some cases, individuals wrote back that they remembered such books in their hospitals but could not find them.

64. WMH, FB, February 20, 1949.

65. Ibid., January 1, 1950.

66. Ibid., March 23, 1949.

67. Ibid., no date, follows May 23, 1950, entry in September 1949 book.

68. Ibid., September 8, 1950.

69. Ibid., May 25, 1952.

70. Ibid., December 9, 1952.

71. Joan Beck, "New Dads Display Agony, Ecstasy," *Chicago Tribune*, June 26, 1972, no page number. Photocopy of this article can be found in the Northwestern Memorial Hospital Archives, Chicago.

72. WMH, FB, February 18, 1960.

73. Sigurd T. Lokken, "Carol's and Sigurd's First Baby—Roald T. Lokken, September 8, 1953" (emphasis in original). I am grateful to Crystal Lokken (then known as Carol) and to Roald T. Lokken for sharing this account with me, on September 10, 2005, AQ, OW.

74. David W. Roberts to author, October 12, 2005, AQ, OW.

75. WMH, FB, October 26, 1949.

76. Ibid., April 19, 1953.

77. Ibid., January 6, 1960.

78. Ibid., October 17, 1950.

79. Ibid., June 2, 1962.

80. In 1950, maternal mortality for all races was 83.3 per 100,000 live births, improved considerably over the 1940 rate, which was 376. Racial differentials were great: in 1950, 61 white women and 223 black women died for every 100,000 live births. See Centers for Disease Control, "Maternal Mortality and Related Concepts," *Vital and Health Statistics*, ser. 3, no. 33 (Washington, D.C.: U.S. Government Printing Office, February 2007), table 1, p. 9. Infant mortality, calculated per 1,000 live births, in 1950 was 19.2 (26.8 for white infants and 43.9 for black infants). See <www.cdc.gov/nchs/data/hus/tables/2001/01hus023.pdf> (accessed February 26, 2008).

81. "Depressed Husband" quoted in Ross, "Bards of the O.B. Floor," 68.

82. WMH, FB, December 4, 1960 (but should be 1961 according to placement).

83. On the cultural authority of medicine, see, for example, Paul Starr, *The Social Transformation of American Medicine* (New York: Basic Books, 1983).

84. WMH, FB, no date, follows May 23, 1950, entry in September 1949 book.

85. Ibid., September 21, 1949.

86. Ibid., January 31, 1950.

87. Ibid., February 9, 1954.

88. George Schaefer, *The Expectant Father*, rev. ed. (New York: Barnes and Noble Books, Division of Harper and Row, 1972), 98.

89. James L. Reycraft, "Induction of Labor," *American Journal of Obstetrics and Gynecology* 61, no. 4 (April 1951): 801–8, quotations from 801, 806.

90. WMH, FB, June 30, 1960. See also January 27, 1951.

91. Ibid., May 26, 1962.

92. Ibid., December 16, 1963.

93. June Stevenson to author, July 24, 1983, AQ, *NYT*.

94. Elinor Kunze to author, no date, AQ, *NYT*.

95. WMH, FB, March 6, 1949.

96. Ibid., August 31, 1950.

97. Ibid., January 20, 1951.

98. Ibid., March 15, 1952.

99. Ibid., October 31, 1954, May 4, 1959.

100. Ibid., November 13, 1963.

101. "Dear Diary," entry undated, but from placement in book seems to be 1974. My thanks to Dr. Susan Davidson and the St. Mary's Medical Center staff for helping me locate and use this book, which is held by the hospital.

102. Quoted in Beck, "New Dads Display Agony."

103. Quoted in ibid. See also the first part of this two-part article, "Doodles by Daddies." Although the extant Fathers' Books at Wesley only date until 1965, this article makes it clear that the books were still out in the waiting room into the 1970s. For other

newspaper articles on the Wesley Stork Club books, see Robert S. Kleckner, "Jottings from 'Stork Room' Diary: Jittery Fathers-to-Be Write Down Their Thoughts While They Wait," *Chicago Sun-Times*, May 4, 1952; Sue Ellen Christian, "Pregnant Pauses," *Chicago Tribune*, July 2, 1999; and Williams, "I Was a Father Once Myself."

104. Quoted in "Nat King Cole Baby," *Ebony*, June 1950, 33.

105. WMH, FB, October 24, 1951.

106. Ibid., May 6, 1952.

107. Ibid., January 13, 1953.

108. Ibid., December 12, 1950.

109. Ibid., April 16, 1951.

110. Ibid., July 6, 1950.

111. Ibid., February 28, 1954.

112. Ibid., March 30, 1949.

113. David Gruener to author, July 7, 2005, AQ, *OW*.

114. WMH, FB, February 28, 1954.

115. Ibid., July 18, 1949.

116. Ibid., April 19, 1953.

117. Marvin D. Muhlhausen to author, June 28 and June 29, 2005, AQ, *OW*.

118. Howard D. Johnson to author, July 8, 2005, AQ, *OW*.

119. Aileen Hogan, "Natural Childbirth," *Child-Family Digest* 4, no. 4 (April 1951): 61–64, quotation on 62.

120. Aileen Hogan, "The Scope of Maternity Nursing," *Child-Family Digest* 5, no. 4 (October 1951): 44–48, quotation on 44–45.

121. Vance Packard, "Now You Can Both Rehearse for Parenthood," *American Magazine*, June 1952, 24–27, 105–10, quotation on 25.

122. Jack Harrison Pollack, "The Case for Natural Childbirth," *Cosmopolitan*, July 1953, 39–43, quotation on 42.

123. Ruth Brecher and Edward Brecher, "How to Get Better Maternity Care," *Redbook*, July 1962, 43, 108–11, quotation on 43.

124. Peter S. Douglas, "A Father Reports on Natural Childbirth," *Child-Family Digest* 3, no. 3 (September 1950): 60.

125. Marion D. Laird and Margaret Hogan, "An Elective Program on Preparation for Childbirth at the Sloane Hospital for Women, May, 1951 to June, 1954," *American Journal of Obstetrics and Gynecology* 72, no. 3 (September 1956): 641–47, quotation on 646.

126. Howard Johnson to author, July 8, 2005, AQ, *OW*.

127. Shirley Zussman, *A Study of Certain Social, Psychological, and Cultural Factors Influencing Husbands' Participation in Their Wives' Labor* (Ann Arbor, Mich.: UMI, 1969), quotations on 146, 147. The author understood some of this attitude to stem from the men feeling that "waiting for someone to bring them the news of the birth of their son or daughter may be . . . to confirm *their* feeling of manliness" (174).

128. Unidentified man is quoted in Sally Olds and Linda Witt, "New Man in the Delivery Room—the Father," *Today's Health*, October 1970, 52–56, quotation on 54.

129. Steven M. Barney, "I Was There When My Son Was Born," *Wisconsin State Journal* (Madison), July 27, 1969. My thanks to Steven Barney and to William Wineke at the *State Journal* for helping me locate this article.

130. John M. Jullien, *Planning the Labor-Delivery Unit in the General Hospital* (Washington, D.C.: U.S. Department of Health, Education and Welfare, Public Health Service, Division of Hospital and Medical Facilities, Architectural and Engineering Branch, 1964), Public Health Service publication no. 830-D-15, quotations on 3. See also Roy Hudenburg, *Planning the Community Hospital* (New York: McGraw-Hill, 1967), 110–23, section on maternity facilities.

131. George Schaefer, "The Expectant Father: His Care and Management," *Postgraduate Medicine* 38 (December 1965): 658–63, quotation on 662.

132. Robert N. Rutherford, "Fathers in the Delivery Room—Long Experience Molds One Viewpoint," *Hospital Topics* 44, no. 1 (January 1966): 97–102, quotation on 100.

133. Earl Withycombe to author, September 3, 2005. Contrast this with Withycombe's next birth experience, related in Chapter 7. I am grateful to Shannon Withycombe for facilitating this communication.

Chapter Three

1. Grantly Dick-Read, *Childbirth without Fear: The Principles and Practice of Natural Childbirth* (New York: Harper and Brothers, 1944). The book, first published in England in 1933 under the title *Natural Childbirth*, went through many American editions beginning in 1944 and including further revised ones in 1970 and 1979. Americans generally refer to Dick-Read as Read, but I will use his name as it appeared in his books, Dick-Read, unless it is in a direct quotation. See also Thomas A. Noyes, *Dr. Courageous: The Story of Dr. Grantly Dick-Read* (New York: Harper, 1957), and A. Susan Williams, *Women and Childbirth in the Twentieth Century: A History of the National Birthday Trust Fund, 1828–1993* (Stroud, England: Sutton Publishing, 1997). Fernand Lamaze became well known in the United States through the writings of Marjorie Karmel, first in an article, "A New Method of Painless Childbirth," *Harper's Bazaar*, June 1957, 72, 120, and then in her book *Thank You, Dr. Lamaze* (Philadelphia: Lippincott, 1959). See also Fernand Lamaze, *Painless Childbirth: The Lamaze Method*, trans. L. R. Celestin (New York: Pocket Books, 1972). That method will be further described in Chapter 4. Both Dick-Read and Lamaze were more popular in the United States than they were in their respective countries.

2. See, for example, Nancy A. Hewitt, ed., *Companion to American Women's History* (Oxford: Blackwell, 2002); Nancy F. Cott, ed., *No Small Courage: A History of Women in the United States* (New York: Oxford University Press, 2000); Elaine Tyler May, *Home-*

ward Bound: American Families in the Cold War Era (New York: Basic Books, 1988) and her *Barren in the Promised Land: Childless Americans and the Pursuit of Happiness* (New York: Basic Books, 1995); Sara Evans, *Born for Liberty: A History of Women in the United States* (New York: Free Press, 1989); and William Chafe, *The Paradox of Change: American Women in the Twentieth Century* (New York: Oxford University Press, 1991).

3. Dale Clark, "A Man's Crusade for Easy Childbirth: A Husband's Place Is Not in the Waiting Room, but Close to His Wife's Side," *Esquire*, October 1949, 51, 151–52, quotations on 51, 152.

4. See, for example, the Chicago Board of Health, "Regulations for the Conduct of Maternity Hospitals, Maternity Divisions of General Hospitals and Nurseries for the Newborn," January 16, 1958, 17, in which it seemed the fathers would only briefly be allowed to see their wives during labor; copy in the Northwestern Memorial Hospital Archives, Chicago. Similar policies can be found for most hospitals at midcentury. Wesley procedures added, "No visitors are permitted while the babies are out of the nursery and in the mothers' rooms. 9:30 AM–10:30 AM; 1:30 PM–2:30 PM; 5:30 PM–6:30 PM; After 9:00 PM." Virtually the same hours held at Passavant Memorial Hospital, across the street. See "Visiting Regulations for the Ninth Floor Obstetrics and Gynecology" and pamphlet "For You and Your Baby," issued by Passavant, no date, in the same archives.

5. Patricia Murphy, "A Nurse-Mother Looks at Natural Childbirth," *Child-Family Digest* 7, no. 4 (December 1952): 55–60.

6. Hazel Corbin, "Maternity Care Today and Tomorrow," *Child-Family Digest* 8, no. 3 (March 1953): 36–45, quotation on 37. The article is taken from Corbin's address to the Fifth American Congress on Obstetrics, April 1, 1952, in Cincinnati, Ohio.

7. Dorothy E. Jump, "Mothers Classes for Preparation for Labor," *Child-Family Digest* 5, no. 2 (August 1951): 97–100, quotation on 99.

8. Mildred W. Hollander to author, June 29, 2005, AQ, *OW*.

9. Joseph B. DeLee and Mabel Carmon, *Obstetrics for Nurses* (Philadelphia: W. B. Saunders, 1937), 196. The phrase is repeated in the 1942 edition (182).

10. J. P. McEvoy, "Our Streamlined Baby," *Reader's Digest* (May 1938): 16–17. On the subject of anesthesia use in this period, see Jacqueline H. Wolf, *Deliver Me from Pain: Anesthesia and Birth in America* (Baltimore: Johns Hopkins University Press, 2009).

11. WMH, FB, March 18, 1961.

12. Ibid., August 31, 1949.

13. On the importance of language to reveal real meanings, see Emily Martin, *The Woman in the Body: A Cultural Analysis of Reproduction* (Baltimore: Johns Hopkins University Press, 1987).

14. Laurance G. Roth, "Natural Childbirth in a General Hospital," *American Journal of Obstetrics and Gynecology* 61, no. 1 (January 1951): 167–72, quotation on 170.

15. Discussant D. J. Bay Jacobs following the talk by Silas Starr, "Prolonged Labor," *American Journal of Obstetrics and Gynecology* 63, no. 2 (February 1952): 333–43, quotation on 339.

16. American College of Obstetricians and Gynecologists, *Manual of Standards in Obstetric-Gynecologic Practice* (Washington, D.C.: American College of Obstetricians and Gynecologists, 1959), 18; copies in the library of the American College of Obstetricians and Gynecologists, Washington, D.C.

17. Josephine H. Kenyon, "Before the Baby Comes," *Good Housekeeping*, August 1945, 185, 199, quotation on 185.

18. The woman delivered four babies between 1946 and 1960 in Milwaukee. (Quoted in an unnamed student paper, Medical History and Women's Studies 431, Spring 2004, University of Wisconsin, and used with the student's permission, without the name.)

19. Constance Ola to author, July 24, 1983, AQ, *NYT*.

20. William H. Genne, *Husbands and Pregnancy: The Handbook for Expectant Fathers* (New York: Association Press, 1956), 19, 74. See also Emma Mai Ewing to author, no date, AQ, *NYT*.

21. Joan Knudson interview, August 26, 1986, MNOHP, 2–3, 9.

22. Joseph B. DeLee, "The Maternity Ward of the General Hospital," *Modern Hospital Yearbook* 6 (1926): 67–72.

23. See, for example, Charles Butler and Addison Erdman, *Hospital Planning* (New York: F. W. Dodge, 1946), chap. 5, "Maternity and Children's Department," 56–67.

24. Sylvia Rinker, "To Cultivate a Feeling of Confidence: The Nursing of Obstetric Patients, 1890–1940," *Nursing History Review* 8 (2000): 117–42, quotations on 120, 126.

25. Anonymous woman to author, September 18, 1983, AQ, *NYT*.

26. Kathleen Lander to author, July 25, 1983, AQ, *NYT*.

27. Mrs. Donald Johnson's story was told in "Report on Mother's Class #8," Public Health Nursing Consultant's Files, 1946–69, Waushara County Expectant Parents, 1953, ser. 2549, box 2, folder 35, WHSA. "Hypo" referred to a hypodermic needle, an injection of a sedative.

28. The differences in opinion are related in "Report on Mother's Class #4," by Mrs. Helmrick, obstetrics nurse from Berlin Hospital, Public Health Nursing Consultant's Files, 1946–69, Waushara County Expectant Parents, 1953, ser. 2549, box 2, folder 35, WHSA. In the same collection, see also "Mothers Demonstration Tape," 1953, box 2, folder 15, ser. 2549.

29. Jean E. Schultz to Rev. J. Lawrence Ainsworth, February 7, 1962. I am very grateful to Rev. Ainsworth for sharing this letter with me and giving permission for me to quote from it.

30. Ibid.

31. Helen F. Callon, Hospital Nursing Consultant, memo, September 22, 1960, Hospital Reports W, ser. 2702, box 1, folder 33, WHSA.

32. Muriel Korn to author, July 24, 1983, AQ, *NYT*. The hospital is now named Maimonides.

33. Marian Tompson, oral history interview with Micaela Sullivan, March 7, 1984, transcript, 3, from a Loyola University Student Oral History Project. I am grateful to Micaela Sullivan-Fowler for sharing this transcript with me.

34. Lois Madsen to author, July 27, 1983, AQ, *NYT*. This woman also wrote about the "elderly, white haired lady" who came to help her through the second stage of her labor by holding her hand and calming her, possibly an example of an early hospital use of a doula, a knowledgeable lay birth attendant.

35. Marian Tompson interview with Micaela Sullivan, 9, 8 of transcript (emphasis in original).

36. Moya Sullivan to author, September 9, 1983, AQ, *NYT*.

37. WMH, FB, November 11, 1951.

38. Ibid., April 9, 1953.

39. Ibid., March 30, 1949.

40. Ibid., February 23, 1952. For hospital regulations, see, for example, Chicago Board of Health, "Regulations for the Conduct of Maternity Hospitals, Maternity Divisions of General Hospitals and Nurseries for the Newborn," January 16, 1958, and the Passavant Memorial Hospital "For You and Your Baby" pamphlet.

41. Erna Ziegel interview, July 9, 1986, MNOHP, 34. Interestingly, Ziegel said that in the 1930s, when she was training in Chicago, "we used heroin. . . . There was heroin available at the hospital and it was used, as I understood this, as it was explained to me, it was used mainly for obstetric patients" (4).

42. Rosemary Stevens, *In Sickness and in Wealth: American Hospitals in the Twentieth Century* (New York: Basic Books, 1989), 252. For more on segregated hospitals, see Vanessa Northington Gamble, *Making a Place for Ourselves: The Black Hospital Movement, 1920–1945* (New York: Oxford University Press, 1995).

43. Elizabeth S. LaPerle, Health Division, Welfare Council of Metropolitan Chicago, "Study of Maternity Facilities in Cook County," May 1954, typescript, 56; copy in the University of Illinois Library, Urbana-Champaign.

44. David Barton Smith, *Health Care Divided: Race and Healing a Nation* (Ann Arbor: University of Michigan Press, 1999), 154.

45. See, for example, WMH, FB, April 20, 1951.

46. Lauretta Scherschel interview, August 12, 1986, MNOHP, 4.

47. Sigurd T. Lokken, "Carol's and Sigurd's First Baby—Roald T. Lokken, September 8, 1953," September 10, 2005, AQ, *OW*.

48. WMH, FB, October 16, 1951.

49. Ibid., June 23, 1953.

50. Ibid., March 13, 1949.

51. Katherine Egan to author, August 25, 1983, AQ, *NYT*.

52. Helen Minton to author, August 11, 1983, AQ, *NYT*.

53. Fred D. Kartchner, "A Study of the Emotional Reactions during Labor," *American Journal of Obstetrics and Gynecology* 60, no. 1 (July 1950): 19–29, quotation on 26.

54. Jack Harrison Pollack, "The Case for Natural Childbirth," *Cosmopolitan*, July 1953, 39–43, quotations on 42.

55. Dick-Read, *Childbirth without Fear*. See also the photo essay by Dick-Read, "Are You Afraid of Childbirth?" *Parents Magazine*, July 1953, 34–39. His visit to New York was reported in "Relates Technique in Painless Births," *New York Times*, January 18, 1947, 9.

56. On this subject, see Margarete Sandelowski, *Pain, Pleasure, and American Childbirth: From the Twilight Sleep to the Read Method, 1914–1960* (Westport, Conn.: Greenwood Press, 1984), and Margot Edwards and Mary Waldorf, *Reclaiming Birth: History and Heroines of American Childbirth Reform* (Trumansburg, N.Y.: Crossing Press, 1984).

57. Bimbetta Coats, "The Most Glorious Experience," *Reader's Digest*, May 1950, 23–27, quotations on 25, 27.

58. Chester Bradley of Newport News, Virginia, to Grantly Dick-Read, September 6, 1949, Grantly Dick-Read Papers, General Correspondence with U.S. Doctors, 1936–57, folder A–B, PP/GDR/D197, Wellcome Library, London. See also ibid., August 29, 1951; September 22, 1951. I am grateful to Lesley A. Hall for easing my way through the library archives.

59. Angela Wyse to author, June 14, 2005, AQ, *OW*. In 1952, she had her second child at St. Mary's Hospital in Madison, Wisconsin: "It was an entirely different experience. A totally unfriendly nurse did not even allow my husband in the labor room." For her fourth delivery in 1961, Wyse remembers that the doctor and her husband were watching a college basketball game during her labor.

60. The hospitals are named by Herbert Thoms of Yale in a letter to Grantly Dick-Read, April 3, 1950, Grantly Dick-Read Papers, folder Herbert Thoms 1947–54, PP/GDR/D196, Wellcome Library, London.

61. His fuller story was related in Chapter 2.

62. Marian Tompson interview with Micaela Sullivan, March 3, 1984.

63. Untitled and undated page in box 1, folder 3, of ser. 2702, Dane County 1952–59, Wisconsin Bureau of Community Health, General Records 1916–79, WHSA. The page was connected to a letter dated August 25, 1952.

64. Anonymous woman to author, September 18, 1983, AQ, *NYT* (emphasis in original). Palmeri was possibly Anthony F. Palmeri, who received his M.D. from Georgetown University School of Medicine and practiced in New Jersey beginning in 1943. See *American Medical Directory*, 20th ed. (Chicago: American Medical Association, 1958), 917.

65. Marguerite Ball, "Without Pain," *Woman's Home Companion*, May 1943, 16, 82, 85, quotations on 82, 85.

66. WMH, FB, August 6, 1961. He was referring to caudal anesthesia.

67. "Awake and Aware" was the title of a popular natural childbirth manual: Irwin Chabon, *Awake and Aware* (New York: Delacorte Press, 1969). The second quotation is from Herbert Thoms and Robert H. Wyatt, "A Natural Childbirth Program," *American Journal of Public Health* 40 (July 1950): 787–91, quotation on 788.

68. Ethel Cates to author, July 26, 1983, AQ, *NYT*. See also, for example, Frederick W. Goodrich and Herbert Thoms, "A Clinical Study of Natural Childbirth: A Preliminary Report from a Teaching Ward Service," *American Journal of Obstetrics and Gynecology* 56, no. 5 (November 1948): 875–83.

69. Thoms and Wyatt, "Natural Childbirth Program," 788–89 (emphasis in original). See also Herbert Thoms, *Understanding Natural Childbirth: A Book for the Expectant Mother* (New York: McGraw-Hill, 1950).

70. Thoms and Wyatt, "Natural Childbirth Program," 789–90.

71. Herbert Thoms in collaboration with Laurence G. Roth, *Understanding Natural Childbirth: A Book for the Expectant Mother* (New York: McGraw-Hill, 1950), 8.

72. Woman quoted in Morton Sontheimer, "Miracle in the Delivery Room," *Woman's Home Companion*, December 1948, 4, 164, Quotation on 164. For more on the Yale program, see "Painless Childbirth at Yale," *Newsweek*, November 7, 1949, 51.

73. Albert M. Vollmer, "Clinical Experiences and Observations on the Use of Relaxation Methods in Obstetrical Practice," *Child-Family Digest* 1, no. 4 (September 1949): 17–23, quotation on 20.

74. Floyd Sterling Rogers, "Dangers of the Read Method in Patients with Major Personality Problems," *American Journal of Obstetrics and Gynecology* 71, no. 6 (June 1956): 1236–41. The author suggested that women undergo psychological assessments of their ability to deal with stress before their physician agreed to attend at a natural childbirth.

75. Thoms and Wyatt, "Natural Childbirth Program," 789–90.

76. Mary Ann Grant, "Letter from a Mother," *Child-Family Digest* 7, no. 3 (November 1952): 102–3, quotations on 103.

77. Vollmer, "Clinical Experiences and Observations," 22.

78. Joan Gerver to author, August 30, 1984, AQ, *NYT*.

79. [Doris Haire], "Natural Childbirth," *Life*, January 30, 1950, 71–77, quotations on 73.

80. Peter S. Douglas, "A Father Reports on Natural Childbirth," *Child-Family Digest* 3, no. 3 (September 1950): 60–62, quotation on 61.

81. Woman who wishes to remain anonymous to author, September 3, 1983, AQ, *NYT*.

82. Mary Naoum to author, August 10, 1983, AQ, *NYT*.

83. Corbin, "Maternity Care Today and Tomorrow," 37.

84. Herbert Thoms and Robert H. Wyatt, "One Thousand Consecutive Deliveries under a Training for Childbirth Program," *American Journal of Obstetrics and Gynecology* 61, no. 1 (January 1951): 205–9, quotation on 206.

85. Hazel Corbin, "Changing Maternity Service in a Changing World," *Child-Family Digest* 4, no. 3 (March 1951): 28–39, quotation on 36.

86. William B. D. Van Auken and David R. Tomlinson, "An Appraisal of Patient Training for Childbirth," *American Journal of Obstetrics and Gynecology* 66, no. 1 (July 1953): 100–105, quotation on 101.

87. "Report of Parent Education Workshop — Racine and Kenosha, November 30 and December 1, 1953," Public Health Nursing Consultant's Files, 1946–69, ser. 2549, box 2, WHSA.

88. Glenna Crooks Richardson, "Portrayal of Birth in an American Medium: Non-Fiction Content in Popular Women's Magazines" (Ph.D. diss., School of Education, Indiana University, 1978; copy in the Library of the American College of Obstetricians and Gynecologists, Washington, D.C.).

89. Jan Ruby, Mary Taylor, Mary S. Foerster, and Mrs. Arnold Brawner, "We Had Our Babies without Fear," *Parents Magazine*, June 1950, 38–39, 78–83, quotations on 38, 78.

90. Lawrence Galton, "What Every Husband Should Know about Childbirth Pain," *Better Homes and Gardens*, November 1950, 14–15, 226–27, 229–31, quotation on 230–31.

91. Leigh Smith to author, July 24, 1983, AQ, NYT.

92. "I Want a Thousand Babies," letter to instructor from mother trained for childbirth, *Child-Family Digest* 6, no. 1 (January 1952): 94–99, quotation on 96.

93. Joan Ernst Wagner and Lavern John Wagner, *Pick Up Your Feet: A Family's Music and Mirth, Living and Loving* (Quincy, Ill.: Lavern Wagner Publishing, 2003), 193. I am grateful to Lavern Wagner for sending me a copy of this book, a moving story of his family, which records every delivery and adoption.

94. Galton, "What Every Husband Should Know," 230. See also Richardson, "Portrayal of Birth in an American Medium," 89, who notes that "husbands were described in 1950's articles as participating in labor by rubbing the woman's back and helping with contractions."

95. Dorothy Barclay, "'Natural Childbirth': A Progress Report," *New York Times*, January 29, 1950, 148. See also her *New York Times* articles "Father's Aid Asked in Birth of Baby," May 19, 1950, and "What Every Father Should Know," June 11, 1950, 170.

96. Hazel Corbin, "Natural Childbirth: The Basic Philosophy behind Natural Childbirth Is as Old as the Human Race," a condensed form of the address as published in *Child-Family Digest* 2, no. 12 (May 1950): 41–50, quotation on 42. See Corbin's obituary in the *New York Times*, May 20, 1988, B6. For a full account of the Maternity Center Association and its training men for childbirth, consult Laura E. Ettinger, *Nurse-Midwifery: The Birth of a New American Profession* (Columbus: Ohio State University Press, 2006).

97. Harvey Graham [pseud.], "Expectant Mothers Go into Training," *Child-Family Digest* 3, no. 1 (July 1950): 60–64, quotation on 62–63.

98. Laurence G. Roth, "Natural Childbirth in a General Hospital," *American Journal of Obstetrics and Gynecology* 61, no. 1 (January 1951): 167–72.

99. A study completed in the 1970s looking at popular women's magazines and their portrayal of birth found that the articles published during the 1950s described husbands' participation in terms of back rubbing, whereas in the 1960s attention turned to concerns of men wanting to be in the delivery room. Back rubbing fit with notions that action was masculine while just being there could be seen as feminine passivity. By the 1970s men seemed to focus more on experiencing the momentous occasion. Richardson, "Portrayal of Birth in an American Medium," found 1,152 articles about birth in 144 different magazines between January 1, 1947, and December 21, 1976 (89). See also Morton Sontheimer, "Miracle in the Delivery Room," *Child-Family Digest* 4, no. 1 (January 1951): 65–71.

100. Silas Starr, "Prolonged Labor," *American Journal of Obstetrics and Gynecology* 63, no. 2 (February 1952): 333–43, quotations on 339, 343.

101. May, *Homeward Bound*, quotation on 146, but see also 145–49.

102. *Father's Little Dividend*, written by Albert Hackett and Frances Goodrich, produced by Pandro S. Berman, directed by Vincente Minnelli, 1951. *I Love Lucy* was discussed in the Introduction to this book. See also *My Blue Heaven* (1950), *Monika* (1952), *Westward the Women* (1952), *The Eddie Cantor Story* (1953), *Giant* (1956), and *Tunnel of Love* (1958).

103. Corbin, "Changing Maternity Service," 29. See also, for example, Hazel Corbin quoted in "Highlights of American Congress on Obstetrics and Gynecology," *Child-Family Digest* 7, no. 1 (September 1952): 64–67. On 64, Corbin is quoted: "The security of the family is shattered at one of the most important moments of life when husband and wife are separated."

104. Corbin, "Changing Maternity Service," 36.

105. Vance Packard, "Now You Can Both Rehearse for Parenthood," *American Magazine*, June 1952, 24–27, 105–10, quotations on 105, 25.

106. Aileen Hogan, "Natural Childbirth," *The Grail*, December 1950, 12–16, quotations on 14–15.

107. Aileen Hogan, "Natural Childbirth," *Child-Family Digest* 4, no. 4 (April 1951): 61–64, quotation on 63.

108. Quoted in Barbara Francis, *Childbirth Is Natural* (Notre Dame, Ind.: Ave Maria Press, 1952), 15–16; copy in ser. 2702, box 2, folder 15, WHSA.

109. Mabel Fitzhugh, "The Role of Abdominal Breathing during Labor," *Child-Family Digest* 5, no. 5 (November 1951): 73–79, quotation on 76.

110. Mabel Fitzhugh, "How to Be Comfortable While Pregnant," reprinted from *My Baby* in *Child-Family Digest* 8, no. 2 (February 1953): 93–98, quotation on 98.

111. Mrs. O. E. is quoted in Milton J. E. Senn, "Let's Be Sensible about Natural Childbirth," *Woman's Home Companion*, May 1953, 30–31, quotation on 31.

112. Man and woman quoted in Margaret Hickey, "Training for Childbirth . . . in Seattle, Washington," *Ladies' Home Journal*, May 1953, 28, 146, 148–49, quotations on 146.

113. Edward Davis and Mabel Carmon, *Obstetrics for Nurses*, 15th ed. of DeLee's textbook (Philadelphia: W. B. Saunders, 1951), 253, 261.

114. Edward Davis and Catherine Sheckler, *Obstetrics for Nurses*, 16th ed. of DeLee's textbook (Philadelphia: W. B. Saunders, 1957), 220–21. On emotional responses, see, for example, Kartchner, "Study of the Emotional Reactions during Labor."

115. Davis and Sheckler, *Obstetrics for Nurses*, 220.

116. Charles D. Kimball, "An Evaluation of Family Centered Obstetrical Care," *Western Journal of Surgery, Obstetrics, and Gynecology* 62, no. 4 (April 1954): 216–21, quotations on 217, 220.

117. Patricia Knowlton, "Childbirth Is a Family Affair," reprinted from *Minneapolis Sunday Tribune*, February 8, 1953, in *Child-Family Digest* 8, no. 5 (May 1953): 75–79, quotations on 76.

118. Helen Glixon to author, September 22, 1983, AQ, *NYT*.

119. Memo dated June 6, 11, 12, 13, and 14, 1952, ser. 2702, box 1, folder 23, Wisconsin Bureau of Community Health, General Records, 1916–79, WHSA.

120. Robert N. Rutherford, Daniel C. More, John Dare, and Patricia A. Rose, "Coordinated Obstetric Care," *Obstetrics and Gynecology* 8, no. 5 (November 1956): 581–90, quotation on 586.

121. "A Father Sees His Child Born," *Life*, June 13, 1955, 133–38, quotations on 133, 134.

122. California Department of Public Health, *Conclusions and Recommendations of the Conferences on Maternity Practices*, 1955, 16, 30, 50; copy at the National Library of Medicine, Bethesda, Maryland.

123. See, for example, ibid., 18.

Chapter Four

1. Vance Packard, "Now You Can Both Rehearse for Parenthood," *American Magazine*, June 1952, 24–27, 105–10, quotations on 25, 105, 107. Packard's book *The Hidden Persuaders* was published in 1957.

2. Packard, "Now You Can Both Rehearse," 110. The man was not with his wife during the delivery but was able to spend time with both his wife and new baby soon thereafter.

3. Ibid., 109.

4. Laura E. Ettinger, "'The Forgotten Man': New York City's Maternity Center Association Educates Expectant Fathers" (paper presented to the History of Science Society Annual Meeting, Milwaukee, November 8, 2002), 1. I am grateful to Laura E. Ettinger for sending me a copy of the unpublished paper. See also her book *Nurse-Midwifery: The Birth of a New American Profession* (Columbus: Ohio State University Press, 2006). See, too, Anne A. Stevens and the Maternity Center Association of New York City, *Maternity Handbook: For Pregnant Mothers and Expectant Fathers* (New York: G. P. Putnam's Sons, 1932).

5. Ettinger, "'Forgotten Man,'" 9.

6. Hazel Corbin, *Getting Ready to Be a Father* (New York: Macmillan, 1945), 46. The book was first published in 1939, and it was dedicated to the men in the first class at the Maternity Center.

7. Frances Porter, R.N., to Elizabeth Sapp, R.N., March 21, 1956, Public Health Nursing Consultant's Files, 1946–69, ser. 2549, box 1, folder 10, WHSA.

8. See, for example, Mildred Skaff to Frances Porter, September 18, 1958, and Lucile Pohl to Frances Porter, February 21, 1957, Public Health Nursing Consultant's Files, 1946–69, County Correspondence, Fond du Lac-Lincoln, 1951–69, ser. 2549, box 1, folder 12, WHSA.

9. Margaret R. Montgomery and G. Elsie Will, "The Maternity Nurse Evolves: An Historical Study of Nursing Education and Parent Education [at] the Chicago Lying-In Hospital and Dispensary, 1896–1970," 39, 40, typescript at the University of Chicago Hospital, Chicago.

10. Judith Chase Churchill, "The Paternal Instinct," *Good Housekeeping*, November 1946, 42–43, 172–76, quotation on 42, listing of classes on 173.

11. See, for example, County Correspondence in the Public Health Nursing Consultant's Files, ser. 2549, WHSA.

12. See, for example, notes on a meeting in the Medford-Taylor County Nursing Office, July 24, 1969, in the County Correspondence, Public Health Nursing Consultant's Files, ser. 2549, box 1, folder 15, WHSA.

13. See Narrative Report, Conference of MCH and Hospital Consultant Nurses, March 1–3, 1950, Public Health Nursing Consultant's Files, ser. 2549, box 1, folder 22, WHSA.

14. Philip A. Bearg, M.D., and Eleanor L. Wood, R.N., "Community Planning for Parent Education," *Public Health Nursing* 39 (1947): 256–57, quotation on 257.

15. Ibid., 257.

16. Catherine Mackenzie, "Schools for Fathers," *New York Times Sunday Magazine*, January 4, 1948, 24.

17. Ruth Davis, "*Cum Laude* for Dad and Baby Too," *American Home*, April 1948, 28–29, quotations on 28.

18. Ibid.

19. Herbert Thoms, "A Program of Training for Motherhood," *Child-Family Digest* 2, no. 10 (March 1950): 31–35, quotation on 33–34.

20. Herbert Thoms, "Preparation for Parenthood in the Childbirth Program," *Obstetrics and Gynecology* 10, no. 4 (October 1957): 434–36, quotation on 434.

21. Edward A. Graber, "A Doctor Looks at Parents' Classes," *Child-Family Digest* 1, no. 2 (July 1949): 46–52, quotation on 50.

22. Workshop on Parent Education, Sheboygan [Wisconsin] Child Hygiene Association panel, County Reports 1951, Public Health Nursing Consultant's Files, ser. 2549, box 1, folder 23, WHSA.

23. See, for example, class notes, Dane County Expectant Parents 1952–53, Public Health Nursing Consultant's Files, ser. 2549, box 1, folder 27, WHSA.

24. Workshop on Expectant Parent Groups, July 1963, Public Health Nursing Consultant's Files, ser. 2549, box 2, folder 18, WHSA.

25. Conference on Prenatal Class on Maternity Department Tour, June 22, 1953, Public Health Nursing Consultant's Files, 1946–69, ser. 2549, box 2, folder 35, WHSA.

26. See, for example, Montgomery and Will, "Maternity Nurse Evolves," 42, where they note that attendance at classes fell when the community around the University of Chicago changed demographically in the 1960s.

27. See, for example, Doris Haire, "Focal Point on Childbirth Education: A History of Childbirth Education," *International Journal of Childbirth Education* 14, no. 4 (December 31, 1999): 26–28.

28. Lawrence Galton, "Motherhood without Misery," *Collier's*, November 16, 1946, 13, 88, 90, quotation on 88.

29. Hazel Corbin, "Natural Childbirth: The Basic Philosophy behind Natural Childbirth Is as Old as the Human Race," *Child-Family Digest* 2, no. 12 (May 1950): 41–50, quotation on 44.

30. Sloan Wilson, "The American Way of Birth," *Harper's Magazine*, July 1964, 48–54, quotations on 49, 51.

31. Ann Onymous, "Letter to the Editors," *Child-Family Digest* 2, no. 13 (June 1950): 77–80, quotation on 80.

32. Harvey Graham [pseud.], "Expectant Mothers Go into Training," *Child-Family Digest* 3, no. 1 (July 1950): 60–64, quotation on 62.

33. Lawrence Galton, "What Every Husband Should Know about Childbirth Pain," *Better Homes and Gardens*, November 1950, 14–15, 226–27, 229–31, quotation on 226.

34. Sue Frazier interview, September 2, 1986, MNOHP, 2.

35. Ann Gunderson interview, August 6, 1986, MNOHP, 5.

36. Galton, "What Every Husband Should Know," 230.

37. Ibid.

38. Grantly Dick-Read, *Childbirth without Fear: The Principles and Practice of Natural*

Childbirth, 2nd rev. ed. of 1944 book (New York: Harper and Row, 1959), 27. For early experiences with childbirth education in Madison, Wisconsin, see Mary Rogers interview, August 26, 1986, MNOHP. See also the nurse who remained uncomfortable teaching men and women in the same classes in memo from Helen F. Callon, R.N., Hospital Nursing Consultant, Bureau of Maternal and Child Health, Wisconsin State Health Department, Hospital Reports C–D, 1960–64, ser. 2702, box 1, folder 27, WHSA.

39. Packard, "Now You Can Both Rehearse," 107.

40. George Kosmak was quoted in "Highlights of American Congress on Obstetrics and Gynecology," *Child-Family Digest* 7, no. 1 (September 1952): 64–67, quotation on 67. Reprinted from *My Baby*.

41. Mabel L. Fitzhugh, "How to Be Comfortable While Pregnant," *Child-Family Digest* 8, no. 2 (February 1953): 93–98, quotation on 98.

42. Louise Zabriskie, *Nurses Handbook of Obstetrics*, 9th ed. (Philadelphia: Lippincott, 1952), 186, and 11th ed. (1966), quotation on 7 of the latter.

43. "Prospective Parents Are Offered Classes," *New York Times*, March 3, 1956, 22.

44. Patricia Murphy, "Expectant Mothers Organize for Natural Childbirth," *American Journal of Nursing* 56, no. 10 (October 1956): 1298–1301, quotation on 1299.

45. Ibid., 1301.

46. Marion D. Laird and Margaret Hogan, "An Elective Program on Preparation for Childbirth at the Sloane Hospital for Women, May, 1951 to June, 1953," *American Journal of Obstetrics and Gynecology* 72, no. 3 (September 1956): 641–47, quotation on 643.

47. Richard Gehman (with photos by Don Hunter), "Education for Motherhood," *Cosmopolitan*, November 1956, 50–53, quotations on 50, 52.

48. "Queens Center Offers Course for Parents," *New York Times*, October 3, 1957, 34.

49. Fred D. Kartchner, "Active Participation in Childbirth: A Psychosomatic Approach to Pregnancy and Parturition," *American Journal of Obstetrics and Gynecology* 75, no. 6 (June 1958): 1244–54, quotation on 1246.

50. American College of Obstetricians and Gynecologists, *Manual of Standards in Obstetric-Gynecologic Practice* (Washington, D.C.: American College of Obstetricians and Gynecologists, 1959), 17; copies in the library of the American College of Obstetricians and Gynecologists, Washington, D.C. See, similarly, the 1965 standards, 25.

51. Virginia Senders, "An Academic Psychologist Looks at Natural Childbirth," *Obstetrics and Gynecology* 14, no. 6 (December 1959): 817–24, quotation on 823.

52. William B. D. Van Auken and David R. Tomlinson, "An Appraisal of Patient Training for Childbirth," *American Journal of Obstetrics and Gynecology* 66, no. 1 (July 1953): 100–105, quotation on 101.

53. The Mount Sinai program was described in "Parents' School Ending First Year," *New York Times*, December 31, 1953, 12.

54. Margaret Hickey, "Training for Childbirth . . . in Seattle, Washington," *Ladies' Home Journal*, May 1953, 28, 146, 148–149, quotation on 146.

55. Sue Ernst, ed., "Father Participation Guide," ICEA, 1975, 8; copy at the library of the American College of Obstetricians and Gynecologists in Washington, D.C. My thanks to Debra Scarborough and her associates, who welcomed me to the collection.

56. Dialogue from *Happy Days* taken from watching a tape of the episode "Little Baby Cunningham," which first aired on ABC on November 3, 1981.

57. "When Mother Went from Home to Hospital," *Child-Family Digest* 3, no. 6 (December 1950): 47–52, quotation on 51.

58. Claire Terse, "Aid for False Labor," *Child-Family Digest* 5, no. 3 (September 1951): 87–91, quotation on 90–91.

59. Mabel L. Fitzhugh, "Bill of Rights for Expectant Mothers," *Child-Family Digest* 4, no. 1 (January 1951): 54–64, quotation on 56–57.

60. Nathan Hurvitz, "Group Counseling in Private Obstetric Practice," *Obstetrics and Gynecology* 16, no. 6 (December 1960): 724–29, quotation on 726.

61. O. Spurgeon English, M.D., and Constance J. Foster, "What's Happening to Fathers?" *Better Homes and Gardens*, April 1952, 200, 202, 205, 228–29, quotation on 205.

62. H. Lloyd Miller and Francis E. Flannery, "Education for Childbirth in Private Practice: 585 Consecutive Cases," *Child-Family Digest* 6, no. 4 (April 1952): 33–44, quotation on 36–37.

63. Milton J. E. Senn, "Let's Be Sensible about Natural Childbirth," *Woman's Home Companion*, May 1953, 30–31, quotation on 30.

64. Jack Harrison Pollack, "The Case for Natural Childbirth," *Cosmopolitan*, July 1953, 39–43, quotations on 40, 43. The use of the phrase "we're pregnant" by men has become common at the turn of the twenty-first century, but it was rare at the middle of the twentieth century.

65. Morris Osofsky, "Natural Childbirth," *Child-Family Digest* 9, no. 1 (September 1953): 97–104, quotations on 104, 103.

66. Alice Young Kohler, "The Place of the Public Health Nurse in Private Medical Practice," *Nursing Outlook* 1, no. 9 (September 1953): 528–29. I am grateful to Susan L. Smith for calling my attention to this reference and for her book *Japanese American Midwives: Culture, Community, and Health Policies, 1880–1950* (Urbana: University of Illinois Press, 2005).

67. "School for Expectant Fathers," *Ebony*, December 1955, 112–17, quotations on 112, 113.

68. William H. Genne, *Husbands and Pregnancy: The Handbook for Expectant Fathers* (New York: Association Press, 1956), 70.

69. Ibid., 74, 88.

70. Eleanor Waddell interview, July 1, 1986, MNOHP, 18–19.

71. Lloyd H. Miller, "Education for Childbirth," *Obstetrics and Gynecology* 17, no. 1 (January 1961): 120–23, quotation on 120–21.

72. Ruth Brecher and Edward Brecher, "How to Get Better Maternity Care," *Redbook*, July 1962, 43, 108–11, quotations on 43.

73. See Fernand Lamaze, *Painless Childbirth* (Chicago: Henry Regnery, 1970), and Robert A. Bradley, *Husband-Coached Childbirth* (1965; New York: Harper and Row, 1981). For more on various childbirth methods, see Margarete Sandelowski, *Pain, Pleasure, and American Childbirth: From the Twilight Sleep to the Read Method, 1914–1960* (Westport, Conn: Greenwood Press, 1984), and Margot Edwards and Mary Waldorf, *Reclaiming Birth: History and Heroines of American Childbirth Reform* (Trumansburg, N.Y.: Crossing Press, 1984). For a critique of the Lamaze method, see Barbara Katz Rothman, "Awake and Aware, or False Consciousness? The Cooption of Childbirth Reform in America," in *Childbirth: Alternatives to Medical Control*, ed. Shelly Romalis (Austin: University of Texas Press, 1981), and Rothman's *In Labor: Women and Power in the Birthplace* (New York: Norton, 1982), esp. chap. 3. See also Robbie E. Davis-Floyd, *Birth as an American Rite of Passage* (Berkeley: University of California Press, 1992). Both Rothman and Davis-Floyd conclude that the Lamaze method was more popular than Dick-Read's in the United States because it fit most easily into hospital practices and did not fundamentally challenge physician authority; this book has demonstrated that Dick-Read was popular in an earlier period, during the late 1940s and 1950s.

74. Edward Davis and Reva Rubin, *Obstetrics for Nurses*, 17th ed. (Philadelphia: W. B. Saunders, 1962), 156; see also 489, and the 18th ed. (1966), in which the same words are repeated.

75. Sloan Wilson, "The American Way of Birth," *Harper's Magazine*, July 1964, 48–54.

76. Hal Higdon, "Dad Had It!" *Parents Magazine*, June 1960, 103–5, 107–8, quotation on 107.

77. Ibid., 108.

78. Connie Mattson, "How Not to Have a Lamaze Baby," *ASPON*, December 1967–January 1968.

79. Sandra Eiseman, interview with author, July 8, 2005, Madison, Wisconsin.

80. Elizabeth King, "The Pregnant Father," *Bulletin of the American College of Nurse Midwives* 13 (February 1968): 19–25, quotation on 21.

81. Robert Allen Fein, "Men's Experiences before and after the Birth of a First Child: Dependence, Marital Sharing, and Anxiety" (Ph.D. diss., Harvard University, 1974), 171.

82. Teresa Modzelewski, "Fathers in the Delivery Room," *The Nevadan* (Sunday supplement to the *Las Vegas Review-Journal*), May 26, 1974, 6. My thanks to Rima Apple for this reference.

83. T. J. Blasing, with the consent of his wife, Carolyn, to author, August 21, 2005, AQ, OW.

84. George Schaefer, "The Expectant Father: His Care and Management," *Postgraduate Medicine* 38 (December 1965): 658–63, quotations on 658, 659.

85. Irwin Chabon, *Awake and Aware: Participating in Childbirth through Psychoprophylaxis* (1966), quoted in Deborah Ruth Wolf Tanzer, *The Psychology of Pregnancy and Childbirth: An Investigation of Natural Childbirth* (Ann Arbor, Mich.: UMI, 1967), 385.

86. Heinrich E. Beernink, "The Doctor's Corner," *ASPON*, November–December 1971.

87. Mr. Petretti quoted in Errol G. Rampersad, "Expectant Fathers Join in 'Natural Births,'" *New York Times*, April 2, 1978, WC14.

88. *Mary Tyler Moore Show*, September 25, 1976, CBS. I watched the show in reruns in 2004. My thanks to Kendra Smith-Howard and Abby Markwyn for their assistance with this video. See discussion of this show in Judy Kutulas, "'Do I Look Like a Chick?': Men, Women, and Babies on Sitcom Maternity Stories," *American Studies* 39, no. 2 (Summer 1998): 13–32, esp. 21–23. See also Bonnie J. Dow, *Prime-Time Feminism: Television, Media Culture, and the Women's Movement since 1970* (Philadelphia: University of Pennsylvania Press, 1996), esp. chap. 1, and Serifina Bathrick, "The Mary Tyler Moor Show: Women at Home and at Work," in *Mary Tyler Moore Quality Television* (London: BFI, 1984). On the changing demographics of television audiences and the business of television in this period, see Julie D'Acci, *Defining Women: Television and the Case of Cagney and Lacey* (Chapel Hill: University of North Carolina Press, 1994).

89. *ASPON*, June 1967; excerpt is from Richard Marchick's address to the annual meeting.

90. See Joan Beck series from May 23, 1972, to June 27, 1972, in the *Chicago Tribune*, quotation from "Dauntless Is the Domesticated Dad," June 13, 1972, 2.

91. Edith B. Wonnell, "The Education of Expectant Father for Childbirth," *Nursing Clinics of North America* 6, no. 4 (December 1971): 591–603, quotation on 592.

92. "Natural Childbirth Classes Offered," *Oakland (Calif.) Post*, March 12, 1975, 9.

93. James C. Sasmor, "The Role of the Father," in *Childbirth Education: A Nursing Perspective*, ed. Jeannette L. Sasmor (New York: John Wiley and Sons, 1979), 149–59.

94. Wonnell, "Education of Expectant Father," 595.

95. Shirley Tighe Frank, "The Effect of Husbands' Presence at Delivery and Childbirth Preparation Classes on the Experience of Childbirth" (Ph.D. diss., Michigan State University, 1973), see esp. 45.

96. Linda R. Cronenwett and Lucy L. Newmark, "Fathers' Responses to Childbirth," *Nursing Research* 23, no. 3 (1973): 210–17, quotation on 215.

97. Branko Terzic to author, March 15, 2005, in response to my author's query in the *New York Times* Book Review, March 6, 2005. Terzic also fainted after his third child was born in 1985 as he went through the report with the nurse after the birth. But he became more comfortable with labor and delivery over the three births.

98. Sloan Wilson, "The American Way of Birth," *Harper's Magazine*, July 1964, 48–54, quotation on 52.

99. Wonnell, "Education of the Expectant Father," 595.

100. *The Story of Eric*, American Society for Psychoprophylactic Obstetrics of Los Angeles, 1973. There is a copy of this film in the National Library of Medicine, Bethesda.

101. *Through a Father's Eye* (Boston: Polymorph Films, 1976). There is a copy of this film at the Martin County Library, Fairmount, Minnesota.

102. James Heise [pseud.], "Toward Better Preparation for Involved Fatherhood," *Journal of Obstetrics and Gynecology Nursing* (September/October 1975): 32–35, quotations on 32.

103. Leslie D. Atkinson, "Is Family-Centered Care a Myth?" *American Journal of Maternal Child Nursing* (July/August 1976): 256–59, quotation on 258.

104. Jacqueline Rose Hott, "The Crisis of Expectant Fatherhood," *American Journal of Nursing* 76 (September 1976): 1436–40, quotations on 1439.

105. E. Rick Beebe, "Expectant Parent Classes: A Case Study," *Family Coordinator* 27, no. 1 (January 1978): 55–58.

106. Judith Roehner, "Fatherhood: In Pregnancy and Birth," *Journal of Nurse-Midwifery* 21, no. 1 (1976): 13–18, quotation on 18.

107. Georgia Dullea, "Parents-To-Be Get Word on Babies from Those Who Know," *New York Times*, November 10, 1982, C1.

108. John Wapner, "The Attitudes, Feelings and Behaviors of Expectant Fathers Attending Lamaze Classes," *Birth and the Family Journal* 3, no. 1 (Spring 1976): 5–13, quotations on 13, 11, 13.

109. Andree Brookes, "Awaiting Fatherhood: The Strain," *New York Times*, December 20, 1982, D12.

110. Jo Griffiths, "Prenatal, Postpartum Classes Are Big Business These Days Series: Birthing Options Available in South-Central Pennsylvania," *Sunday Patriot-News* (Harrisburg, Pa.), November 6, 1988, E1. See also Nicole R. Hampton, "Preparing Couples for Childbirth Classes Help Mothers-to-Be Learn to Relax," *Providence (R.I.) Journal*, August 30, 1988, Z-01. An early twenty-first-century example of men's reactions to prenatal classes appeared on Badger Nation Off Topic Water Cooler Board, March 23–24, 2006 (<www.badgermaniac.com>). Of twenty-one men answering the query "Birthing Class—worth it?" nine gave some positive responses, and the majority were negative or at best neutral. My thanks to David I. Leavitt for sending me this citation.

111. See, for example, Philip E. Sumner, "Six Years Experience of Prepared Childbirth in a Home-Like Labor-Delivery Room," *Birth and the Family Journal* 3, no. 2 (Spring 1976): 79–82.

Chapter Five

1. The term "masculine domesticity" is Margaret Marsh's, in *Suburban Lives* (New Brunswick, N.J.: Rutgers University Press, 1990), xiv. See also Stephanie Coontz, *The*

Way We Never Were: American Families and the Nostalgia Trap (New York: Basic Books, 1992), and Jessica Weiss, *To Have and to Hold: Marriage, the Baby Boom and Social Change* (Chicago: University of Chicago Press, 2000).

2. David Barton Smith, *Health Care Divided: Race and Healing a Nation* (Ann Arbor: University of Michigan Press, 1999), 103.

3. Edward H. Beardsley, "Good-Bye to Jim Crow: The Desegregation of Southern Hospitals, 1945–1970," *Bulletin of the History of Medicine* 60, no. 3 (Fall 1986): 367–86, quotation on 382. Beardsley argues that hospital integration in the South was relatively smooth: "Hospitals were in fact the first vital social institution, apart from the armed forces, to implement full scale integration" (377). Before integration, African American women in the South often delivered at home, attended by midwives; also, black hospitals and segregated wards of general hospitals offered birth options. See, for example, David T. Beito, "Black Fraternal Hospitals in the Mississippi Delta, 1942–1967," *Journal of Southern History* 65, no. 1 (February 1999): 109–40, and Wilson O. Elkins, "A History of L. Richardson Memorial Hospital," *North Carolina Medical Journal* 30, no. 1 (December 1969): 146–51.

4. Detroit Commission on Community Relations, "Report 6: Racial Factors in Policy and Practice: Hospital Bed Utilization," 1954; copy in the National Library of Medicine, Bethesda, Maryland; see 4–5 for birth statistics.

5. Patricia Murphy, "Expectant Mothers Organize for Natural Childbirth," *American Journal of Nursing* 56, no. 10 (October 1956): 1298–1301, quotation on 1301.

6. Ibid., 1301.

7. Reverend David W. Roberts (who was a seminary student at the time) to author, October 12, 2005, AQ, OW.

8. Editors, "Doctors Can't Do It Alone," *Ladies' Home Journal*, April 1960, 80–81, 116, 118, quotation on 116.

9. Roberta Scaer and Diana Korte, "A Survey of Maternity Options," © authors, 1977, Boulder, Colorado, typescript. The study was funded in part by the March of Dimes, Northern Colorado Chapter, and distributed locally. I am very grateful to the authors for sending me a copy of the study. The table of findings about women's wishes concerning husbands in the labor room is on 11; about friends is on 39. See also an article about the study: Elizabeth Jean Pascoe, "How Women Want to Have Their Babies," *McCall's*, October 1977, 109–10. La Leche League was founded in the 1950s; its mission was (and is) to support breast-feeding mothers through mother-to-mother engagement and education. See Jule DeJager Ward, *La Leche League: At the Crossroads of Medicine, Feminism, and Religion* (Chapel Hill: University of North Carolina Press, 2000).

10. "How Women Want to Have Their Babies: A Study of Consumers' Attitudes on Maternal Health Care, Conducted by the Committee on Maternal Alternatives," Baltimore, 1978, 1980, typescript in the National Library of Medicine and in the Library of Congress; statistics on 37, 39, quotation on 140.

11. Muriel Goldfarb and Robert W. Goldfarb, "We Shared Our Baby's Birth . . . ," *Ladies' Home Journal*, December 1958, 140, 142, quotation on 140.

12. Dale Clark, "A Man's Crusade for Easy Childbirth: A Husband's Place Is Not in the Waiting Room, but Close to His Wife's Side," *Esquire*, October 1949, 51, 151–52, quotation on 51; Catharine Baldwin Hoffmann, "The Perils of Pauline—1941," *Herald* (monthly from Junior Woman's Club of Orange, N.J.), November 1941, 10–12. A copy of Hoffman's article was included in her letter to author, August 8, 1983, AQ, *NYT*.

13. E. Todd Wheeler, *Hospital Design and Function* (New York: McGraw-Hill, 1964), 136. See also Roy Hudenburg, *Planning the Community Hospital* (New York: McGraw-Hill, 1967).

14. George Schaefer, "The Expectant Father: His Care and Management," *Postgraduate Medicine* 38 (December 1965): 658–63, quotation on 662.

15. Marjorie Karmel, *Thank You, Dr. Lamaze: A Mother's Experience in Painless Childbirth* (Philadelphia: Lippincott, 1959).

16. Ibid., 93–94.

17. Elisabeth Bing, interview with Elaine Zwelling, *Journal of Perinatal Education* 9 (March 31, 2000): 15–21.

18. Sandra Eiseman, interview with author, July 8, 2005, Madison, Wisconsin.

19. See Elisabeth Bing, *Six Practical Lessons for an Easier Childbirth* (New York: Grosset and Dunlap, 1967).

20. Bing interview with Zwelling. See also Elly Rakowitz, "ASPO: Birth and Growth of an Ideal," *Mother's Manual* (January–February 1978): 29–35, and Margot Edwards and Mary Waldorf, *Reclaiming Birth: History and Heroines of American Childbirth Reform* (Trumansburg, N.Y.: Crossing Press, 1984).

21. Rakowitz, "ASPO," 30, 31.

22. Ibid., 31 (emphasis in original).

23. Sue Ernst, ed., "Father Participation Guide," ICEA, 1975, iii; copy at library of American College of Obstetricians and Gynecologists in Washington, D.C.

24. See, for example, Edwards and Waldorf, *Reclaiming Birth*.

25. Catholic Hospital Association of the U.S. and Canada, "Family Centered Maternity Care at St. Mary's Hospital Evansville, Indiana," 1960; copy at the American College of Obstetricians and Gynecologists, Washington, D.C.

26. "Fathers-to-Be Don't Always Pace the Floor," *New York Times*, June 19, 1961, 32.

27. For an accounting of New York hospitals' practices, see Phyllis Ehrlich, "Father's Role at Baby's Birth Disputed," *New York Times*, February 13, 1962, 30. See also "Delivery Room 'Invader' Fined," *American Medical Association News*, January 4, 1965, 11. See also Edward Davis and Reva Rubin, *Obstetrics for Nurses*, 17th ed. (Philadelphia: W. B. Saunders, 1962), 156. See the same statement in the 18th ed. (1966).

28. Quoted in Deborah Ruth Wolf Tanzer, *The Psychology of Pregnancy and Childbirth: An Investigation of Natural Childbirth* (Ann Arbor, Mich: UMI, 1967), 341–42.

29. Ibid.

30. William Hazlett is quoted in Elisabeth King, "The Pregnant Father," *Bulletin of the American College of Nurse Midwives* 13 (February 1968): 19–25, quotation on 22–23.

31. Shirley Zussman, *A Study of Certain Social, Psychological, and Cultural Factors Influencing Husbands' Participation in Their Wives' Labor* (Ann Arbor, Mich.: UMI, 1969), 144–45, 147.

32. Ron Goodman, "Diary of a Lamaze Father," *American Baby*, June 1974, 37, 42, 43, 50, 53, quotations on 41–42, 43.

33. Julie Harris, as told to Betty Friedan, "I Was Afraid to Have a Baby," *McCall's*, December 1956, 68, 72, 74, quotation on 72, 74.

34. For another story of a man's support during labor in a widely read magazine, see "The First Baby: Georgette Mapes and a Million Others Share a Rich Experience," *Life*, December 24, 1956, 57–63; photographs by Suzanne Szasz. Georgette was medicated, although the particulars were not provided in the story. In the *Life* story, smoking figured significantly; on cigarettes during labor, see, for example, WMH, FB, November 1, 1960. On the question of audience and *Life*, see James L. Baughman, "Who Read *Life*? The Circulation of America's Favorite Magazine," in *Looking at Life Magazine*, ed. Erika Doss (Washington, D.C.: Smithsonian Institution Press, 2001), 41–51, and other essays in the book.

35. Marion D. Laird and Margaret Hogan, "An Elective Program on Preparation for Childbirth at the Sloane Hospital for Women, May, 1951 to June, 1953," *American Journal of Obstetrics and Gynecology* 72, no. 3 (September 1956): 641–47, quotation on 642.

36. William H. Genne, *Husbands and Pregnancy: The Handbook for Expectant Fathers* (New York: Association Press, 1956), 16.

37. Ibid., 66.

38. Ibid., 72.

39. Ibid., 74. For another example of how important the husband could be, see Emmy B. interview, May 7, 1996, BP, about her 1956 delivery at Mt. Sinai Hospital in New York. In that case, when the husband left briefly, he came back to find his wife wandering the hospital corridors.

40. Peter Browne, "I Saw My Son Born," *Readers' Digest*, November 1957, 61–64, quotations on 62, 63.

41. Gladys Denny Shultz, "Journal Mothers Report on Cruelty in Maternity Wards," *Ladies' Home Journal*, May 1958, 44–45, 152–55, quotation on 153. See also her "Journal Mothers Testify to Cruelty in Maternity Wards," *Ladies' Home Journal*, December 1958, 58–59, 135, 137–39.

42. Shultz, "Journal Mothers Report," 153.

43. Ibid., 155.

44. Ibid. (emphasis in original).

45. Ibid., see esp. 59.

46. Muriel Goldfarb and Robert W. Goldfarb, "We Shared Our Baby's Birth . . . ," *Ladies' Home Journal*, December 1958, 140, 142, quotations on 140.

47. James Watts, "A New Father Speaks Up and Says It's His Baby Too," *Parents Magazine*, August 1959, 52–53, 76–77, quotation on 76.

48. American College of Obstetricians and Gynecologists, *Manual of Standards in Obstetric-Gynecologic Practice* (Washington, D.C.: American College of Obstetricians and Gynecologists, 1959), 18. See also the manual of 1965, 26. Copies in the library of the American College of Obstetricians and Gynecologists, Washington, D.C.

49. David N. Danforth, *Textbook of Obstetrics and Gynecology* (New York: Harper and Row, 1966), 526. The exact same sentences are repeated in the second edition of this text (1971, 590), in the fourth edition (1982, 648), and the fifth edition (1986, 653–54).

50. Herbert Thoms and Bruce Bliven Jr., "The Challenge to American Obstetrics," *Ladies' Home Journal*, April 1960, 81.

51. Margaret Hickey, "Too Many Babies Die," *Ladies' Home Journal*, May 1961, 43, 140, quotation on 140. See also Louise Zabriskie, *Nurses Handbook of Obstetrics*, 10th ed. (Philadelphia: J. B. Lippincott, 1960), and Schaefer, "Expectant Father."

52. Elisabeth D. Bing, ed., *The Adventure of Birth: Experiences in the Lamaze Method of Prepared Childbirth* (New York: Simon and Schuster, 1970), quotations on 14–16, 19.

53. Paul Messling to author, August 13, 2005, AQ, *OW*.

54. Trina B. interview, July 13, 1996, BP.

55. Anita D. interview, May 5, 1996, BP.

56. Ronnie Rae R. interview, June 6, 1996, BP.

57. Unnamed woman quoted in Shultz, "Journal Mothers Report," 45. For an experience a decade later, see Steven M. Barney, "I Was There When My Son Was Born," *Wisconsin State Journal* (Madison), July 27, 1969.

58. Sally Olds and Linda Witt, "New Man in the Delivery Room—the Father," *Today's Health*, October 1970, 52–56, quotation on 53.

59. Jerry Martin is quoted in *ASPON*, November–December 1971.

60. Quoted in Joan Beck, "Doodles by Daddies: A Waiting Room Diary," *Chicago Tribune*, June 17, 1972, 11.

61. Pat Evansizer quoted in *ASPON*, Winter 1972.

62. Ludmilla Alexander, "Fathers in the Delivery Room," *American Baby*, January 1972, 24, father quoted on 25.

63. Ruth Forbes, "A New Role for Expectant Fathers," *Midwife and Health Visitor* 8 (May 1972): 166–68, quotation on 168.

64. Jeannette L. Sasmor, "The Role of the Father in Labor and Delivery," in *Psychosomatic Medicine in Obstetrics and Gynaecology*, 3rd International Congress, London, 1971 (New York: Karger, Basel, 1972), 277, 178.

65. Donald Sutherland, "Childbirth Is Not for Mothers Only," *Ms.*, May 1974, 47–51, quotation on 47. His wife's name is Francine Racette.

66. Robert Allen Fein, "Men's Experiences before and after the Birth of a First Child: Dependence, Marital Sharing and Anxiety" (Ph.D. diss., Harvard University, 1974), quotation on 184.

67. Nicholas Vick and Lewis Leavitt, who were medical students at the University of Chicago from 1961 to 1965, personal communication, May 2008.

68. To follow hospital integration debates, see Vanessa Northington Gamble, *Making a Place for Ourselves: The Black Hospital Movement, 1920–1945* (New York: Oxford University Press, 1995), and David Barton Smith, *Health Care Divided: Race and Healing a Nation* (Ann Arbor: University of Michigan Press, 1999). See also Edward H. Beardsley, "Good-Bye to Jim Crow: The Desegregation of Southern Hospitals, 1945–1970," *Bulletin of the History of Medicine* 60, no. 3 (Fall 1986): 367–86, and Edward C. Halperin, "Desegregation of Hospitals and Medical Societies in North Carolina," *New England Journal of Medicine* 318, no. 1 (January 7, 1988): 58–63. See also some individual hospital histories, for example, Claude W. Munger, "Report of a Study of the Lincoln Hospital, Durham, North Carolina," 1947, typescript at Duke University, Durham, North Carolina, and Wilson O. Elkins, "A History of L. Richardson Memorial Hospital," *North Carolina Medical Journal* 30, no. 1 (December 1969): 146–51, or some individual city hospital histories, for example, J. C. Brierre, "History of Medicine in Shreveport: The Black Experience," *Journal of North Louisiana Historical Association* 17, nos. 2–3 (Spring–Summer 1986): 91–96, or regional studies such as David T. Beito, "Black Fraternal Hospitals in the Mississippi Delta, 1942–1967," *Journal of Southern History* 65, no. 1 (February 1999): 109–40. Without a hospital-by-hospital survey it is impossible to know the extent of continuing discrimination over these and later decades, although recent studies showed clear differences in practices. See, for example, the classic study by Kevin A. Schulman et al., "The Effect of Race and Sex on Physicians' Recommendations for Cardiac Catheterization," *New England Journal of Medicine* 340, no. 8 (February 25, 1999): 618–26.

69. Charlotte Bonds and Ozell Bonds, "Initiation into Parenthood," *Essence*, September 1973, 58–59, 72, 74, 78–79, 85, quotation on 72, 74.

70. Ibid., 78.

71. Patricia Patterson, "Childbirth: The Total Experience," *Essence*, November 1976, 13, 124, 130, 152, quotations on 130.

72. Ernst, "Father Participation Guide."

73. At Manchester Memorial Hospital in Manchester, Connecticut, husbands' participation during labor had became increasingly popular in the 1960s and "put new demands on the hospital." The hospital realized that "the father's support is invaluable, but fathers vary in the ability and inclination to verbalize during labor," so it also provided a birthing monitrice—a labor assistant—to help the couples through. Billie Carlson and Philip E. Sumner, "Hospital 'at Home' Delivery: A Celebration," *Journal of Obstetric, Gynecologic, and Neonatal Nursing* (March/April 1976): 21–27, quotations on 22, 25.

74. Lee H. interview, BP, describing 1974 and 1977 deliveries.

75. Brian D. Best, "Comparative Obstetrics: Address of the President," *American Journal of Obstetrics and Gynecology* 75, no. 5 (May 1958): 957–63, quotation on 960.

76. Ruth Brecher and Edward Brecher, "How to Get Better Maternity Care," *Redbook*, July 1962, 43, 108–11, quotation on 109.

77. Jacqueline Hott, "An Investigation of the Relationship between Psychoprophylaxis in Childbirth and Changes in Self-Concept of the Participant Husband and His Concept of His Wife" (Ph.D. diss., New York University, 1972), 107.

78. Allan T. Moss, "Childbirth Education: The Physician's Dilemma and the Patient's Response," *ASPON*, March–April 1969.

79. Brecher and Brecher, "How to Get Better Maternity Care," 110.

80. Robert H. Stewart, "Natural Childbirth, Father Participation, Rooming-In, or What-Have-You," *Medical Times* 91, no. 1 (November 1963): 1065–68, quotations on 1067.

81. Robert H. Barter, "Should 'Natural Childbirth' Be Encouraged? No! Ridiculous and Foolhardy," *American Medical News*, October 7, 1974, 19 (emphasis added).

82. John B. Franklin, "Should 'Natural Childbirth' Be Encouraged? Yes! Begins Healthy Family Life," *American Medical News*, October 7, 1974, 19.

83. Letters to the editor, *American Medical News*, November 4, 1974, 6.

84. Edgar L. Engel, "Family-Centered Hospital Maternity Care," *American Journal of Obstetrics and Gynecology* 85, no. 2 (January 1963): 260–66, quotation on 261.

85. Robert A. Bradley, "Father's Place during Childbirth," *Medical Opinion and Review* (December 1966): 72–77, quotation on 73.

86. Elizabeth P. Rice, "Social Aspects of Maternity Care," *Obstetrics and Gynecology* 23, no. 2 (February 1964): 307–15.

87. Helen Freedman, "Diary of My Baby's Birth," *Parents Magazine*, August 1965, 44, 99–100, quotation on 99.

88. John S. Miller, "'Return the Joy of Home Delivery,' with Fathers in the Delivery Room," *Hospital Topics* 44, no. 1 (January 1966): 105–9, quotation on 107.

89. In 1970, only 7.2 percent of obstetricians were women. This increased to 12.6 percent in 1980. Based on the fact that not until the 1990s did the number of women residents in training exceed 50 percent, it is projected that 2014 will be the year when there will be more women practicing obstetrics and gynecology than men. See Erica Frank, John Rock, and Danielle Sara, "Characteristics of Female Obstetrician-Gynecologists in the United States," *Obstetrics and Gynecology* 94, no. 5 (1999): 659–65.

90. Carolyn Conant Van Blarcom and Erna Ziegel, *Obstetrical Nursing*, 4th ed. (New York: Macmillan, 1957), 297.

91. Mickie Schmudlach interview, June 5, 1986, MNOHP, 11. See also Sally Berliot interview, August 8, 1986, MNOHP. She thought the men wanted to leave when any procedures were being conducted.

92. Sloan Wilson, "The American Way of Birth," *Harper's Magazine*, July 1964, 48–54, quotation on 53.

93. See, for example, John S. Miller, "Fathers in the Delivery Room," *Child and Family* 3, no. 4 (1964): 3–11.

94. Patricia A. Huprich, "Assisting the Couple through a Lamaze Labor and Delivery," *American Journal of Maternal Child Nursing* (July/August 1977): 245–53, quotations on 252–53.

95. See, for example, Linda Leonard, "The Father's Side: A Different Perspective on Childbirth," *Canadian Nurse* 73, no. 2 (1977): 16–20.

96. Carolyn Splett interview, April 24, 1986, MNOHP, 8–9.

97. Ibid., 17.

98. Hazel Corbin is quoted in "New Fathers Get Briefing," *New York Times*, January 9, 1958, 39.

99. Minutes of the Community Nursing Committee for Expectant Parent Classes, January 12, 1965, Public Health Nursing Consultant's File, 1946–69, Kenosha Expectant Parents, 1964–68, ser. 2549, box 2, folder 10, WHSA.

100. Bonnie Miller interview, August 20, 1986, MNOHP.

101. Kathleen Dicker, "Husbands in the Labour Ward," *Nursing Times*, March 27, 1969, 416–17, quotation on 417.

102. Florence E. Hoff, "Natural Childbirth: How Any Nurse Can Help," *American Journal of Nursing* 49, no. 7 (July 1969): 1451–53, quotation on 1452.

103. Sarah Jane Williams, "Caught in the Middle: Maternity Nurses and the Natural Childbirth Movement" (M.S. thesis, University of Wisconsin, Madison, School of Nursing, 1987).

104. Susan Gould Tidyman to author, December 9, 1983, AQ, *NYT*.

105. Jeanette D. Hines, "Father—the Forgotten Man," *Nursing Forum* 10, no. 2 (1971): 177–200, quotation on 193–94.

106. M. Pawson and N. Norris, "The Role of the Father in Pregnancy and Labour," *Psychosomatic Medicine in Obstetrics and Gynecology*, Third International Congress, London, 1971 (New York: Basel, Karger, 1972), 273–75. See also Max Deutscher, "First Pregnancy and Family Formation," in *Psychoanalytic Contributions to Community Psychology*, ed. Donald S. Miller and George D. Goldman (Springfield, Ill.: Charles C. Thomas, 1971), 233–55.

107. Hott, "Investigation of the Relationship," 107.

108. Beatrice Liebenberg, "Expectant Fathers," in *Psychological Aspects of a First Pregnancy and Early Postnatal Adaptation*, ed. P. M. Shereshefsky and L. J. Yarry (New York: Raven Press, 1974), 109.

109. Jo Manion, "A Study of Fathers and Infant Caretaking," *Birth and the Family Journal* 4, no. 4 (1977): 174–79, quotation and figures on 175.

110. George Schaefer, *The Expectant Father*, rev. ed. (New York: Barnes and Noble Books, Division of Harper and Row, 1972), 82, 84.

111. Ibid., 97.

112. Nirvana K. interview, May 28, 1996, BP.

113. Celeste R. Phillips and Joseph T. Anzalone, *Fathering: Participation in Labor and Birth* (St. Louis, Mo.: Mosby, 1978); the unnamed men are quoted on 82, 92–93, 105.

114. Anonymous father in conversation with author, 2005.

115. Phillips and Anzalone, *Fathering*, 66.

116. Ibid., 64.

117. Ibid., 92–93. Other men felt "helpless" and "disappointed"; see 105, 112.

118. Sally Langendoen, "To Expectant Fathers: What to Do If She Panics during Labor," *American Baby*, November 1978, 16, 19.

119. Ibid.

120. Charen Elsherif, Garnet McGrath, and Joyce Thies Smyrski, "Coaching the Coach," *Journal of Obstetric, Gynecologic, and Neonatal Nursing* (March/April 1979): 87–89, quotation on 89.

121. Jack Pritchard and Paul MacDonald, *Williams Obstetrics*, 16th ed. (New York: Appleton-Century, 1980), 453. The same advice is repeated in the following editions in 1989 and 1997.

122. Judith A. Maloni, "The Birthing Room: Some Insights into Parents' Experiences," *Maternal Child Nursing* 5 (September/October 1980): 314–19, quotations on 318.

123. Branko Terzic to author, March 6, 2005, in response to my author's query in the *New York Times* Book Review, March 6, 2005.

124. Robert P. Klein et al., "A Study of Father and Nurse Support during Labor," *Birth and the Family Journal* 8, no. 3 (Fall 1981): 161–64, quotations on 161, 162. See also Stephanie MacLaughlin, "First-Time Fathers' Childbirth Experience," *Journal of Nurse-Midwifery* 25, no. 3 (May/June 1980): 17–21. For routine suggestions for nurses to welcome and support fathers, see William Kunst-Wilson and Linda Cronenwett, "Nursing Care for the Emerging Family: Promoting Paternal Behavior," *Research in Nursing and Health* 4 (1981): 201–11.

125. Celeste R. Phillips and Joseph T. Anzalone, *Fathering: Participation in Labor and Birth*, 2nd ed. (St. Louis, Mo.: Mosby, 1982), 154–55. A study in 1992 identified three major roles men played (coach, teammate, and witness): Linda L. Chapman, "Expectant Fathers' Roles during Labor and Birth," *Journal of Obstetric, Gynecologic, and Neonatal Nursing* 21, no. 2 (March/April 1992): 114–20.

126. Anne Campbell and Everett L. Worthington Jr., "Teaching Expectant Fathers How to Be Better Childbirth Coaches," *Maternal Child Nursing* 7, no. 1 (January/February 1982): 28–32, quotations on 28, 31.

127. Philip Taubman, "Doubts in the Delivery Room," *New York Times*, October 21, 1984, SM 72.

128. Pam L. interview, BP.

Chapter Six

1. Quoted in Robert A. Bradley, "Fathers' Presence in Delivery Rooms," *Psychosomatics* 3 (November–December 1962): 474. The same story was noted in a sidebar in *Hospital Topics* (January 1966): 106, in which the hospital was identified as the Redwood Empire Hospital in California.

2. Joan Gerver to author, August 30, 1984, AQ, *NYT*. When Gerver delivered again in 1954, "my husband was stopped at the door to the delivery room. The door had a glass window, and I think he watched from there."

3. Bertie Livingston to author, July 24, 1983, AQ, *NYT*.

4. Doris Conway to author, no date, AQ, *NYT*.

5. Moya Sullivan to author, September 9, 1983, AQ, *NYT*.

6. Mildred Cherry to author, August 7, 1983, AQ, *NYT*.

7. Julianne Trychta to author, June 16, 2005, AQ, *OW*. My thanks to Beth Black for encouraging this exchange.

8. Charles A. Lindbergh, *The Wartime Journals of Charles A. Lindbergh* (New York: Harcourt Brace Jovanovich, 1970), 695–96. I am grateful to David Courtwright for calling my attention to this reference.

9. See also, for example, Claire Terse, "Aid for False Labor," *Child-Family Digest* 5, no. 3 (September 1951): 87–91.

10. Joanna Long, R.N., "Let's Count the Fathers In," in "Letters from Readers," *American Journal of Nursing* 45, no. 5 (1945): 313–14.

11. Rosemarie Braatz to author, November 2, 2005, AQ, *OW*.

12. Nurse Barrington's Mothers' Class, March 20, 1952, Public Health Nursing Consultant's Files, 1946–69, ser. 2549, box 1, folder 27, WHSA.

13. Robert N. Rutherford, "Fathers in the Delivery Room—Long Experience Molds One Viewpoint," *Hospital Topics* 44 (January 1966): 97, 100–102, quotation on 97.

14. Ibid., 101–2.

15. Gail Ravitts to author, in response to author's query in *New York Times* Book Review, July 30, 1983. See also Elizabeth Austin Lindsay, "The Old Way Is New: Natural Childbirth Plus Rooming-In," *Parents' Digest*, June 1949, 23–28.

16. Joseph MacLeod to author, March 10, 2005, in response to my author's query in the *New York Times* Book Review, March 6, 2005.

17. Muriel Korn to author, July 24, 1983, AQ, *NYT*, referring to her deliveries of 1939 and 1941.

18. Albert M. Vollmer, "Clinical Experiences and Observations on the Use of Relax-

ation Methods in Obstetrical Practice," *Child-Family Digest* 1, no. 4 (September 1949): 17–23, quotation on 22–23.

19. See, for example, James A. Gunn, M.D., to author, November 21, 2005, AQ, *OW*. My thanks to Jennifer Gunn for facilitating this correspondence.

20. Herbert Thoms, *Understanding Natural Childbirth: A Book for the Expectant Mother* (New York: McGraw-Hill, 1950). See also Doris Haire, "Natural Childbirth," *Life*, January 30, 1950, 71–77.

21. Peter S. Douglas, "A Father Reports on Natural Childbirth," *Child-Family Digest* 3, no. 3 (September 1950): 60–62, quotation on 61–62.

22. Char Glashagel to author, June 15, 2005, AQ, *OW*, about her 1969 delivery. My thanks to Beth Black for facilitating this correspondence.

23. Owen's account, dated May 7, 1947, can be found in the Edith Banfield Jackson Papers at the Arthur and Elizabeth Schlesinger Library on the History of Women in America, Radcliffe College, Harvard University Library, Cambridge, Massachusetts, box 3, folder 52, quotations on 2, 1. I am extremely grateful to Rebecca Jo Plant for alerting me to this source.

24. Parent Class Project, District 8, January 20, 1955, Public Health Nursing Consultant's File, 1946–69, Racine-Kenosha Nurses Workshop, ser. 2549, box 2, folder 25, WHSA.

25. Robert A. Bradley, *Husband-Coached Childbirth: The Bradley Method of Natural Childbirth*, 4th ed., rev. and ed. with Marjie and Jay Hathaway (New York: Bantam Books, 1996), 52–53. Stories of women traveling from California to Denver to birth with Bradley are reminiscent of women traveling long distances home to mother.

26. Robert Bradley and Herbert Thoms quoted in the appendix of ICEA, "Husbands in the Delivery Room: Recommendations to Hospital Administrators and Physicians on the Desirability and Safety of the Practice," April 1965, typescript available in the City College of New York Library, New York, 25, 23.

27. Mary Rogers interview, August 26, 1986, MNOHP, 10.

28. Dorothy Barclay, "Father's Aid Asked in Birth of Baby," *New York Times*, May 19, 1950, no page number. See also Barclay's "What Every Father Should Know," *New York Times*, June 11, 1950, Parent and Child Section, 170.

29. Marguerite Ball, "Without Pain," *Woman's Home Companion*, May 1943, 16, 82, 85, quotation on 85.

30. Robert J. Hawkins, "Essential Delivery Room Equipment," *Proceedings of the First American Congress on Obstetrics and Gynecology*, Cleveland, September 11–15, 1939 (Evanston, Ill.: Mumm Print Shop, 1941), 656–62. See also M. Edward Davis, "Delivery Room Safeguards," *Hospitals* 12, no. 6 (June 1938): 68–69; "Proposed Plan for Labor and Delivery Room Set-Up in Hospitals," *Bulletin of the University Hospital* (Augusta, Ga.) 5, no. 6 (1943–44): 11–15; Gertrude Armstrong, "Delivery Room Technique," *Canadian Nurse* 43, no. 5 (May 1947): 349–52; and various state standards for maternity hos-

pitals, such as *Standards for Maternity Hospitals of Minnesota* (Saint Paul: State Board of Control Children's Bureau, 1928), or *Standards for Maternity Hospitals of Montana* (Helena: Montana State Board of Health in cooperation with the U.S. Children's Bureau, 1942).

31. Charles Butler and Addison Erdman, *Hospital Planning* (New York: F. W. Dodge, 1946), 58.

32. Edward F. Stevens, *The American Hospital of the Twentieth Century* (New York: F. W. Dodge, 1928), 21.

33. Elizabeth Diringer quoted in *ASPON*, August–September, 1969.

34. I did not see explicit discussion of curtains, but if they were considered, hospitals would have worried about keeping them clean.

35. Robert N. Rutherford, Daniel C. More, John Dare, and Patricia A. Rose, "Coordinated Obstetric Care," *Obstetrics and Gynecology* 8, no. 5 (November 1956): 581–90, quotation on 586.

36. Hazel Corbin, "Changing Maternity Service in a Changing World," *Child-Family Digest* 4, no. 3 (March 1951): 28–39, quotation on 36.

37. Woman quoted by Corbin in ibid., 36.

38. Nonette Hanko, "Well Trained for Childbirth," *Child-Family Digest* 6, no. 6 (June 1952): 57–63, quotation on 61.

39. Paul A. Bowers, "Husbands in the Delivery Room," *Child-Family Digest* 6, no. 4 (April 1952): 3–6, quotation on 4. See also an example from Milwaukee, Patricia Murphy, "Expectant Mothers Organize for Natural Childbirth," *American Journal of Nursing* 56, no. 10 (October 1956): 1298–1301. The group called itself the Natural Childbirth Association of Milwaukee, and its advisory board included two obstetricians, a general practitioner, a pediatrician, a lawyer, a sociologist, and representatives of the city health department, the Visiting Nurse Association, and the Milwaukee Adult and Vocational School. The Maternity Center Association of New York City had offered expectant father education classes beginning in the 1930s, focusing on teaching the men how to be good fathers and making no argument for allowing fathers into the delivery room. See, for example, Hazel Corbin, *Getting Ready to Be a Father* (New York: Macmillan, 1939; reprinted in 1945).

40. Man quoted in Bowers, "Husbands in the Delivery Room," 5–6.

41. WMH, FB, October 20, 1959. He may actually have been referring to the fact that men cannot physically share women's pain, rather than to his exclusion from the delivery room.

42. Patricia Murphy, "A Nurse-Mother Looks at Natural Childbirth," *Child-Family Digest* 7, no. 4 (December 1952): 55–60, quotation on 59–60.

43. Woman who wished to remain anonymous to author, July 24, 1983, AQ, *NYT*.

44. Kathleen Lander to author, July 25, 1983, AQ, *NYT*.

45. California Department of Public Health, *Conclusions and Recommendations of*

the Conferences on Maternity Practices, 1955, quotations on 18, 51; copy at the National Library of Medicine, Bethesda, Maryland.

46. "Fathers-to-Be Don't Always Pace the Floor," *New York Times*, June 19, 1961, 32.

47. Margaret Hickey, "Training for Childbirth . . . in Seattle, Washington," *Ladies' Home Journal*, May 1953, 28, 146, 148–49, quotations on 146, 149.

48. Jack Harrison Pollack, "The Case for Natural Childbirth," *Cosmopolitan*, July 1953, 39–43, quotation on 43.

49. "A Father Sees His Child Born," *Life*, June 13, 1955, 133–38.

50. Julie Harris, as told to Betty Friedan, "I Was Afraid to Have a Baby," *McCall's*, December 1956, 68, 72, 74, quotation on 74 (emphasis in original). For practices of obstetrical anesthesia, see Jacqueline H. Wolf, "'Mighty Glad to Gasp in the Gas': Perceptions of Pain and the Traditional Timing of Obstetrical Anesthesia," *Health: An Interdisciplinary Journal for the Social Study of Health, Illness and Medicine* 6, no. 3 (2002): 365–87.

51. Wisconsin Administrative Code, 1956, chap. H29, rule H29.14; available in the University of Wisconsin Law Library, Madison.

52. William H. Genne, *Husbands and Pregnancy: The Handbook for Expectant Fathers* (New York: Association Press, 1956), 73.

53. Ibid.

54. Peter Browne, "I Saw My Son Born," *Readers' Digest*, November 1957, 61–64, quotations on 62, 61.

55. Ibid., 63–64.

56. Muriel Goldfarb and Robert W. Goldfarb, "We Shared Our Baby's Birth . . . ," *Ladies' Home Journal*, December 1958, 142. There are other such stories of the period. For example, "(Question: Do you think anyone could help you during labor?) 'Oh, my husband! I know I'd feel a lot better if he could come upstairs with me. Just knowing he was there. He could hold my hand, you know,'" quoted in Marion S. Lesser and Vera R. Keane, *Nurse-Patient Relationships in a Hospital Maternity Service* (St. Louis, Mo.: Mosby, 1956), 103. Men's roles in delivery, as prescribed by the natural childbirth movement, changed in these years from emotional supporter to active labor coach. This changing role is described in Linda L. Chapman, "Expectant Fathers' Roles during Labor and Birth," *Journal of Obstetric, Gynecologic, and Neonatal Nursing* 21 (March 1992): 114–20.

57. Goldfarb and Goldfarb, "We Shared our Baby's Birth," 142.

58. Grantly Dick-Read, "Childbirth without Fear and without Pain," *Ladies' Home Journal*, June 1957, 72–73, 138–39, 141–43, 148–50, quotation on 149–50.

59. Fred D. Kartchner, "Active Participation in Childbirth: A Psychosomatic Approach to Pregnancy and Parturition," *American Journal of Obstetrics and Gynecology* 75, no. 6 (June 1958): 1244–54, quotation on 1251.

60. Gladys Denny Shultz, "Journal Mothers Report on Cruelty in Maternity Wards," *Ladies' Home Journal*, May 1958, 44–46, 152–55, quotation on 155.

61. Gladys Denny Shultz, "Journal Mothers Testify to Cruelty in Maternity Wards," *Ladies' Home Journal*, December 1958, 58–59, 135, 137–39, quotations on 59, 137. See a medical response to this exposé agreeing that physicians needed to be more sensitive to women's emotional needs during labor and delivery, "Letter," *Ladies' Home Journal*, March 1959, 55. See also "New Fathers Get Briefing," *New York Times*, January 9, 1958, 39.

62. Jane C. Maher to author, June 10, 2005, AQ, *OW*.

63. See, for example, William D. Feeny to author, June 21, 2005, AQ, *OW*. Feeny was excluded from his wife's delivery but did get to observe and photograph the birth of his first grandchild in 1989.

64. WMH, FB, October 6, 1959. Or see the February 9, 1960, entry: "I stood with her most of the time she labored."

65. George G. Greene, "A General Survey of Maternal Care in a Navy Hospital," *American Journal of Obstetrics and Gynecology* 53, no. 4 (April 1947): 669–73, quotation on 671. The hospital, nonetheless, had a high record of interventions of forceps and episiotomies, including midforceps.

66. Bonnie Miller interview, August 20, 1986, MNOHP, 13.

67. Ibid., 14. See also a similar story, Larry Eriksson to author, June 9, 2005, AQ, *OW*.

68. Malcolm S. Allan, "After Office Hours: Husband-Attended Deliveries," *Obstetrics and Gynecology* 27 (January 1966): 146–48, quotations on 147, 148.

69. Holy Cross Hospital, Merrill, Wisconsin, July 23, 1962, report by Helen F. Callon, Hospital Nursing Consultant, box 1, folder F28, ser. 2702, WHSA.

70. Jean E. Schultz, M.D., Principal Public Health Physician, Nassau County Department of Health, to Rev. J. Lawrence Ainsworth, February 7, 1962. I am grateful to Reverend Ainsworth for sending me a copy of this letter, following my talk at the University of Michigan in April 2003.

71. ICEA, "Husbands in the Delivery Room: Recommendations to Hospital Administrators and Physicians on the Desirability and Safety of the Practice," ed. Fay Stender, 1965, bound typescript available at the City College of New York Library, New York, and at the American College of Obstetricians and Gynecologists, Washington, D.C., 30–31.

72. Glen E. Hayden et al., "Maternity Care Should Be Family Centered," *Modern Hospital* 102, no. 2 (February 1964): 105. See also ICEA, "Husbands in the Delivery Room," 27.

73. Bonnie Miller interview, MNOHP, 12–13.

74. Joan Knudson interview, August 26, 1986, MNOHP, 18.

75. Lauretta Scherschel interview, August 12, 1986, MNOHP, 11–12.

76. Ibid., 12–13.

77. Ann Gunderson interview, August 6, 1986, MNOHP, 7–9. See also Patricia Alm interview, July 1, 1986, MNOHP.

78. Jane C. Maher to author, June 17, 2005, AQ, *OW*.

79. Bradley, "Fathers' Presence in Delivery Rooms," 477–79. See also Letter from "A Denver Physician" [possibly Robert Bradley without attribution], *Child-Family Digest* 19 (July–August 1960): 97.

80. Charles W. Aldridge, "Initial Experiences with Fathers in the Delivery Room," *Michigan Medicine* 69 (June 1970): 489–91.

81. Catholic Hospital Association of the United States and Canada, "Family Centered Maternity Care at St. Mary's Hospital Evansville, Indiana," 1960, no page numbers, available at the American College of Obstetricians and Gynecologists Library, Washington, D.C.

82. Phyllis Ehrlich, "Father's Role at Baby's Birth Disputed," *New York Times*, February 13, 1962, 30.

83. Stuart Price to author, June 29, 2005, AQ, *OW*. Price felt he could share the story after so many years.

84. Roger W. Hoag, Berkeley, California, quoted in ICEA, "Husbands in the Delivery Room," 29–30.

85. Allan Barnes, "Reducing the Hazards of Birth," *Harper's Magazine*, January 1964, 31–37, quotation on 32.

86. John S. Miller, "Fathers in the Delivery Room," *Child and Family* 3, no. 4 (1964): 3–11, quotation on 5–6.

87. An editorial in *Modern Hospital* agreed that hospitals needed to find ways to allow the fathers to attend delivery because "medical fashions and practices change, and it is the responsibility of administrators and trustees to keep up with changing practices." "Fashion Notes," *Modern Hospital* 104, no. 2 (February 1965): 85–86, quotation on 86.

88. American College of Obstetricians and Gynecologists, *Manual of Standards in Obstetric-Gynecologic Practice*, 2nd ed. (Chicago, 1965), 26; a copy can be found in the library of the American College of Obstetricians and Gynecologists, Washington, D.C.

89. "Delivery Room 'Invader' Fined," *American Medical Association News*, January 4, 1965, 11. Unfortunately, I was unable to determine what happened during the appeal.

90. "Surgeons and Nurses Discuss Whether Fathers Should Be in Delivery Room," *Modern Hospital* 106 (April 1966): 32.

91. Malcolm S. Allan, "Husband-Attended Deliveries," *Obstetrics and Gynecology* 27, no. 1 (January 1966): 146–48, quotations on 146–47.

92. Donald L. Sheaffer to author, February 21, 2005, in response to my author's query in Book World, *Washington Post*, February 20, 2005.

93. Robert N. Rutherford, "Fathers in the Delivery Room—Long Experience Molds One Viewpoint," *Hospital Topics* 44, no. 1 (January 1966): 97–102.

94. John S. Miller, "'Return the Joy of Home Delivery' with Fathers in the Delivery Room," *Hospital Topics* 44, no. 1 (January 1966): 105–9, quotations on 106, 107.

95. Ibid., 108.

96. Carl Goetsch, "Fathers in the Delivery Room—'Helpful and Supportive,'" *Hospital Topics* 44, no. 1 (January 1966): 104–5, quotations on 104.

97. John H. Morton, "Fathers in the Delivery Room—an Opposition Standpoint," *Hospital Topics* 44, no. 1 (January 1966): 103–4, quotation on 103.

98. Ibid., 103–4.

99. See, for example, the father claiming the opposite (in response to this point of view) in Sally Olds and Linda Witt, "New Man in the Delivery Room—the Father," in *Today's Health*, October 1970, 56.

100. See "Father-Attended Deliveries: Pros, Cons on the New Trend," *Medical Tribune* 7 (March 12–13, 1966): 12. Husbands' lack of interest was revealed in Cleveland when a survey of husbands of maternity patients demonstrated that more than 59 percent had no desire to be present in the delivery room. See "Surgeons and Nurses Discuss Whether Fathers Should Be in Delivery Room," *Modern Hospital* 106 (April 1966): 32.

101. Schaefer is quoted in "Father-Attended Deliveries: Pros, Cons on the New Trend," 12.

102. Robert H. Stewart is quoted in Deborah Ruth Wolf Tanzer, *The Psychology of Pregnancy and Childbirth: An Investigation of Natural Childbirth* (Ann Arbor, Mich: UMI, 1967), 388, and in Robert H. Stewart, "Natural Childbirth, Father Participation, Rooming-In, or What-Have-You," *Medical Times* 91, no. 11 (November 1963): 1065–68, quotations on 1066, 1067.

103. I am grateful to Professor Claire Wendland of the University of Wisconsin for forwarding me, with his permission, a copy of an email letter she received from her father, Dan Wendland, May 30, 2005.

104. E. Todd Wheeler, *Hospital Design and Function* (New York: McGraw-Hill, 1964), 136.

105. Ruth Brecher and Edward Brecher, "How to Get Better Maternity Care," *Redbook*, July 1962, 43, 108–11, quotation on 108. See also ICEA, "Husbands in the Delivery Room." For a full look at the Boston area activities of ICEA, see Boston Association for Childbirth Education 1934–93 records at the Arthur and Elizabeth Schlesinger Library on the History of Women in America, Radcliffe Institute for Advanced Study, Harvard University, Cambridge, Mass.

106. Walden B. Crabtree, "A Father's Experience," *Bulletin of the American College of Nurse-Midwifery* 7, no. 2 (1962): 52–53.

107. David R. Downs, M.D., to author, June 12 and 16, 2005, AQ, OW. Downs did not think husbands' presence was necessarily tied to natural childbirth. See also Terry Woster, "Happy Birthday, Andrew, You've Come a Long Way," *Sioux Falls Argus Leader*, January 27, 2008, in which the author recounts his son's 1969 birth when the doctor encouraged his attendance in the delivery room.

108. ICEA, "Husbands in the Delivery Room."

109. Ibid., 6.

110. Ibid., 13.

111. Bradley quoted in ibid., 26.

112. Newton is quoted in ibid., 27. See also Joseph P. Whitlatch quoted in ibid., 29. Whitlatch admitted that he was slow to admit fathers, but now he encourages the practice: "I have never ceased to be thrilled at their spontaneous expression of elation at having been present at the culmination of the pregnancy. I feel sure this experience has knit the family unit much closer together than it could have been without their complete sharing at the birth of the fruits of their love."

113. Sister M. Clarice was quoted in ibid., 32–33.

114. The list is in ibid., 14–18. For experience in Seattle at the same time, see also Glen E. Hayden, Daniel C. Moore, and L. Donald Bridenbaugh, "Maternity Care Should Be Family Centered," *Modern Hospital* 102 (February 1964): 104–5. See more about the ICEA report in "Father-Attended Deliveries: Pros, Cons on the New Trend," 12.

115. The opinion of the attorney general of California, February 27, 1964, is quoted in ICEA, "Husbands in the Delivery Room," 12. See also "Hospital Deliveries," *American Medical Association News*, October 12, 1964, 8. The full opinion can be found in *Opinions of the Attorney General of California*, March 1964, February 27, 1964, opinion number 64-52. See also Miller, "'Return the Joy of Home Delivery,'" 105–9.

116. 77ILL.Adm.Code 250.1830ILL Admin.Code Tit77 250.1830. Interestingly the law was written to include "the presence of the father or individual selected by the mother." See also C. Y. Shu, "Husband-Father in Delivery Room?" *Hospitals: Journal of the American Hospital Association* 47, no. 18 (September 16, 1973): 90, 92–94.

117. Novelist Sloan Wilson wanted to be with his wife through labor and delivery. He admitted, "I wasn't at all sure I would have the guts to stand by her calmly while she writhed in labor, and I was terrified that I would faint when the child actually started to emerge. . . . Above all, I did not want to lose my wife's lovely concept of me as a calm and wise man." Risking all that, he persisted in arranging it all with the doctors. See Sloan Wilson, "The American Way of Birth," *Harper's Magazine*, July 1964, 48–54. In the end, he could not accompany his wife into the delivery room because of a complicated presentation.

118. Miller, "Fathers in the Delivery Room," 3.

119. Ibid., 6, 9.

120. Jane Kavanau to author, February 27 and March 4, 2005, in response to my author's query in the *New York Times* Book Review, March 6, 2005.

121. Robert A. Bradley, "Father's Place during Childbirth," *Medical Opinion and Review* (December 1966): 72–77, quotations on 73, 77.

122. The women were quoted in Tanzer, *Psychology of Pregnancy and Childbirth*, 348, 359 (emphasis in original).

123. Ibid., 374.

124. Elisabeth D. Bing, ed., *The Adventure of Birth: Experiences in the Lamaze Method of Prepared Childbirth* (New York: Simon and Schuster, 1970), 21.

125. Edgar L. Engel, "Family-Centered Hospital Maternity Care," *American Journal of Obstetrics and Gynecology* 85, no. 2 (January 1963): 260–66, quotations on 264.

126. W. A. Regan, "Delivery Room Spectators and the Law: Regan Report on Nursing Law," *Colorado Nurse* 68 (May 1968): 8.

127. Charles W. Aldridge Jr., "Initial Experiences with Fathers in the Delivery Room," *Michigan Medicine* 69 (June 1970): 489–91, quotation on 489.

128. Ibid., 491. But see also a contradictory position by an unnamed physician quoted in Shirley Zussman, *A Study of Certain Social, Psychological, and Cultural Factors Influencing Husbands' Participation in their Wives' Labor* (Ann Arbor, Mich.: UMI, 1969), 72.

129. See Maternity Hospital Codes, Wisconsin Administrative Code, 1956–60, chap. H29.14, p. 67, which read: "Visitors shall not have contact with nursery infants at any time and shall not be admitted to the delivery room or nursery." For the codes in effect in later years, see, 1960–68 code, chap. H26.032, and 1968–84, chap. H24, both of which seem to allow hospitals to set their own regulations.

130. James Lindblade, interview with author, University of Wisconsin, December 27, 2001; quoted with permission. For a slightly different perspective, see Mary McCool interview, May 9, 1986, MNOHP. This obstetrics nurse at the same hospital thought that physicians' egos made them resist the new practice when it was first suggested: "Their authority is being challenged, their territory is being invaded by another male," she said. "Their authority is on the line. They have to watch what they say. Papa's watching. And for a lot of these men who are used to being the absolute, the be all and end all, God in the delivery room, it took them a long time before [they agreed to the father's presence]" (12).

131. Mary McCool interview, May 9, 1986, MNOHP, 11.

132. Steven M. Barney, "I Was There When My Son Was Born," *Wisconsin State Journal* (Madison), July 27, 1969. Barney thought the hospital policy changed to admit the men in July 1969.

133. John A. Roberts, "I Watched My Baby Being Born," *Parents Magazine*, January 1969, 60–61, 74, quotation on 74. See also "The Role of Fathers," *Science News* 93, no. 23 (June 15, 1968): 567–68. For more on physician attitudes to fathers in delivery rooms, see Michael Newton, "Dad's Role in Delivery," *Health* 14, no. 1 (January 1982): 11–12, and Sherwin A. Kaufman, "Before the Baby Comes: New Roles and Responsibilities for the Expectant Father," *Parents Magazine*, April 1978, 37–38.

134. "Oscar Brown Jr. Watches as His, Jean's Baby Is Born," *Jet*, May 1, 1969, 24.

Chapter Seven

1. *All in the Family*, dialogue from episode 115, October 6, 1975.

2. In "intentionally creat[ing] a character [Archie] whose prejudices would be revealed as illogical and senseless . . . [and making him] a ridiculous figure, [producer Norman] Lear hoped that viewers would see how stupid their own prejudices were and change their attitudes," writes Richard Butsch in "A Half Century of Class and Gender in American TV Domestic Sitcoms," *Cercles* 8 (2003): 16–34, quotation on 23. See also Sari Thomas and Brian P. Callahan, "Allocating Happiness: TV Families and Social Class," *Journal of Communications* (Summer 1982): 184–90, and Nancy L. Buerkel-Rothfuss et al., "Learning about the Family from Television," in the same issue, 191–201.

3. *ASPON*, 1970. See January through September issues of that year, quotations from the April–May and August–September issues, no page numbers.

4. Earl Withycombe to author, September 3, 2005, AQ, *OW*. Withycombe similarly attended and played a role in two subsequent births. My thanks to Shannon Withycombe for arranging this correspondence.

5. Tom Clark, "'Til Delivery Room Do Us Part," *ASPON*, September–October 1971.

6. Ibid.

7. Gloria Sarto, M.D., oral history interview with Ann Peckham, University of Wisconsin Oral History Program, July 26, 2005. I am grateful for the permission of Dr. Sarto to attend the interview and tell the story here.

8. Jean Truesdale to author, July 1, 2005, AQ, *OW*.

9. Alvin J. Berndt to author, no date, AQ, *OW*. See also the story told by "Jean" (who did not want her last name to be used), whose husband was allowed to be with her in a small town in northern Wisconsin in 1972 because the physician was a family friend: "Jean" to author, June 14, 2005, AQ, *OW*.

10. Inez Carter interview, June 12, 1986, MNOHP, 18.

11. Sandra Eiseman, interview with author, July 8, 2005, Madison, Wisconsin.

12. Alice Robbin to author, August 22, 2005, AQ, *OW*.

13. Anonymous to author, June 17, 2005, AQ, *OW*.

14. Sue Ernst, ed., "Father Participation Guide," ICEA, 1975, 4–6; copy in the library of the American College of Obstetricians and Gynecologists, Washington, D.C.

15. Daniel P. B. Smith to author, June 18, 2005, AQ, *OW*.

16. Narinder N. Sehgal, "The Potential for Problems When Husbands Are in the Delivery Room," *Resident and Staff Physician*, March 1973, 33–35, quotations on 33.

17. Ibid., 34.

18. Ibid., 35. See also Narinder N. Sehgal, "Husbands in the Delivery Room: Potential for Problems," *Medical Times* 102, no. 2 (February 1974): 56–58.

19. Eleanor Waddell interview, July 1, 1986, MNOHP, 19.

20. Carolyn Splett interview, April 24, 1986, MNOHP, 17.

21. Anonymous to author, August 21, 2005, AQ, *OW*.

22. Eric V. D. Luft to author, May 21, 2003.

23. Male and female obstetricians, for example, used forceps at significantly different rates. See Karen D. Bonar, Andrew M. Kaunitz, and Luis Sanchez-Ramos, "The Effects of Obstetric Resident Gender on Forceps Delivery Rate," *American Journal of Obstetrics and Gynecology* 182, no. 5 (2000): 1050–51.

24. Mike Bitney interview, August 25, 1986, MNOHP, 10. There was also the factor that residents, instead of attending physicians, might do the actual delivery, and physicians did not want the fathers to see that. See, for example, Dr. Gloria Sarto, who alluded to it briefly in her oral history interview with Ann Peckham (Wisconsin Oral History Program, July 26, 2005). It makes sense that physicians who wanted the birthing woman to think she was delivered by the person she had been expecting (and paying for) might not be happy to learn that a resident in training in fact did the work.

25. Margaret Gamper, *Preparation for the Heirminded* (Hammond, Ind.: Sheffield, 1971), 61, as quoted in Margot Edwards and Mary Waldorf, *Reclaiming Birth: History and Heroines of American Childbirth Reform* (Trumansburg, N.Y.: Crossing Press, 1984), 26.

26. *A Bill to Provide for Hospitals to Allow the Biological Father to Attend the Birth of His Child If the Woman Consents*, HR 1504, 93rd Cong., 1st sess. (January 9, 1973), *Congressional Record* 119, pt. 1, 577. A copy of the bill is reprinted in Rosalyn Baxandall and Linda Gordon, eds., *Dear Sisters: Dispatches from the Women's Liberation Movement* (New York: Basic Books, 2000), 130. The bill was reintroduced two more times during the Ninety-fourth Congress session in 1975: as HR 6694 by Representative James C. Corman of California and as HR 10497 by Representative Richard M. Nolan of Minnesota.

27. Baxandall and Gordon, *Dear Sisters*, 130, suggest that the bill introduced in Congress was "evidence of women's political power."

28. Kathy Linck, "Legalizing a Woman's Right to Choose," in *Proceedings of the First International Childbirth Conference*, coordinated by Dorothy Tennov and Lolly Hirsch, June 2, 1973, Cloonan Middle School, Stamford, Connecticut (emphasis in original).

29. Quoted in "Thoughts on Women's Liberation," *ASPON*, November–December 1971. Seemingly in response to the notion of rights, the author of an article in the journal *Hospitals* assured his readers, "It must be clearly understood that the presence of the husband-father in the delivery room is a privilege to be granted and not a right to be demanded." C. Y. Shu, "Husband-Father in Delivery Room?" *Hospitals: Journal of the American Hospital Association* 47, no. 18 (September 16, 1973): 90, 92–94, quotation on 94.

30. Barbara Kaiser and Irwin H. Kaiser, "The Challenge of the Women's Movement to American Gynecology," *American Journal of Obstetrics and Gynecology* 20, no. 5 (November 1, 1974): 652–65, quotation on 653.

31. Elizabeth Jean Pascoe, "How Women Want to Have Their Babies," *McCall's*, October 1977, 109–10, quotation on 109.

32. Suzanne Arms, *Immaculate Deception: A New Look at Women and Childbirth in America* (New York: Bantam Books, 1977). See also its sequel: *Immaculate Deception II: Myth, Magic, and Birth* (Berkeley, Calif.: Celestial Arts, 1994). For other influential books on this subject during the 1970s, see Irvin Chabon, *Awake and Aware: Participating in Childbirth with Prophylaxis* (New York: Dell Books, 1977); Sheila Kitzinger, *The Experience of Childbirth* (London: Gollancz, 1972); and Elizabeth D. Bing, ed., *The Adventure of Birth: Experiences in the Lamaze Method of Prepared Childbirth* (New York: Simon and Schuster, 1970). Some used more feminist rights arguments than others, but they all fostered natural childbirth and having the father attend the delivery.

33. The story and many of the documents about the campaign are told and reproduced in Ernst, "Father Participation Guide."

34. Roberta Scaer and Diana Korte, "A Survey of Maternity Options," © authors, 1977, Boulder, Colorado, typescript, study funded in part by the March of Dimes, Northern Colorado Chapter, distributed locally. I am extremely grateful to Roberta Scaer for sending me a copy of this booklet and for describing the activity in a letter to me, September 23, 2004. See also Diana Korte and Roberta Scaer, *A Good Birth, a Safe Birth*, 3rd rev. ed. (Boston: Harvard Common Press, 1992). See also Pascoe, "How Women Want to Have Their Babies."

35. Such cases are discussed in Howard Moss and Jeffrey Brown, "Dilemma in the Delivery Room," *Beverly Hills Bar Journal* 16 (Winter 1982): 35–40. See also Karen Koppel Kaunitz, "Point of Law: Fathers in the Delivery Room," *Hospital Medical Staff* 9 (December 1980): 17–22.

36. Decision is quoted in Kaunitz, "Point of Law," 21. See the full case, *Justus v. Atchison*, 139 Cal. Rptr. 97 (Cal. 1977). In a 1979 case, however, the judge ruled that because the husband observed the fetal death with his hand over his wife's abdomen, he could recover for the emotional damage (*Austin v. Regents of the University of California*, 152 Cal. Rptr. 420 [Cal. App. 1979]).

37. Barry Gross quoted in Sally Olds and Linda Witt, "New Man in the Delivery Room—the Father," *Today's Health*, October 1970, 52–56, quotations on 52, 56. On Barry Gross, see also "Judge Lets Father into Delivery Room," *Chicago Tribune*, June 2, 1970, A5, and Franklin D. Yoder, "Husbands in the Delivery Room," *ICEA News* 10, no. 1 (Spring 1971): 8–11, esp. 10.

38. Kaunitz, "Point of Law," 17.

39. *Hulit v. St. Vincent's Hospital*, 520 P.2d 99 (Montana 1974), 14. My thanks to attorney Jessica Feierman for her help in locating this decision.

40. Ibid., 13, 15.

41. *Fitzgerald v. Porter Memorial Hospital*, 523 F.2d 716 (7th Cir. 1975), *Federal Reporter*,

2nd ser., 716–24. The judge was John Paul Stevens (now U.S. Supreme Court justice). See also Moss and Brown, "Dilemma in the Delivery Room," 40; Kaunitz, "Point of Law" and "Hospital's Refusal to Allow Husbands in Delivery Room Upheld," *The Citation* 29, no. 6 (July 1974): 85–86; and Eric M. Newman, "Family Law—Constitutional Right of Privacy: The Father in the Delivery Room," *North Carolina Law Review* 54, no. 6 (September 1976): 1297–1308.

42. *Fitzgerald v. Porter Memorial Hospital*, 721. Two judges dissented. See also Moss and Brown, "Dilemma in the Delivery Room."

43. *Fitzgerald v. Porter Memorial Hospital*, 722. See also Harvey E. Pies, "The Right of the Father to Be Present in the Delivery Room," *American Journal of Public Health* 66 (July 1976): 688–89, quotations on 688. In *Baier v. Woman's Hospital Foundation* in the Court of Appeals of Louisiana the following year, the court found that federal funds used for hospital construction was not sufficient to allow for state action invoking the Equal Protection Clause of the Fourteenth Amendment. *Fitzgerald* was part of the justification. See *Baier v. Woman's Hospital Foundation*, November 15, 1976, 340 So.2d 360.

44. The form presented here is from the medical record of Nancy M. Smith, who delivered a baby at Lakeland Hospital on May 2, 1983. It was signed by David Smith, Nancy Smith, and their physician Dr. B. Kolar, in addition to a nurse (name not legible) as a witness. I quote from it with Nancy Smith's permission, and I thank her for it. See also Ernst, "Father Participation Guide," 14, where other wordings and forms are suggested. For an earlier version, see Helen F. Callon to Robert Houfek, November 10, 1964, copy in Hospitals Reports E–G, box 1, folder 26, ser. 2702, WHSA.

45. Max Deutscher, "First Pregnancy and Family Formation," in *Psychoanalytic Contributions to Community Psychology*, ed. Donald S. Miller and George D. Goldman (Springfield, Ill.: Charles C. Thomas, 1971), 233–55, quotation on 249.

46. J. P. Greenhill and Emanuel Friedman, *Biological Principles and Modern Practice of Obstetrics* (Philadelphia: W. B. Saunders, 1974), 152.

47. George Schaefer, *The Expectant Father*, rev. ed. (New York: Barnes and Noble Books, Division of Harper and Row, 1972), 86.

48. Ibid., 87.

49. Joan Beck, "Dauntless Is the Domesticated Dad," *Chicago Tribune*, June 13, 1972, sec. 2, 4.

50. Joan Beck, "Childbirth: An Experience to Be Shared," *Chicago Tribune*, June 20, 1972, sec. 2, 1.

51. Joan Beck, "Opening Delivery Room to Dads," *Chicago Tribune*, June 22, 1972, sec. 2, 1.

52. "Dear Diary," February 9, 1971. I am grateful to Dr. Susan Davidson and the St. Mary's Hospital staff for facilitating access to this set of fathers' books.

53. Ibid., February 16, 1978. See also entries for April 18 and August 31, 1971.

54. Ibid., October 27, 1971.

55. Ibid., February 13, 1972. See also May 12, 1972, where a man advised others, "Don't miss it guys!!"

56. Lee Epperson, "Love: To See a Grown Man Cry," *ASPON*, May–June 1971.

57. Donald Sutherland, "Childbirth Is Not for Mothers Only," *Ms.*, May 1974, 47–51, quotation on 47.

58. Susan Gould (Tidyman) to author, September 9, 1983, AQ, *NYT*.

59. Barbara Grizzuti Harrison, "Men Don't Know Nuthin' 'bout Birthin' Babies," *Esquire*, July 1973, 109–11, 133, 170, 172–73, quotation on 109.

60. Katherine Wolff, "Birth Report," *ASPON*, Spring 1972.

61. Marilyn Wood (Oakland, Calif.), *ASPON*, Summer 1972.

62. Linda Leonard, "The Father's Side: A Different Perspective on Childbirth," *Canadian Nurse* 73, no. 2 (1977): 16–20, quotation on 17.

63. The men are quoted in Jacqueline Hott, "An Investigation of the Relationship between Psychoprophylaxis in Childbirth and Changes in Self-Concept of the Participant Husband and His Concept of His Wife" (Ph.D. diss., New York University, 1972), 106.

64. Shirley Tighe Frank, "The Effect of Husbands' Presence at Delivery and Childbirth Preparation Classes on the Experience of Childbirth" (Ph.D. diss., Michigan State University, 1973), quotations from abstract and 38. See also Linda R. Cronenwett and Lucy L. Newmark, "Fathers' Responses to Childbirth," *Nursing Research* 23, no. 3 (1973): 210–17.

65. Teresa Modzelewski, "Fathers in the Delivery Room," *The Nevadan* (Sunday supplement to the *Las Vegas Review-Journal*), May 26, 1974, 6.

66. Charlotte Bonds and Ozell Bonds, "Initiation into Parenthood," *Essence*, September 1973, 58–59, 72, 74, 78–79, 85, quotations on 59, 78.

67. Ludmilla Alexander, "Fathers in the Delivery Room," *American Baby*, January 1972, 24–25, quotations on 24.

68. Quoted in ibid., 25.

69. Martin Greenberg and Norman Morris, "Engrossment: The Newborn's Impact upon the Father," *American Journal of Orthopsychiatry* 44 (1974): 520–31, quotations on 522, 524, 525.

70. Jo Manion, "A Study of Fathers and Infant Caretaking," *Birth and the Family Journal* 4, no. 4 (1977): 174–79. See also Toba Korenblum, "Probing the Father-Child Connection," *Maclean's*, June 22, 1981, 40–41.

71. Robert Allen Fein, "Men's Experiences before and after the Birth of a First Child: Dependence, Marital Sharing, and Anxiety" (Ph.D. diss., Harvard University, 1974), quotations on 187.

72. David Lynn, *The Father: His Role in Child Development* (Monterey, Calif.: Brooks/Cole, 1974), 228.

73. Jeannette L. Sasmor, "The Role of the Father in Labor and Delivery," *Psychosomatic Medicine in Obstetrics and Gynecology*, Third International Congress, London, 1971 (New

York: Karger, Basel, 1972), 279. See also Ron Goodman, "Diary of a Lamaze Father," *American Baby*, June 1974, 37, 42–43, 50, 53.

74. Shirley A. Oswald to author, July 8, 2005, AQ, *OW*.

75. William James Henneborn and Rosemary Cogan, "The Effect of Husband Participation on Reported Pain and Probability of Medication during Labor and Birth," *Journal of Psychosomatic Research* 19 (1975): 215–22.

76. Mickie Schmudlach interview, June 5, 1986, MNOHP, 16.

77. See, for example, Jeanette D. Hines, "Father — the Forgotten Man," *Nursing Forum* 10, no. 2 (1971): 177–200, quotation on 196.

78. Steven Strassberg, "Paternal Involvement with First-Borns during Infancy" (Ph.D. diss., Boston University, 1978), 83.

79. Man quoted in Eileen DeGarmo, "Fathers' and Mothers' Feelings about Sharing the Childbirth Experience," in *Current Practice in Obstetric and Gynecologic Nursing*, vol. 2, ed. Leota Kester McNall and Janet Trask Galeener (St. Louis, Mo.: Mosby, 1978), 164.

80. Robert Price, "A Father's Labor Pains," *Essence*, December 1975, 52–53, 77, 79, quotations 53. The couple took a natural childbirth class together, planned a hospital delivery, but ultimately had the baby at home with a midwife attending.

81. Patricia Patterson, "Childbirth: The Total Experience," *Essence*, November 1976, 13, 124, 130, 152, quotations on 13, 152.

82. Lynn Meyer, "More Fathers Witnessing the Birth of Their Children," *Eau Claire (Wis.) Leader-Telegram*, January 8, 1975, 1B. I am grateful to Bethany Relyea for showing me this story. See also Rita Kramer, "Revolution in the Delivery Room," *New York Times*, July 11, 1976, 167.

83. Man quoted in Celeste R. Phillips and Joseph T. Anzalone, *Fathering: Participation in Labor and Birth* (St. Louis, Mo.: Mosby, 1978), 99.

84. Mark Bernheim to author, April 16, 2005, in response to author's query in the *New York Review of Books*, April 7, 2005.

85. Leslie D. Atkinson, "Is Family-Centered Care a Myth?" *American Journal of Maternal Child Nursing* (July–August 1976): 256–59, quotation on 258.

86. Marcia Gollober, "A Comment on the Need for Father-Infant Postpartal Interaction," *Journal of Obstetric, Gynecologic, and Neonatal Nursing* (September–October 1976): 17–20, quotation on 17.

87. Robert A. Fein, "The First Weeks of Fathering: The Importance of Choices and Supports for New Parents," *Birth and the Family Journal* 3, no. 2 (Summer 1976): 53–59, quotation on 57. See also his "Men's Entrance to Parenthood," *Family Coordinator* 25, no. 4 (October 1976): 341–48, and his "Consideration of Men's Experiences and the Birth of a First Child," in *The First Child and Family Formation*, ed. Warren B. Miller and Lucile F. Newman (Chapel Hill: Carolina Population Center, University of North Carolina, 1978), 327–39.

88. Men were quoted in Phillips and Anzalone, *Fathering*, 105, 121. See also a review

of this book by Eugene Declercq in *Birth and the Family Journal* 7, no. 4 (Winter 1980): 274–75. Declercq thought the authors had described fathers in delivery as still "controversial," whereas he thought the issue was essentially settled by that time.

89. Jacqueline Rose Hott, "The Crisis of Expectant Fatherhood," *American Journal of Nursing* 76 (September 1976): 1436–40, quotations on 1439.

90. DeGarmo, "Fathers' and Mothers' Feelings," 167.

91. Lonnie Schlein, "Photographing the Birth of Your Own Celebrity," *New York Times*, October 31, 1976, D37.

92. Terri F. interview, May 8, 1996, BP.

93. See, for example, Marshall Klaus, *Maternal-Infant Bonding: The Impact of Early Separation or Loss on Family Development* (New York: Mosby, 1976), and Marshall Klaus and John Kennell, *Parent-Infant Bonding*, 2nd ed. (New York: Mosby-Yearbook, June 1981).

94. Elly Rakowitz, "ASPO: Birth and Growth of an Ideal," *Mother's Manual*, January–February 1978, 29–35, quotation on 32. But see Julia Kagan, "What Newborn Babies Need," *McCall's*, June 1978, 54–55, for the view that most hospitals still did not include the husbands.

95. "'Family-Centered' Birth Urged," *American Medical News*, August 4, 1978, 14. See also, for example, Errol G. Rampersad, "Expectant Fathers Join in 'Natural Births,'" *New York Times*, April 2, 1978, WC14.

96. Committee on Maternal Alternatives, "How Women Want to Have Their Babies: A Study of Consumers Attitudes on Maternal Health Care," Baltimore, ca. 1978, 1980, 39; typescript in the National Library of Medicine, Bethesda, Maryland, and the Library of Congress. More than 97 percent thought husbands should be there.

97. This and the next paragraph from Helen Gabel, "Childbirth Experiences of Unprepared Fathers," *Journal of Nurse-Midwifery* 27, no. 2 (March–April 1982): 5–8, quotations on 6 and 7.

98. Bing, *Adventure of Birth*, 10.

99. Gail H. Peterson, Lewis E. Mehl, and Herbert Leiderman, "The Role of Some Birth-Related Variables in Father Attachment," *American Journal of Orthopsychiatry* 49, no. 2 (April 1979): 330–38, quotation on 330.

100. Sheila M. Bowen and Brent C. Miller, "Paternal Attachment Behavior As Related to Presence at Delivery and Preparenthood Classes: A Pilot Study," *Nursing Research* 29, no. 5 (September–October 1980): 307–11, quotation on 307. See also Margaretha Rodholm, "Effects of Father-Infant Postpartum Contact on Their Interaction Three Months after Birth," *Early Human Development* 5 (1981): 79–85.

101. See, for example, Colette Jones, "Father to Infant Attachment: Effects of Early Contact and Characteristics of the Infant," *Research in Nursing and Health* 4 (1981): 193–200. But see also Antoinette S. Cordell, Ross D. Parke, and Douglas B. Sawin, "Fathers' Views on Fatherhood with Special Reference to Infancy," *Family Relations* 29 (1980):

331–38, which found that men who were already committed to greater participation with their children were the ones who sought out participation in delivery. See also H. K. Heggenhougen, "Father and Childbirth: An Anthropological Perspective," *Journal of Nurse-Midwifery* 25, no. 6 (November–December 1980): 21–26.

102. This was up from 32 percent of married women in the workforce in 1960 and 40 percent in 1970. Bruce A. Chadwick and Tina B. Heaton, *Statistical Handbook on the American Family*, 2nd ed. (Westport, Conn.: Oryx Press, 1999), 206, table G1-1. See also U.S. Census Bureau, *Statistical Abstract of the United States: 2007* (Washington, D.C.: Department of Commerce, October 2006), 379, table 583.

103. Sorvillo is quoted in Georgia Dullea, "Fatherhood: Expanding Role and Expanding Joys," *New York Times*, June 20, 1982, 52. The question of whether father-infant bonding was related to the men holding their newborns immediately after delivery is explored in Linnie Toney, "The Effects of Holding the Newborn at Delivery on Paternal Bonding," *Nursing Research* 32, no. 1 (January–February 1983): 16–19. For some fathers' concerns, see Stephanie MacLaughlin, "First-Time Fathers' Childbirth Experience," *Journal of Nurse-Midwifery* 25, no. 3 (May–June 1980): 17–21.

104. Dialogue from *Happy Days* taken from watching a tape of the episode, "Little Baby Cunningham," which first aired on ABC on November 3, 1981.

105. See, for example, Frederick C. Irving, "Ten Years of Cesarean Section at the Boston Lying-In Hospital," *American Journal of Obstetrics and Gynecology* 50, no. 6 (December 1945): 660–80, and Anthony D. D'Esoro, "A Review of Cesarean Section at Sloane Hospital for Women, 1942–1947," *American Journal of Obstetrics and Gynecology* 59, no. 1 (January 1950): 77–95. D'Esoro believed that African Americans had genetic differences that led to cephalo-pelvic disproportion; he did not mention higher rates of rickets that might have led to pelvic distortions. See also Robert Kistner, "An Analysis of Ten Years of Cesarean Section at the Cincinnati General Hospital," *American Journal of Obstetrics and Gynecology* 61, no. 1 (January 1951): 109–20; William Dieckmann, "The Place of Operative Obstetrics," *American Journal of Obstetrics and Gynecology* 69, no. 5 (May 1955): 1005–18; and Charlotte G. Borst, "Teaching Obstetrics at Home: Medical Schools and Home Delivery Services in the First Half of the Twentieth Century," *Bulletin of the History of Medicine* 72 (1998): 220–45. Borst noted that "normal presentations were sometimes converted to breech ones for the benefit of teaching interns" and that racial segregation affected access to and quality of care.

106. WMH, FB, June 1, 1953. See also September 7, 1953.

107. Ibid., December 15, 1953. See also December 1, 1961.

108. Ibid., October 8, 1949.

109. Ibid., April 2, 1954.

110. Ibid., November 18, 1963.

111. Bonds and Bonds, "Initiation into Parenthood," 78. See the description of the Bonds' labor experience in Chapter 5.

112. The parents and the physician are quoted in Olive Evans, "Caesarean: A Husband Plays a Role," *New York Times*, August 18, 1976, 65.

113. Woman quoted in Committee on Maternal Alternatives, "How Women Want to Have Their Babies," 146.

114. The two are quoted in Rita E. Watson, "Making a Cesarean a Birth," *New York Times*, March 6, 1977, 475.

115. "Father's Presence at C-Section 'No Safety Risk,'" *Obstetrics and Gynecology News*, July 1, 1977, 14.

116. Jill Smolowe, "Fathers Help Out in Delivering Cesarean Babies," *New York Times*, January 8, 1978, CN9.

117. "Delivery-Room Ban Is Upheld by Court," *American Medical News*, October 20, 1978, 25. The case was a Seventh Circuit Court decision, *Praetz v. Peterson*.

118. Barbara Mason to author, January 23, 2006, AQ, *OW*.

119. Jane Qualle to author, June 25, 2005, AQ, *OW*.

120. "MDs Urged to Change on Cesareans," *American Medical News*, October 10, 1980, 20. See also Jacqueline Rose Hott, "Best Laid Plans: Pre- and Postpartum Comparison of Self and Spouse in Primiparous Lamaze Couples Who Share Delivery and Those Who Do Not," *Nursing Research* 29, no. 1 (January–February 1980): 20–27.

121. Sheryl Thalman Body and Patricia Mahon, "The Family-Centered Cesarean Delivery," *American Journal of Maternal Child Nursing* 5 (1980): 176–80, quotation on 176.

122. *Praetz v. Peterson*, 577 F.2d 745 (7th Cr 1978). See a discussion of this decision in Kaunitz, "Point of Law," 18–19.

123. The physicians are quoted in Andrea Jolles, "Classes on Childbirth," *New York Times*, August 2, 1981, L116.

124. I am grateful to Martin Pernick for this suggestion about the possible hiding of medical errors. The quotation about throwing instruments is the closest to direct evidence to corroborate this possible motivation that I have found, but it is nonetheless plausible.

125. Cyndy Sandberg to author, July 14, 2005, AQ, *OW*.

126. See, for example, Sally C. Curtin and Lola Jean Kozak, "Decline in U.S. Cesarean Delivery Rate 'Appears to Stall,'" *Birth* 25, no. 4 (1998): 259–62.

127. Celeste R. Phillips and Joseph T. Anzalone, *Fathering: Participation in Labor and Birth*, 2nd ed. (St. Louis, Mo.: Mosby, 1982), see esp. 17 and 35–36. See also Linda Leonard and Lori Witherspoon, "And Father Makes Three . . . ," *Canadian Nurse*, March 1982, 38–41.

128. Marc Williams to author, June 14, 2005, AQ, *OW*. His wife had labored for twenty-four hours, during which time he had been with her.

129. "Fathers Attending Cesarean Births," *New York Times*, July 11, 1985, C1, C9, quotation on C9. In 2006, there was still some controversy about men's attendance at cesarean section deliveries. According to the *Women's Health News*, January 25, 2006,

"Fathers who are anxious during a caesarean operation may increase the pain experienced by the mother after the delivery of their baby." <http://www.news-medical.net/print_article.asp?id=15612> (February 16, 2006).

130. For legal cases on the issue, see George James Stephan and Barry D. Silbermann, "Father in Delivery Room Wins Decision That Could Land You in Court," *Legal Aspects of Medical Practice* 7, no. 7 (July 1979): 49–50. The case was *Austin v. The Regents of the University of California*. See also *Blackwell v. Oser*, 436 S. 2d 1293 (La. App. 4th Circuit 1983), and *Schram v. Herkimer Memorial Hospital*, 115 A.D.2nd 882, 496 N.Y.S.2nd 577. On fathers and cesarean sections, see, for example, G. H. Nolan, "Dads Now Attending at Cesareans," *Medical World News*, October 3, 1977, and D. Lush, "Description of Family Centered Cesarean Section by a Father," *C/SEC Newsletter* (Cesarean/Support, Education, and Concern of Boston) (Fall 1976): 3.

131. Freestanding birth centers grew during the 1970s, and by 1987 there were 240 in the United States. See Pamela S. Eakins, "Freestanding Birth Centers: Prospects and Problems," *Birth* 15, no. 1 (March 1988): 25–30, and Judith P. Rooks et al., "Outcomes of Care in Birth Centers," *New England Journal of Medicine* 321 (December 1989): 1801–11. Many couples chose to be in these centers because hospitals would not provide their specific labor and delivery wishes.

132. Patricia A. Huprich, "Assisting the Couple through a Lamaze Labor and Delivery," *American Journal of Maternal Child Nursing* (July–August 1977): 245–53, quotation on 251. See also Barbara E. Bishop, "Editorial: Paying Lip Service . . . ," *Maternal Child Nursing* 3, no. 1 (January–February 1978): 7.

133. See, for example, Charen Elsherif, Garnet McGrath, and Joyce Thies Smyrski, "Coaching the Coach," *Journal of Obstetric, Gynecologic, and Neonatal Nursing* (March–April 1979): 87–89.

134. William Kunst-Wilson and Linda Cronenwett, "Nursing Care for the Emerging Family: Promoting Parental Behavior," *Research in Nursing and Health* 4 (1981): 201–11, quotation on 202.

135. See, for example, Roy Hudenberg, *Planning the Community Hospital* (New York: McGraw-Hill, 1967), 110–23, section on maternity patient facilities.

136. Fred Steinhagen, whose wife delivered at Manchester Memorial Hospital in Manchester, Connecticut, quoted in Philip E. Sumner and Celeste R. Phillips, *Birthing Room: Concept and Reality* (St. Louis, Mo.: Mosby, 1981), 49. There is a helpful graph on 42. See also Roslyn Lindheim, "Birthing Centers and Hospices: Reclaiming Birth and Death," *Annual Reviews of Public Health* 2 (1981): 1–29, esp. 12–15.

137. Certified nurse-midwife Lois Olsen, who delivered 180 babies at the hospital between 1973 and 1976, to author, August 8, 2005, AQ, OW.

138. Michael L. Bahn, with assistance of Joan Dickson Gammell Bahn, to author, July 24, 2005, AQ, OW. After the delivery, with the newborn still fussy, they handed her to the seated (toddler) Elizabeth "and let her hold the precious bundle. Amazingly, Ericka

[newborn] calmed down and relaxed. It was amazing to watch Elizabeth make her first observations of her baby sister." In Phoenix, Arizona, a hospital allowed siblings, relatives, and friends to watch the delivery in new birthing suites that opened in 1976. See Athia Hardt, "In Phoenix Hospital, Birthing Room Offers Home-Style Delivery," *New York Times*, July 12, 1977, 30. See also a description of a home birth with children attending: "Unity, Growth, 'Respectability' Highlight Home Birth," *American Medical News*, June 23, 1978, 16–18.

139. See, for example, "A Better Way," *American Medical News*, March 13, 1978, 5.

140. Woman is quoted in Committee on Maternal Alternatives, "How Women Want to Have Their Babies," 131.

141. Woman quoted in ibid., 163.

142. Judith Schmidt, "The First Year at Stanford's University's Family Birth Room," *Birth and the Family Journal* 7, no. 3 (Fall 1980): 169–74, quotation on 169.

143. Judith A. Maloni, "The Birthing Room: Some Insights into Parents' Experiences," *American Journal of Maternal Child Nursing* 5 (September–October 1980): 314–19, quotations on 318.

144. Robert A. Block, "We've Let 1,500 Fathers Deliver Their Own Babies," *Medical Economics*, August 9, 1982, 181, 189, 193, 197, quotations on 181, 197.

145. Leah Yarrow, "Fathers Who Deliver," *Parents Magazine*, June 1981 62–66, quotation on 63.

146. Elin McCoy, "Birthing Rooms: Maternity Care's Newest Option," *New York Times*, May 1, 1980, C1 and C4. They were not yet, in the 1980s, available in all hospitals.

147. Patrizia Romito, "The Humanizing of Childbirth: The Response of Medical Institutions to Women's Demand for Change," *Midwifery* 2, no. 3 (1986): 135–40. Romito concluded that including the men occurred because of wide consumer demands and did not challenge traditional medical hierarchies.

148. See, for example, Shu, "Husband-Father in Delivery Room?"

149. Herman L. Allen, "Fathers in the Delivery Rooms — Survey Results of Anesthesia Departments," *Anesthesiology* 59 (1983): 152. See also Elmar P. Sakala and Richard A. Henry, "Fathers in the Cesarean Section Room and Maternal/Neonatal Outcomes," *Journal of Perinatology* 8, no. 4 (Fall 1988): 342–46.

150. American College of Obstetricians and Gynecologists, *Manual of Standards for Obstetric-Gynecologic Services* (Washington, D.C.: American College of Obstetricians and Gynecologists, 1985), 37; copies are available at the National Library of Medicine, Bethesda, Maryland, and the library of the American College of Obstetricians and Gynecologists, Washington, D.C.

151. *Karen E. Whitman and Edward T. Coch v. Mercy-Memorial Hospital v. Department of Civil Rights, Intervenor*, 128 Mich. App. 155, 339 N.W. 2d 730. On this case, see also "Delivery Room 'Husband Only' Rule Found to Discriminate against Unmarried," *Hospital Progress* 65, no. 3 (March 1984): 66–67.

152. "Fathers Attending Cesarean Births," C1.

153. Gary Cunningham, Paul MacDonald, and Norman Gant, *Williams Obstetrics*, 18th ed. (Norwalk, Conn.: Appleton and Lange, 1989), 328.

Epilogue

1. On lesbian and gay couples, who have not been the particular subject of this book, see, for example, David Usborne, "Gay with Children," *New York Magazine*, November 3, 2003, 28–33, 44, and Gina Kolata, "Lesbian Partners Find the Means to Be Parents," *New York Times*, June 30, 1989, A13. See also Nancy A. Naples, "Queer Parenting in the New Millennium," *Gender and Society* 18, no. 6 (2004): 679–84; Susan E. Buchholtz, "Experiences of Lesbian Couples during Childbirth," *Nursing Outlook* 48, no. 6 (November 2000): 307–11; Boston Women's Health Book Collective, *Our Bodies Ourselves: Pregnancy and Birth* (New York: Simon and Schuster, 2008); and "Gay Dads and a Life of Surprising Turns," GAYTWOGETHER <http://gaytwogether.typepad.com/> (accessed March 31, 2008).

2. Jodi Kantor, "Move Over, Doc, the Guests Can't See the Baby," *New York Times*, September 11, 2005, A10.

3. Cynthia Haq, M.D., to author, November 6, 2006, quoted with permission.

4. Private parent to Prudie, *Wisconsin State Journal* (Madison), January 10, 2005. My thanks to Susan Friedman for alerting me to this column.

5. Riverview Hospital in Noblesville, Indiana, renamed its fathers' waiting room "Dad's Retreat Room." See Steven Furlow, "Taking Baby Steps in Education," *Noblesville Daily Times*, September 24, 2007.

6. See, for example, "Boot Camp for New Dads," started in 1990 by Greg Bishop and going strong in 2005. See Greg Bishop, *Hit the Ground Crawling: The Essential Guide for New Fathers* (Irvine, Calif.: Dad's Adventure, 2005). See also the group's Web site, <www.newdads.com>. Classes associated with this movement are held at various hospitals around the country; see, for example, on Saturday morning classes at Meriter Hospital in Madison, Wisconsin, Rick Larson, "A Boot Camp Approach Can Arm New Dads with Basic Baby Training," *Wisconsin State Journal* (Madison), November 20, 2005, I1.

7. Of course, as this is written, we still have a long way to go to reach equality in this regard. But the period covered in this book began to see some changes as hospitals integrated racially and as some basic practices were incorporated into some public hospitals. Those hospitals that served middle-class African Americans incorporated these practices much earlier than did public hospitals serving poor blacks and whites.

8. Philip Taubman, "Doubts in the Delivery Room," *New York Times*, October 1984, SM72.

9. Elisabeth D. Bing, "Letter to the Editor," *New York Times*, November 25, 1984, SM 134.

10. Stephen Harrigan, "It's a . . . Father!" *Reader's Digest*, March 1979, 9–14, quotations on 10, 12–13, 14.

11. Richard K. Reed, *Birthing Fathers: The Transformation of Men in American Rites of Birth* (New Brunswick, N.J.: Rutgers University Press, 2005), 23.

12. Ibid., 134 (emphasis in original).

13. Ibid., 31.

14. Ibid., 195, 207.

15. <http://mrdad.com/qa/expectant/excluded-by-ob.html> (accessed September 27, 2005). See also Armin Brott, *The Expectant Father: Facts, Tips and Advice for Dads-to-Be* (New York: Abbeville Press, 2001). A childbirth educator from Fond du Lac, Wisconsin, agrees and said that in her classes, "we don't want dads to be coaches, instead we teach them to be fathers." See Sharon Roznik, "Birthing Moms Find New Methods of Pain Relief," *Fond du Lac Reporter*, April 16, 2008. See also "Your Role as an Expectant Father," InfoMean Blog, <http://blog.infomean.com/your-role-as-an-expectant-father/> and also <http://www.thefunkystork.com> (accessed September 1, 2007).

16. Reed, *Birthing Fathers*, 12.

17. Jessica Weiss, "A Drop-In Catering Job: Middle Class Women and Fatherhood, 1950–1980," *Journal of Family History* 24, no. 3 (July 1999): 374–90, quotations on 382.

18. Rosemary Mander, *Men and Maternity* (London: Routledge, 2004), 82.

19. Ibid., 85.

20. Keith Ablow, "A Perilous Journey from Delivery Room to Bedroom," *New York Times*, August 23, 2005, D5.

21. Elizabeth Lebid, Yorktown Heights, New York; Lisa Phillips Mead, Woodstock, New York; and Richard Reed, San Antonio, Texas, letters to the editor, *New York Times*, August 30, 2005, D6. Richard Reed noted that most men find attending delivery to be rewarding, but he repeated the point he had made elsewhere, that "the experience is traumatic for some and that American medicine exacerbates the problem. . . . American dads benefit from sharing this life-changing experience with mothers, but both need support and reassurance though the process."

22. Alison Rubin, Guilford, Connecticut, letter to the editor, *New York Times*, September 6, 2005, D2.

23. Meghan O'Rourke, "It's a Jerk!" *Slate*, <http://www.slate.com/id/2125227/> (accessed August 31, 2005). My thanks to Marnie R. Leavitt and David I. Leavitt for this link.

24. See, for example, Ann Althouse, who posted thirty-nine comments to her post, <http://althouse.blogspot.com> (accessed August 30, 2005). My thanks to Lewis A. Leavitt for this link. See also John & Belle, <http://examinedlife.typepad.com/johnbelle/

2005/08/would_it_hurt_if I_called_you . . . >, August 23, 2005 (accessed September 5, 2005), and Crookedtimber, <http://crookedtimber.org/2005/08/23/childbirth-porn/> (accessed September 5, 2005).

25. Mander, *Men and Maternity*, 94–95, and Michel Odent, "Is the Participation of the Father at Birth Dangerous?" *Midwifery Today* (Autumn 1999): 23–24, quotations on 23, 24.

26. Odent was interviewed on "Head to Head: Fathers and Childbirth," *BBC News*, January 17, 2000, <http://news.bbc.co.uk/1/hi/health/607005.stm> (accessed May 25, 2004). See also, for example, Anthea Rowan, "Should Dads Be in the Delivery Room?" *FairLady Magazine*, May 2008, which quotes Odent saying his views have been consistent over time: "I am convinced that one of the main reasons for long and difficult births is the participation of the father." He repeated his belief that a couple's sexual relationship would be adversely affected. See also Murray Enkin et al., *A Guide to Effective Care in Pregnancy and Childbirth* (Oxford: Oxford Medical Publications, 2000), and Henci Goer and Rhonda Wheeler, *The Thinking Woman's Guide to a Better Birth* (New York: Perigee Trade, 1999). A "cascade of interventions" may start when birthing women are anxious, beginning with the use of an electronic fetal heart monitor, which precludes moving around and can itself lead to a diminution of labor. Then birth attendants might feel it necessary artificially to rupture the membranes to get labor to progress or use Pitocin to increase contractions, which can lead to more pain and discomfort for the woman. That, in turn, might necessitate increasing pain medication or anesthesia, which might affect fetal heart rate patterns, and ultimately lead to the use of forceps or the vacuum extractor, or even to cesarean section. Epidurals, which have increased significantly in the past fifteen years, have been shown to lengthen the time of labor. See Ellice Lieberman and Carol O'Donoghue, "Unintended Effects of Epidural Anesthesia during Labor: A Systematic Review: The Nature and Management of Labor Pain," *American Journal of Obstetrics and Gynecology* 186, no. 5 (May 2002), supplement: S31–S68; James Alexander et al., "The Course of Labor with and without Epidural Analgesia," *American Journal of Obstetrics and Gynecology* 178, no. 3 (March 1998): 516–20; and Sigrid Johnson and JoAnn Rosenfeld, "The Effect of Epidural Anesthesia on the Length of Labor," *Obstetrics and Gynecological Survey* 50, no. 11 (November 1995): 770–71.

27. "Dads in the Delivery Room," *Dr. Phil*, January 28, 2004, <www.drphil.com/advice/advice.jhtml?contentld=par_raising_dadsdeliveryroom.xml&section=Parenting&subsection=Raising%20kids> (accessed January 29, 2004). My thanks to Sarah A. Leavitt for this link.

28. Doulas' history has not been systematically followed in this book, but these laywomen birth attendants have been very important in changing hospital practices in recent years. See, for example, Amy Gilliland, "Beyond Holding Hands: The Modern Role of the Professional Doula," *Journal of Obstetric, Gynecologic, and Neonatal Nursing* 31 (2002): 547–54.

29. For example, see Ruma Kumar, "'Camp' Shows Dads the Rope," *Baltimore Sun*, March 12, 2008, about a "Boot Camp for New Dads" offered once a month at the Annapolis Hospital, at a cost of fifty dollars.

30. Joyce is quoted and photographed in James Estrin, "Lens," *New York Times*, October 19, 2005, B2.

31. On nurses' tensions between their obligations to physicians and their connection to women, which was not examined in this book, see Judith Walzer Leavitt, "'Strange Young Women on Errands': Obstetric Nursing between Two Worlds," *Nursing History Review* 6 (1998): 3–24.

ACKNOWLEDGMENTS

I could not have written this book without the help of a lot of people, many of whom I do not know. I am very grateful to all those who shared their birth stories with me and who got excited when they heard about this project and encouraged me to write this book. When I first presented this material to the American Association of the History of Medicine, men came forward with their own personal birth stories and commentary; this outpouring of interest and help prompted me to continue to pursue the men's side of the story. I appreciate all the eager cooperation of the hundreds of people, men and women, who took the time to communicate with me.

My mother, Sally H. Walzer, whose accounts of her harrowing taxicab ride while in labor with me during my premature arrival, first sparked my interest in this subject. Two of her childbirth stories (one real, one not) that I heard repeatedly as I was growing up are included in this book. My father, Joseph P. Walzer, who was sent home to await his children's arrivals, did not get to witness birth itself but modeled men's connections to their families and helped me understand "masculine domesticity" in the mid-twentieth-century period. My husband, Lewis A. Leavitt, partner extraordinaire, provided encouragement and support at each step in the lives of our two children, including attending their deliveries, and in the development of this project. To all my family members I owe my greatest thanks for support and encouragement over the years.

Susan Sacharski, the archivist at Northwestern Memorial Hospital Archives in Chicago, deserves special thanks. She opened the door for me to use the hospital's fathers' books and first led me to this subject. I received financial support from the University of Wisconsin Foundation, the University of Wisconsin Rupple Bascom Chair Professorship, and the Women's Studies Feminist Scholar Fellowship.

Many researchers, during their graduate-student years, helped the project along. I am grateful for the efforts of Katie Benton, Bridget Collins, Hilary Domush, Elizabeth Evans, David Herzberg, Judy Kaplan, Abigail Markwyn, David Meshoulam, Camilo Quinteros, Kendra Smith-Howard, and Karen Walloch. Other friends and colleagues gave generously of their time—and kept their eyes out for birth accounts. I am happy to thank those who added important contributions: Rima Apple, Beth Black, Charlotte Borst, Jay Chervenak, David Courtwright, Susan Davidson, Robert Domush, Sandra Eiseman, Laura Ettinger, Jessica Feierman, Susan Friedman, Vanessa Northington Gamble, Linda Gordon, David I. Leavitt, Lewis A. Leavitt, Marnie R. Leavitt, Sarah A. Leavitt, Gerda Lerner, Russell F. Lewis, James Lindblade, Kari Niedermaier, Ronald Numbers, Ann Peckham, Rebecca Jo Plant, Leslie Reagan, Naomi Rogers, Gloria Sarto, Susan Smith, Micaela Sullivan-Fowler, Andrea Tone, and Jackie Wolf. I appreciate the collegiality and insights provided by the faculty members in the Departments of Medical History and Bioethics, History of Science, and Gender and Women's Studies at the University of Wisconsin. I am grateful for the help of the staff in the Medical History and Bioethics Department led by the cheerful assistance of Jean von Allmen and including Lorraine Rondon and Sharon Russ. I acknowledge the University of Wisconsin Institutional Review Board for its evaluation of my project and its granting of exemption status. Joan Mathys, of MJM Picture and Film Research in Washington, D.C., took over the job of securing permission rights for the illustrations, and I am extremely grateful for all her efforts.

A particular thanks is due to the hundreds of men and women who answered my call for birth experiences in the New York Times Sunday Book Review section, the New York Review of Books, On Wisconsin, and the Washington Post. These personal stories, many of which are quoted in this book, added depth and breadth to my understanding of laymen's activities in American hospital waiting, labor, and delivery rooms. The respondents generously offered their accounts in a spirit of cooperation and support for the project that spurred me on; at the same time it let me know that there were other people who felt as passionately as I do about the significance of childbirth.

Parts of this book previously appeared in print. I am grateful for permission to reprint a significant portion of Chapter 1, which appeared as "The Medicalization of Childbirth in the Twentieth Century," Transactions and Studies of the College of Physicians of Philadelphia, ser. 5, 11, no. 4 (December 1989): 299–319. Portions of the Introduction and chapters 2, 3, 5, and 6 appeared as "What Do Men Have to Do with It? Fathers and Mid-Twentieth Century Childbirth," Bulletin of the History of Medicine 77, no. 2 (2003):

235–62, © The Johns Hopkins University Press, reprinted with permission of the Johns Hopkins University Press. Finally, I am grateful to the University of North Carolina Press for its enthusiasm and work on this project. Sian Hunter first encouraged me to make my initial project into a book. Kate Douglas Torrey has been a perceptive and encouraging critic as she guided the text to completion. The readers of the manuscript offered extremely helpful suggestions for revisions.

INDEX

Note: Page numbers in italics refer to illustrations.

Ablow, Keith, 292
African Americans, 12, 16–17, 32, 65, 66, 97, 176–78, 204, 234, 235, 258–59, 261–62, 267
Ainsworth, Reverend John Lawrence, 94
Alabama, 12
Aldridge, Dr. Charles, 218
Allen, Steve, 59, 61–62
All in the Family (television show), 236–38, *237*
Alta Bates Community Hospital (Berkeley, Calif.), 228
Ambrose, Stephen, 101
Ambrose, Dr. Thomas, 101
American Association of Psychiatry, 266
American Baby (magazine), 165, 190

American College of Nurse Midwives, 266
American College of Obstetricians and Gynecologists (ACOG), 91, 220, 266; manual of standards, 133, 282; support for shared labor, 171
American College of Surgeons, 221
American Hospital Association, 8, 44, 134–35, 266
American Journal of Obstetrics and Gynecology, 131, 220
American Magazine, 121
American Medical News, 180–81
American Nursing Association, 266
American Red Cross, 140
American Society for Psychoprophylaxis

in Obstetrics (ASPO), 150, 238, 295; Bay Area Chapter, 146; origin, 162

Anesthesia, 25, 30, 36–37, 39, 99, 105, 130, 188; caudal, 103, 117, 198, 208, 212, 226, 243; epidural, 90

Anesthesiologists, 281–82

Antibiotics, 34

Anzalone, Joseph, 192

Arkansas, 111

Arms, Suzanne, 250

Army of Expectant Fathers (Genne), 168–70, 210

Arnaz, Desi, 1–7, 19

Atomic bomb, x, 47, 68

Ave Maria Press, 114

Bacteriology, 26–28; fear of infection from father, 83–84, 94–95, 201, 217–18, 254; fear of infections in delivery room, 93, 196, 217–18; understanding of germ transmission in 19th century, 26

Bahn, Michael and Joan, 277–78

Baker, Dr., 225

Baker, Russell, 59

Ball, Lucille, 1–7

Baltimore, 159, 266

Bang, Ensign and Mrs., 121–22

Barnes, Allan, 220

Barnes, Charles and Jean, 106

Barney, Steve, 81, 234

Barter, Dr. Robert H., 181–82

Baxandall, Rosalyn, 248

Bayly, Dr. Melvyn, 270

Beardsley, E. H., 157

Beaver Dam Hospital (Beaver Dam, Wis.), 274

Beck, Joan, 146, 254

Bellin Methodist Hospital (Green Bay, Wis.), 219

Benaron, Dr. Harry, 73, 270

Berkeley Night School, 146

Berlin Hospital (Waushara County, Wis.), 93

Berndt, Alvin, 240–42

Bernheim, Mark, 263

Best, Brian, 179

Beth David Hospital (New York City), 96, 196

Better Homes and Gardens (magazine), 110, 129

Betts, Dr., 214

Bing, Elizabeth, 162, 164, 171, 232, 268, 288

Birth experience. See Childbirth; Fathers; Women

Birthing rooms, 10–11, 275–83, 277, 280, 282; physicians' resistance to, 278

Birth plans, 21

Black masculinity, 16

Blasing, T. J. and Carolyn, 144

Block, Robert, 279–80

Bloodletting, 24–25, 30

Board of Commissioners of North Broward Hospital District (Broward County, Calif.), 250

Bonds, Charlotte and Ozell, 176–77, 258–59, 271

Booth Memorial (Cleveland, Ohio), 276

Boston Lying-In Hospital, 46, 85

Bradburn, Dr. G. B., 70, 73

Bradley, Robert, 100, 142, 182, 200, 201, 217–18, 228, 231; influenced by Dick-Read, 201

Bradley method: increasing popularity of, 200; in labor and delivery, 191; in prenatal classes, 100, 142, 144

Brandt, Allan, 59

Brew, Dr. Barbara, 217

Brooklyn Jewish Hospital, 197

Brown, Oscar, Jr., 234–35

Browne, Peter, 170, 211

Bryn Mawr Hospital (Bryn Mawr, Pa.), 246

Buckley, Dr. Daniel J., Jr., 181

Bureau of Maternal and Child Health (Wisconsin), 123

Byrd, William, 22

California, 93, 117, 145, 146, 150, 174, 188, 207, 223; Berkeley, 228; Broward County, 250; Los Angeles, 41; Sacramento, 244; San Luis Obispo, 124–25, 229, 230, 238, 239

Cameras. *See* Fathers: photographing childbirth

Cameron, Dr. Daniel, 24

Carmon, Mabel, 89, 115

Cates, Ethel, 104

CBS (Columbia Broadcasting System), 1

Cesarean sections, 30, 90, 150, 226, 270–75; in fathers' books, 270; Lucille Ball's, 7; rates of, 274

Chabon, Irwin, 145

Charles, Allan, 251

Cherry, Mildred, 197

Chicago, 12, 154, 174

Chicago Board of Health, 196, 251–52

Chicago Lying-In Hospital, 50, 54, 66, 124, 140, 158

Chicago Maternity Center, 66, 197

Chicago Tribune, 146, 254

Childbirth, 8–9; in 18th century, 22–24, 156; in 19th century, 23–27; in early 20th century, 32–47; in 1940s, 48–59, 62–64, 74, 80–81, 83, 89, 101, 103–6, 196–200; in 1950s, 59–62, 64–74, 75–78, 79–81, 87–100, 102–3, 106–19, 121–22, 124–34, 139–41, 161–62, 166–73, 197, 200–202, 206–15; in 1960s, 67, 78–79, 84–85, 141–45, 146, 158, 164–65, 173–74, 183–86, 201, 215, 216–35; in 1970s, 134–37, 145–55, 159–61, 174–79, 180–83, 186–91, 236–68, 270–81; in 1980s, 191–94, 268–70, 281–83; in 2000s, 285, 294; complications in, 30, 196; fathers' experience of in 1940s and 1950s, 196–202; fear of, 24–25, 27, 37; health professionals' response to shared labor, 179–86; home births, 22–23, 39; hospital-based, xi, 8–14, 21, 32–47, 222; increasing popularity of shared labor, 164; intimacy during, 11, 170–73, 192; loneliness during, 34, 37–38, 44–47, 63–64, 95, 137, 159, 166; men's participation in, xi, 22; moves to hospital, 27–34; negative male experience of, 193, 260; physician-assisted home births, 23–27; positive male experience of, 165, 171, 206–7, 227, 231–32, 234–35, 240–43, 255; privacy during, 88, 95, 205, 223; privilege in, 11–13; psychological aspects of, 38–39, 46, 137–38, 153, 164–71, 187, 254; statistics on, 8, 187; traditional histories of, 7–8; transition stage in, 225–26, 276; undesired medication during, 99; unmedicated, 161; women's preference for husbands' presence during, 45–46, 93, 99, 159, 166–67, 170, 173–75, 196–97, 250–51. *See also* Hospitals; Medicalization of childbirth; Natural childbirth

Childbirth Education Association (Wisconsin), 143

Childbirth reform movement, 13; accommodation of medical authority, 17, 287; beginnings of, 98–100; overlap with women's movement, 17. *See also*

Bradley method; Dick-Read method; Lamaze method; Natural childbirth

Childbirth without Fear (Dick-Read), 70, 100, 102, 104, 114, 128, 166, 199

Children's Clinic (Black Mountain, N.C.), 228

Chung, Dr. J. T., 73, 89

Cigarettes. *See* Smoking

Cigars. *See* Smoking

Civil Rights Act (1964), 12, 157

Clarice, Sister M., 229

Clark, Dale, 49, 64, 74, 79, 87, 97, 100, 160

Clark, Tom, 239–40, 244

Class, socioeconomic, 86, 88, 109, 128, 131, 146, 156–57, 265–67, 282, 287; effect on childbirth options, 11–13, 96–97, 157, 160, 205, 266–67; white middle-class ideal, 15

Classes, prenatal. *See* Prenatal classes

Coats, Bimbetta, 101

Cold War, xi, 47, 69, 79, 121

Cole, Nat King, 75, 76

Colorado, 159, 217, 229, 232, 250

Columbia Hospital (Milwaukee, Wis.), 132, 158

Columbia Presbyterian Hospital (New York City), 63, 116, 283

Columbia University, 274

Columbus Community Hospital (Columbus, Wis.), 242

Committee on Maternal Alternatives (Baltimore), 159

Community Hospital (Boulder, Colo.), 159, 250

Connecticut, 81, 104, 106, 228, 248, 272, 276

Consent forms, 253

Cook County Hospital (Chicago), 12, 66, 97

Cooley, Chester L., 118

Coontz, Stephanie, 15

Corbin, Hazel, 108–9, 111, 113, 122–23, 128, 163, 185, 205

Cornell University Medical College, 101, 224

Cosby, Bill, xi

Cosby Show, The (television show), 17

Cosmopolitan (magazine), 80, 139, 208

Crabtree, Walden, 227

Crouse-Irving Hospital (Syracuse, N.Y.), 95

Crowly, Michael and Michele, 252

Daniel Freeman Hospital (Los Angeles, Calif.), 41

Davis, Dr. M. Edward, 115

Davis-Floyd, Robbie, 39, 43

Decision making, 13–14, 99–100; in birthing room, 279; conflict over, 179–82; conflicts between father and physician, 188–89; by father and physician, 89–91, 177, 246, 270; female, 22–25; giving up, 32, 34, 37, 74; by medical personnel, 73–74, 91, 179–80

DeGarmo, Eileen, 265

Delaware, 234

DeLee, Dr. Joseph, 38, 50, 55, 66, 89, 115

Delivery rooms, 10–11, 14, 93, 95, 195–235, 202, 240; description of, 202–5; early example of husbands in, 196–202; fathers barred from, 202, 209–10; policies barring visitors from, 195–96, 199, 204–5, 207–8, 210; promotion of fathers' presence in, 211–13; statistics on fathers' presence in, 232; visitors in, 284–85; women opposed to men's presence in, 197

Demerol, 36

Deutscher, Max, 254

DeVault, Spencer, 52

Dewees, William Potts, 25

Dick-Read, Grantly, 70, 98, 100–102, 130, 182, 199, 212; influence on Bradley, 201; visit to United States, 100, 129, 200. See also *Childbirth without Fear*

Dick-Read method, 100; growth in United States, 129–30; in labor and delivery, 100–104, 108–11, 114, 117, 119, 126, 129, 147, 158, 161, 166, 191; physician support for, 117–18; popularity of, 200–202; in prenatal classes, 128–32, 140–42, 147, 162, 164. *See also* Grace–New Haven Hospital; Natural childbirth; Physicians

Dilks, Dr. Robert, 280

Doctor's Hospital (New York City), 164

Dorr, Dr., 71

Douglas, Peter, 80–81, 106–8, 200

Doulas, 293

Downs, Dr. David R., 227–28

Eau Claire (Wis.) Leader-Telegram, 262

Ebony (magazine), 140

Education, prenatal. *See* Prenatal classes

Egan, Katherine, 46, 62, 99

Eiseman, Sandra, 143, 242

Eisenhower, Dwight D., 7

Episiotomy, 39, 42–43, 141, 226, 233, 246

Epperson, Lee, 255

Equipment, 31, 202, *203*, 239, *241*, 276

Esquire (magazine), 49, 56, 87, 95, 256

Essence (magazine), 176–78, 258, 261–62

Ethnicity, 124; in *I Love Lucy*, 4–6; immigrants, 65–66

Ettinger, Laura E., 123

Fainting. *See* Fathers: fainting in delivery room; Fathers: fainting in prenatal classes

Fairmont Hospital clinics (Bay Area, Calif.), 146

Families: anxiety about, 18; changes within, xi, 14–19; strengthened by shared birth experience, 112–19, 137, 229

Family-centered childbirth, 74, 152, 275, 277; beginnings of, 162–63; film promoting, 163

Family Hospital (Milwaukee, Wis.), 277

Fatherhood, 6, 18–19, 47; impending, 3, 68–69; postwar ambiguity over, 18; and war experience, 138–39

Fathering (handbook), 192

Fathers: ambivalence toward natural childbirth, 186–91, 258, 264; anxiety during labor, 141, 153, 189–91; and back rubbing, 112–15; bonding with children, 79, 259, 267–69; changing advice in obstetrics textbooks regarding, 115; clergy as, 219; delivering their own children, 279–80, *281*; dissatisfaction with peripheral role in delivery, 263–64; effect on labor, 260–61; fainting in delivery room, 208, 227, 240, 244, 246, 260; fainting in prenatal classes, 78, 191; gender role expectations, 75–77, 140; ignored by historians, ix–x; photographing childbirth, 206, 265, *280*; physicians as, 95, 199; preference for baby's sex, 3, 74–75, 76, 78; preference for birthing room, 276–78; preference for waiting room, 81; pressured to attend mother, 291–92; psychological effects of birth on, 159–60, 187, 267, 292; reaction to exclusion from delivery room, 200; response to wives' pain, 89–90, 170, 291; ridiculed, 7, 48, 50–51, 59–62, 68; role in childbirth in 18th century,

22–23; role in labor and delivery, 104, 150, 169, 189–91, 286–87; space in defining role, 9–11; support for medication, 89, 170; variety of experiences of shared labor, 192. *See also* Male bonding

Fathers' books, 64–79, 96–98; concern for wives' and babies' health and safety, 69, 71–72; faith in, 69–71; grief in, 71; humor in, 67; military metaphors in, 77; poetry in, 67, 71; praise for doctors in, 72–73, 207; sports metaphors in, 77. *See also* Wesley Memorial Hospital

Father's Day, xi, 251

Father's Little Dividend (film), 112

Fathers Magazine, xi

Fathers' Rooms. *See* Waiting rooms

Feminism. *See* Women's movement

Fetal monitors, 39, 41–42

First International Childbirth Conference, 248

Fishbein, Dr. Morris, 25

Fiske, John, 6

Fitzgerald, Evelyn and Bruce, 252–53

Fitzgerald v. Porter Memorial Hospital (1975), 252–53, 273, 280

Fitzhugh, Mabel, 114, 137

Florentine, Sister, 111

Fonda, Henry, 59, 61–62

Forceps, 24–25, 30, 36, 37, 39, 226, 259

Fourteenth Amendment, 12

Fowler, Carol, 143

Fowler, Mary Louise, 22–23

Fox, Jim, 144, 258

Frank, Shirley Tighe, 148

Franklin, Dr. John B., 181

French Hospital (San Francisco), 139, 183, 239

Friedan, Betty, 16, 166, 209

Friedman, Dr. Emanuel, 43

Friends (television show), 285

Gabel, Helen, 267

Galton, Lawrence, 129–30

Gamper, Margaret, 247

Gender roles, 2, 15, 18, 23; fathers' expectations for children, 75–77; reinforced by Dick-Read method, 100; during shared labor, 164–65. *See also* Masculinity

Genesee Hospital (Rochester, N.Y.), 91, 111

Genne, William, 91, 140–41, 168–70, 210. See also *Army of Expectant Fathers*

Georgetown Hospital (Washington, D.C.), 222

George Washington University, 181

Georgia, 173

Gerber, Dr. William G., 181

Germ theory. *See* Bacteriology

Gerver, Joan, 196

Glixon, Helen, 116

Goetsch, Carl, 223

Goldfarb, Robert and Muriel, 160, 171, 211–12

Good Housekeeping (magazine), 109, 124

Goodman, Ron, 165

Goodwin, Dr. Peter A., 181

Gordon, Linda, 248

Gould, John, 56–57

Grace–New Haven Hospital (New Haven, Conn.), 64, 80, 104, 106, 107, 108, 125, 128, 130, 139, 200, 228; promotion of Dick-Read method, 104–8

Graham, Harvey, 129

Grail (magazine), 113

Grant, Mary Ann, 105

Great Depression, 47

Griffiths, Martha Wright, 17, 236, 248

Gross, Barry and Merle, 174, 251

Gruener, David, 53, 77

Guinn, Dr. J. H., 26

Gunderson, Ann, 217

Happy Days (television show), 135–37, 269–70, *269*

Haq, Dr. Cynthia, 285

Harpers (magazine), 220

Harrigan, Stephen, 288–89

Harris, Julie and Manning, 166, 209–10

Harrison, Barbara Grizzuti, 256–57, *258*

Harvard University, 259

Hawaii, 140

Hempstead Hospital (Long Island), 94, 215

Hickey, Margaret, 208

Hidden Persuaders, The (Packard), 80, 121

Higdon, Hal, 143

Hill-Burton Act (1946), 12, 157

Hoag, Dr. Roger, 215, 219

Holy Cross Hospital (Silver Spring, Md.), 78

Holy Family Hospital (Manitowoc, Wis.), 260

Home births. *See* Childbirth: home births

Horace Harding Hospital (New York City), 133

Hospitals: changing policies, 94, 178–79, 205–7, 229–34; economic reasons for allowing fathers in delivery room, 242; flexible policies, 93–94, 98; funding, 11, 12, 31–32; and geography, 43–44, 52–54, 83–84, 157, 159–61; growth of, 31–34, 97; policies, 84–85, 88–89, 92–98, 102; prep room, 44; private, 10; private rooms in, 86, 158, 162; regional variations in policies, 178–79, 197, 243; regulations, 207, 215, 220–21, 229–32, 236, 248, 251, 252–53; religious, 113–14; rural, 11, 32, 42, 57, 94, 98; sources of power within, 10; spaces within, 10–11; urban, 11, 32–34. *See also* Birthing rooms; Delivery rooms; Labor rooms; Segregation

Hospital Topics, 222

Hott, Jacqueline Rose, 264

House of Representatives Bill 1504 (1973), 17, 248, *249*

Hulit, Dr. Bob E., 252

Hulit v. St. Vincent's Hospital (1974), 252

Husband-Coached Childbirth (Bradley), 142, 201

Husbands' Room. *See* Waiting rooms

Hydrogen bomb, 47

Idaho, 70, 98, 257

Illinois, 53, 88, 95, 96, 97, 98, 181, 251–52, 254

Illinois Hospital Licensing Act (1967), 230

I Love Lucy (television show), 1–7, 59, 112; "Labor Pains," 3; "Lucy Goes to the Hospital," 4, 18

Immaculate Deception (Arms), 250

Indiana, 39, 221, 252, 253

Induction, 35, 39, 41, 73–74

Infant mortality, 71–72

Infection: postpartum, 32, 83–84, 92

International and Fourth American Congress on Obstetrics and Gynecology, 202

International Childbirth Education Association (ICEA), 134, 141–42, 178, 227–30, 295; founding of, 163; reports, 228–30, 242–43

Interventions, 24–25, 30; surgical, 30–31. *See also* Cesarean sections; Episiotomy; Forceps; Induction

Iowa, 98
Israel Zion Hospital (New York City), 95

Javert, Dr. Carl, 106, 196
Jet (magazine), 235
Johns Hopkins University, 101
Johnson, Howard, 78–79, 81
Johnson, Rich and Wendy, 150
Joyce, James, 294
Justus v. Atchison (1977), 251

Kaiser Foundation Hospital (Oakland, Calif.), 239
Kaiser–Walnut Creek (San Francisco), 205
Kansas, 26, 77
Kansas State University, 77
Karmel, Marjorie, 161–62. See also Thank You, Dr. Lamaze
Kartchner, Fred, 212
Kavanau, Jane, 231
Keim, John O., 220–21
Klingenstein Maternity Pavilion (New York City), 134
Knudson, Joan, 216
Koch, Dr. Robert, 28
Kohler, Alice Young, 140
Korean conflict, x
Korte, Diana, 159, 250
Kosmak, George W., 131

Labor rooms, 9–11, 86–87, 89, 91, 93, 95–96, 103, 108, 155–94; described, 160–61; in I Love Lucy, 4; placement of, 160–61; presence of television in, 189; private, 205; reverse visiting, 58, 102, 116; separate access, 84; shared, 11, 171; temporary visiting, 57, 88, 96–97, 174

Ladies' Home Journal (magazine), 39, 44, 80, 109, 134, 158, 170–71, 208, 211, 212
Lakeland Hospital (Elkhorn, Wis.), 101, 253
La Leche League, 159, 250–51
Lamaze, Fernand, 100, 142, 161, 182, 200
Lamaze International. See American Society for Psychoprophylaxis in Obstetrics
Lamaze method: cited in Fitzgerald v. Porter Memorial Hospital, 253; defined, 142; increasing popularity of, 200; in labor and delivery, 153–54, 161–62, 165, 185, 191, 243; in prenatal classes, 100, 131, 143, 145–46, 150, 153–54, 162, 164, 185
Langendoen, Sally, 190
Las Vegas Review-Journal, 258
Laws, 210, 230. See also Hospitals: regulations
Leave It to Beaver (television show), xi
Lenroot, Clara, 27
Levey, Jane E., 18
Levine, Dr. Myron, 280
Lewis, Jerry, 62, 63
Life (magazine), 80, 106, 117, 209
Linck, Kathy, 248
Lindbergh, Charles A., 197
Lindblade, Dr. James, 233
Lindheim, Roslyn, 44
Lithotomy position, 36, 37
Lokken, Sigurd, 70, 98, 102
Long, Joanna, 197–98
Long Island College Medical School, 101
Long Island Jewish Hospital, 273
Louisiana, 58
Luft, Eric, 246

MacDonald, Betty, 35
MacLeod, Joseph, 199

Madison General Hospital. *See* Meriter Hospital

Magee-Women's Hospital (Pittsburgh), 191

Male bonding, 13, 120; between fathers and physicians, 183, 246; through fathers' books, 66–72, 78–79, 85; in prenatal classes, 138–39, 146–48; in waiting room, 9–10, 64, 72, 78–79, 82–83; on Web, 287–88

Maloni, Judith, 191

Manchester Memorial Hospital (Manchester, Conn.), 276

Mander, Rosemary, 291, 292, 294

Manhattan General Hospital (New York City), 46

Man in the Gray Flannel Suit, The (movie), 16

Man in the Gray Flannel Suit, The (novel), 16, 129

Manion, Jo, 187

Mantle, Mickey, 77

March of Dimes, 250

Marital privacy, 253

Marsh, Margaret, 14

Martin, Jerry, 174

Maryland, 78

Mary Tyler Moore Show, The (television show), 145–46

Masculine domesticity, xi, 47, 112–13, 121, 156–57, 254–55, 287; and African American men, 16–17; defined, 15; reinforced by childbirth, 261–64

Masculinity, 18, 79, 121; during childbirth, 174–75, 190, 224, 254–55; in fathers' books, 67–68; in prenatal classes, 123, 140, 146

Massachusetts, 50, 85, 214, 221, 243

Massachusetts Institute of Technology, 84–85

Maternal mortality, 34, 37–38, 71–72, 92

Maternity Center Association of New York, 122–23, 125, 139–40, 163

Maternity Hospital (Minneapolis, Minn.), 116

May, Elaine Tyler, 112

McCalls (magazine), 109, 166, 250

McGraw, Phillip Calvin (Dr. Phil), 293

McKelway, Dr. George, 30

Medical authority, 13–14, 44, 72, 74, 91–92, 207, 287; accommodated by childbirth reform movement, 17; challenged, 99–100, 245; challenged by women's movement, 247–51; fear of challenges to, 213–17, 244–45, 254; and new technology, 30–31; potentially challenged by prenatal classes, 126; reinforced in prenatal classes, 123

Medicalization of childbirth, 8, 21–22, 24, 34–47; transformation of, 112. *See also* Childbirth

Medical Mission Sisters of Philadelphia, 139

Medicare (1966), 12, 157

Men, x–xi, 14–15, 16, 47, 63; clergy, 70; Jewish, 70; Muslim, 70; in postwar America, x–xi. *See also* Fathers

Mercy-Memorial Hospital (Monroe, Mich.), 282

Meriter Hospital (Madison, Wis.), 81–82, 234, 242

Messling, Paul, 173

Methodist Hospital (Madison, Wis.), 102, 217, 273

Metycaine, 103

Michigan, 62, 63, 124, 199, 218, 232, 282

Michigan Nursing Center Association, 111

Michigan Society of Obstetricians and Gynecologists, 272

Midwives, 7, 21–22, 25, 32, 150. *See also*
Nurse-midwives

Miller, Bonnie, 185, 213–14, 215–16

Miller, Dr. John, 220, 222–23, 230–31

Minnesota, 116, 170, 229

Minority Business Enterprise program
(San Francisco), 177

Minton, Helen, 99

Mississippi, 229

Missouri, 229

Montana, 185, 245, 252

Montana Supreme Court, 252

Moore, John, 140

Morphine, 99

Morton, Dr. John H., 223, 224–25

Mother-infant bonding, 265–66

Mt. Sinai Hospital (New York City), 134,
164

Ms. (magazine), 255

Muhlenberg Hospital (Plainfield, N.J.),
221

Muhlhausen, Marvin, 78

My Baby (magazine), 114, 131

Nassau Hospital, 273

National Institutes of Health, 273

Natural childbirth, 12, 80, 98–112;
changing medical opinion of, 115–16,
131, 158–59; effect on nurses, 105, 108,
111; fostering intimacy, 171–79, 192,
254–55; growing acceptance of, 158;
media portrayal of, 208–9, 236–38;
movement for, 9, 86, 103, 165, 182,
236; negative experiences of, 108; physicians' reaction to, 109, 117–18; popularity of different methods, 200–202;
role in family togetherness, 113–19;
women's reaction to, 109–10. *See also*
Bradley method; Dick-Read method;
Lamaze method; Prenatal classes

Natural Childbirth Association of Milwaukee, 132

NBC (National Broadcasting Company),
59

Neal, Mark Anthony, 16

Nebraska, 29

Nelson, Hallie, 29

Nembutal, 35

Newhart, Bob, 67

New Jersey, 102–3, 128, 220–21, 263

New Mexico, 139, 182

Newsweek (magazine), 181

Newton, Michael, 228–29

New York State, 91, 93, 111

New York Academy of Medicine, 37

New York City, x, 46, 63, 94, 95, 122, 132,
134, 202, 219, 231, 268

New York Hospital, 196

New York Lying-In Hospital, 94, 215,
231, 265

New York Maternity Center, 100

New York Times, 111, 164, 193, 208, 273,
288, 292, 294

Nixon, Richard, xi

Nolan, Dr. George H., 272

North Broward Hospital District (Broward County, Calif.), 250

North Carolina, 133, 228

North Dakota, 229

North Shore Hospital (Manhasset, N.Y.),
94, 215

Northwestern University Medical
School, 65

Norwood Hospital (Norwood, Mass.),
243

Nurse-midwives, 140, 144, 277

Nursery, 53, 55

Nurses, 14–15; and family-centered care,
275–76; fathers' presence increases
workload, 108–9, 184, 208; fathers'

presence decreases workload, 105, 111; interaction with fathers, 57, 183–86, 191; involvement in prenatal classes, 124, 126, 131–32; as mothers, 145, 207; negative response to Lamaze method, 185; opposition to fathers in delivery room, 215–17; and physicians, 246–47; role in mothers' isolation, 45; support for shared labor, 185, 191; as instructors in prenatal classes, 124, 131–32; and technology, 42. *See also* Nurse-midwives; Obstetric nurses; Public health nurses

Nurses Association of ACOG, 266

Obstetric nurses, 7, 44, 57, 92, 183, 185, 191, 201, 216, 245–46, 275–76
Odent, Michel, 292–93, 294
Ohio, 39, 124, 229, 276
Oklahoma, 26
Ola, Constance, 91
Opium, 24, 30
Oppenheimer, Jess, 1
Oregon, 231
Oswald, Shirley, 260
Overstreet, Dr. Edmund W., 117
Oxytocin, 39
Ozzie and Harriet (television show), xi

Packard, Vance, 80, 113, 121–22
Palmieri, Dr. Anthony, 102
Parents (magazine), 109, 280
Parkman, Ebenezer, 22
Pasteur, Louis, 28
Patten, Edith, 208
Patterson, Patricia and Jimmy, 177–78, 261–62
Pennsylvania, 116, 124, 139, 153, 246
Perkins, Barbara Bridgman, 42
Philadelphia, 26, 181

Philip Morris, 1
Phillips, Celeste, 192
Physicians: in 18th century, 22–25; in 19th century, 25–27; acceptance of fathers in delivery room, 246; comforting laboring women, 102; debates over shared labor, 179–82, 218–19, 221–25; opinion of birthing room, 278; opinion of fathers' presence in labor room, 84–85, 117–18, 144, 180–83, 187–88; opinion of prenatal classes, 133, 144; punished for allowing fathers in delivery room, 240; resistance to fathers in delivery room, 207–8, 213–15, 218, 220–25, 244–45; support for natural childbirth, 117–18, 181–83, 227; support for shared labor, 167–68, 217–18
Pitocin, 39, 41, 73
Pituitrin, 35
Place, power of. *See* Hospitals: and geography
Planned Parenthood, 147
Pollack, Jack, 80, 139
Porter Hospital (Denver, Colo.), 217
Postpartum recovery, 8, 44
Pregnancy: euphemisms for, 2; portrayal on television, 1–7. *See also* Prenatal classes
Prenatal classes, 9, 78, 106, 120–55; changes in, 152–55; content of, 125, 133–34, 146–47; early, 122–28; fathers' resistance to, 143; use of films in, 149–53, 191; funding of, 126, 128; integrated, 140, 262; natural childbirth classes, 128–55; nurses' response to, 124, 126; opposition to, 134; outside of hospitals, 131–32; physicians' support for, 144–45; portrayal on television, 135–37, 145–46; reducing anxiety,

141, 153; regional differences in, 135; relationship to natural childbirth, 128–31; sex-segregated, 124, 134, 147, 192; statistics on, 126. *See also* Bradley method; Dick-Read method; Lamaze method

Prentice Women's Hospital (Chicago), 285

Presbyterian Hospital (New York City), 274

Presbyterian Medical Center (New York City), 283

Price, Robert, 7, 261, 262

Price, Stuart, 53, 219

Privilege. *See* Class, socioeconomic; Race

Pronatalism, 86, 250

Public health nurses, 123–24

Pyle, Ernie, 70

Queens Education for Childbirth Center (New York City), 132

Race, 12, 205, 266–67; effect on childbirth options, 234–35, 265, 267; in *I Love Lucy*, 4–6; privilege based on, 11–13; whiteness, 50. *See also* Segregation

Radbill, Dr. Samuel X., 26–27

Rakowitz, Elly, 162, 266

Ravitts, Gail, 199

Reader's Digest (magazine), 35, 211, 288

Redbook (magazine), 80, 109, 142, 179–80, 226

Reed, Richard, 289–90, 291, 294

Regulations, hospital. *See* Hospitals: regulations

Religion, 70–71, 113–14

Relyea, Connie and Tim, 262–63

Rex Hospital (Raleigh, N.C.), 157

Ricardo, Lucy. *See* Ball, Lucille

Ricardo, Ricky. *See* Arnaz, Desi

Ricketts, Shirley, 63

Rinker, Sylvia, 92–93

Robbin, Alice, 242

Roberts, David, 158

Roberts, John, 234

Rock-a-Bye Baby (film), 62, *63*

Rockwell, Norman, 50, *52*

Rogers, Mary, 201–2

Rosengren, William, 52

Rosie the Riveter, 15

Rovinsky, Dr. Joseph, 273

Ruby, Jan, 109

Rural hospitals. *See* Hospitals: rural

Rutherford, Dr. Robert, 84, 198–99, 205, 222

Sacramento Medical Center, 244

Sacred Heart Medical Center (Spokane, Wash.), 277–78

St. Alexius Hospital (Bismarck, N.D.), 229

St. Bernard's Hospital (Jonesboro, Ark.), 111

St. Catherine's Hospital (Kenosha, Wis.), 242

St. Croix Valley Memorial Hospital (St. Croix Falls, Wis.), 198

St. Joseph's Hospital (Milwaukee, Wis.), 242

St. Luke's Hospital (Bedford, Mass.), 50

St. Luke's Hospital (Jacksonville, Fla.), 204

St. Mary's Hospital (Evansville, Ind.), 163

St. Mary's Hospital (Grand Rapids, Mich.), 232

St. Mary's Hospital (Madison, Wis.), 64, 233, 243

St. Mary's Hospital (Passaic, N.J.), 102

St. Michael Hospital (Milwaukee, Wis.), 132, 158

Salvation Army Home, 146

Sandberg, William, 274

Sandelowski, Margarete, 42

San Francisco, 181, 183, 205

San Francisco Gynecological Society, 230

Sarto, Dr. Gloria, 240

Saturday Evening Post, 50

Sawyer, Dr. Blackwell, 128

Scaer, Roberta, 159, 250

Schaefer, Dr. George, 84, 187–88, 224, 254

Schultz, Dr. Jean E., 215

Scopolamine, 35–36, 99

Scranton State Hospital (Scranton, Pa.), 196

Segregation: by class, 11–12; of hospitals, 86, 97, 157–58, 204; within hospitals, 11–13; of neighborhoods, 16; by race, 11–13; racial integration of hospitals, 176; regional, 157–58

Sehgar, Dr. Narinder, 244–45

Semmelweis, Dr. Ignaz, 28

Senn, Dr. Milton, 139

Seventh Circuit Court, 252, 273

Sexuality, 173, 211–12, 225, 255, 292–94

Sheaffer, Donald, 222

Sheckler, Catherine, 115

Sheppard-Towner Act (1921), 32

Shobin, Dr. David, 273

Shultz, Gladys Denny, 212–13

Simkins v. Moses H. Cone Memorial Hospital (1963), 12

Sioux Valley Hospital (Sioux Falls, S.D.), 79

Slate (magazine), 292

Sloane Hospital (Columbia University), 41, 81

Smith, Daniel P. B., 243

Smith, David Barton, 12, 97

Smoking, 1, 60, 63, 77, 115; in labor room, 103, 117, 118; in waiting room, 48, 53, 58–59, 61–62

Social childbirth, 22–23, 29

Social Security Act (1935), 32

Sorvillo, Carmen, 268

South Carolina, 88, 181

South Dakota, 57, 79

Splett, Carolyn, 41, 184–85, 245

Spock, Benjamin (Dr. Spock), 15

Stanford University, 117

Stanford University Hospital, 279

Steffen, Dr., 109

Steve Allen Show, The (television show), 59, 61–62

Stevens, Rosemary, 97

Stewart, Jimmy, 59

Stewart, Dr. Robert, 180, 224

Stork Club. See Waiting rooms

Story of Eric, The, 150, 152

Stouffer, John and Mary, 117, 118, 209

Strassberg, Steven, 261

Suburbs, xi, 14–17, 287; segregated, 16

Sullivan, Moya, 196–97

Sunrise Hospital (Las Vegas), 144

Sutherland, Donald, 175–76, 255, 256, 290

Tanzer, Deborah, 164–65

Taubman, Philip, 193, 288

Taylor, Elizabeth, 112

Taylor, Dr. W. Scott, 181

Technocratic birth, 43

Terrace Heights Hospital (New York City), 271

Terzic, Branko and Judy, 149, 191

Texas, 229

Thank You, Dr. Lamaze (Karmel), 161

Thomas Jefferson University (Philadelphia), 181

Thoms, Dr. Herbert, 104–5, 111, 119, 125, 182, 200

Through a Father's Eyes (film), 150

Tompson, Marian, 95–96, 102

Tracy, Spencer, 112

Tropicana Club, 2

Truesdale, Jean, 240

Twilight sleep, 99

U.S. Congress, xi, 17, 236, 248

U.S. District Court for the Northern District of Illinois, 251

U.S. Supreme Court, 272

University Hospital (Madison, Wis.), 130, 217, 240

University Hospital (Minneapolis, Minn.), 213

University of California, 230

University of California Hospital Clinic (Berkeley), 146

University of Chicago Lying-In Hospital (Chicago), 176

University of Kansas Hospital, 199

University of Mississippi School of Medicine, 229

University of Utah Medical Center (Salt Lake City), 274

University of Wisconsin, 285

Utah, 274

Vietnam War, x

Virginia, 22, 29

Virginia Mason Hospital (Seattle, Wash.), 117, *188*, 198, 209, 222

Visiting Nurse Association of New York, 125

Visiting Nurse Association of Brooklyn, 132

Wagner, Joan Ernst, 111

Waiting rooms, 10, 13–14, 46, 48–85, *51*, *52*, *53*, 60, 61, 63, 65, 87–89, 207, 209; access to information in, 56; artistic representation of, 50–51; changing policies in regard to, 88; fathers' discontent with, 79–85, 86–87, 98; in *I Love Lucy*, 4; location within hospital, 52–53, *82–83*, 83–84; obstetric textbook advice on, 55; television in, 48; regional variation in policies, 57–58, 85. *See also* Fathers' books

Washington, D.C., 124, 181, 198, 222, 229

Washington Memorial Hospital (Turnersville, N.J.), 280

Washington State, 205, 208, 209, 222, 277

Wautoma Community Hospital (Wautoma, Wis.), 95

Websites, 291

Wendland, Dan, 225

Weiss, Jessica, 16, 291

Wesley Memorial Hospital (Chicago), 53, 57, 64–66, 69, 70, 88, 96, 97, 98, 207. *See also* Fathers' books

Wesson Maternity Hospital (Springfield, Mass.), 214, 221

Whiting, Helen, 29

Whitman v. Mercy Memorial Hospital (1983), 282

Williams, Marc, 274

Williams, Sarah, 186

Williams Obstetrics (textbook), 283

Wilmington Medical Center (Wilmington, Del.), 234

Wilson, Sloan, 129, 143, 149, 184

Winchell, Walter, 7

Wisconsin, 24, 32–34, 95, 109, 123, 198, 233, 242; Beaver Dam, 274; Clintonville, 116; Dodgeville, 227; Elkhorn,

101, 253; Green Bay, 219; Kenosha, 185; Madison, 36, 64, 82, 92, 102, 162, 216, 225, 240, 243, 273; Manitowoc, 260; Merrill, 214; Milwaukee, 132; Waushara County, 93

Wisconsin Administrative Code, 210

Wisconsin Bureau of Maternal and Child Health, 123

Wisconsin State Journal, 234

Withycombe, Earl, 84–85, 239

Wolff, Katherine, 257–58

Woman's Home Companion (magazine), 80, 103, 139

Women, 15–16; African American, 12–13, 32–34, 66, 97; breakdown of networks for, 29; fear of childbirth, 27–28, 30–31; lesbians, 13, 155, 284; motherhood, 6; negative response to fathers sharing childbirth, 108, 186, 255–56; positive response to fathers sharing childbirth, 109–10, 257–58; supporting each other through childbirth, 22–23, 26–27; unfulfilled, 16; unmarried, 13, 18; women's rights, 137, 248–49; working outside home, 15

Women's movement, x, 15, 17, 141, 236, 247–51, 287

World War I, 32

World War II, x, 15, 34, 97, 123, 287

Wyse, Angela, 101

Yale Grace–New Haven Hospital. *See* Grace–New Haven Hospital

Yale University, 101, 105, 108, 109, 111, 182

Young Women's Christian Association (YWCA), 134

Zabriskie, Louise, 131

Zussman, Shirley, 165